EPILEPTOLOGY - THE MODERN STATE OF SCIENCE

Edited by **Vladimir V. Kalinin**

Epileptology - The Modern State of Science
http://dx.doi.org/10.5772/61409
Edited by Vladimir V. Kalinin

Contributors

Ben Chindo, Bulus Adzu, Karnius Gamaniel, Jolanta Dorszewska, Urszula Lagan-Jedrzejczyk, Marta Kowalska, Katarzyna Wize, Wojciech Kozubski, Anna Staniszewska, Marta Dąbrowska-Bender, Marcin Sobiecki, Grzegorz Juszczyk, Dominik Olejniczak, Magdalena Bujalska-Zdrożny, Aleksandra Czerw, Marta Vázquez, María Carmen Carrascosa-Romero, Carlos De Cabo De La Vega, Vladimir Kalinin, Elena Zheleznova, Lyudmila Sokolova, Anna Zemlyanaya, Kirill Subbotin, Alberto Lazaarowski, Ayse Kutlu, Serap Mulayim, Tamer Rizk, Svetlana Dolina, Ricardo Zavala-Yoe, Ricardo A. Ramirez-Mendoza

Published by InTech

Janeza Trdine 9, 51000 Rijeka, Croatia

Publishing Process Manager Edi Lipovic

Technical Editor SPi Global

Cover InTech Design team

First published October, 2016

Printed in Croatia

Additional hard copies can be obtained from orders@intechopen.com

Epileptology - The Modern State of Science, Edited by Vladimir V. Kalinin

p. cm.

Print ISBN 978-953-51-2698-0
Online ISBN 978-953-51-2699-7

For EU product safety concerns:
IN TECH d.o.o., Prolaz Marije Krucifikse Kozulić 3, 51000 Rijeka, Croatia,
info@intechopen.com or visit our website at intechopen.com.

Meet the editor

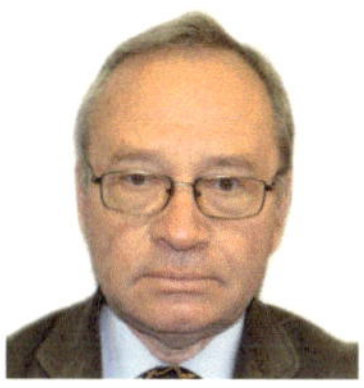

Professor Vladimir V. Kalinin is a psychiatrist and Head of the Department of Brain Organic Disorders and Epilepsy of the Moscow Research Institute of Psychiatry of Ministry of Healthcare of Russian Federation. Vladimir Kalinin, MD, PhD, was born in 1952 in Orenburg, Russian Federation, in a family of physicians. He graduated from Moscow Medical Stomatological University in 1976, and in 1976–1977, he finished an internship in Psychiatry. In 1978, he became a scientific researcher at the Moscow Research Institute of Psychiatry where he is still working as the Head of Department. The scope of his scientific interests concerns a broad range of psychiatry problems, including general psychopathology, psychopharmacology, neuropsychiatry, and epileptology. The topic of his doctoral thesis (1996) concerns the anxiety disorders, psychopathology, and treatment with emphasis on panic disorder. Professor V. Kalinin is an author of 194 publications, including research articles in professional journals (in Russian and English) and 4 monographs and was the editor of the monograph *Anxiety Disorders*, 2011, and *Obsessive-Compulsive Disorder: The Old and the New Problems*, 2014, published by InTech. He is a member of Presidium of Russian Psychiatric Society and a member of the Russian League Against Epilepsy. His biography is included in Marquis' "Who is Who in Medicine and Healthcare 2006-2007," "Who is Who in Science and Engineering 2008-2009," "Who is Who in the World 2010," and "Who is Who in the World 2011" and in Cambridge International Biographical Centre.

Contents

Preface

Epileptology seems to be an example of multidisciplinary integrated science in which many medical and biological disciplines take part in. It is noteworthy, that during several hundreds of years epilepsy represents the disease, which remains the so-called apple of discord between neurologists and psychiatrists. The causes for such situations are multifarious, and here, several factors should be taken into account.

First, epilepsy itself represents interest both for neurologists and psychiatrists, although these specialists look at the same phenomena quite differently. Formally speaking, epilepsy belongs to neurological diseases, although it is characterized by a broad palette of psychiatric comorbid disorders and affective and anxiety disorders seem to be the most prevalent among them.

Unlike neurologists, psychiatrists are very keen to the phenomena of comorbid epilepsy pathology and see in its broad manifestations a subject for proper researches that could shed light on pathogenesis of psychopathology at all. In line with this statement, the fact should be mentioned that Norman Geschwind seriously believed that research of epilepsy patients and temporal lobe epilepsy in particular could help us to understand the nature of mental disorders at all.

It must be stressed that during many years between neurology and psychiatry the principal discrepancies in diagnostic modus existed. Thus, for neurology, the cornerstone in diagnostic algorithm and the mode of the so-called topic diagnostics prevailed. The essence of such a method is thought to be based on the quest for concrete basic locus (focus, tumor, hemorrhage, etc.) that could explain all symptoms presented in patients.

On the contrary, in psychiatry, the topic diagnostics seems not to be so significant at all, and its principal diagnostic algorithm is based mainly on the so-called matrix (multidimensional) thinking. Such approach implies that some psychopathological symptoms may appear along with definite other symptoms, that is, to be correlated with them positively. In such a case, the steady symptom constellations (syndromes) of complex structure can be formed. On the other hand, there are symptoms that can exclude each other, that is, to be correlated with them negatively, and this implies the existence of strictly concrete syndrome in concrete patients.

Moreover, the causes of mental disorders are thought to be also multifactorial, and from this point of view, there is no need to seek the single cause of any psychiatric disorder. Such attitude from psychiatrist has resulted in that psychopathological method has become good enough and independent from other basic research data, including neurological results, and additional data of patient investigations, such as CT, MRT, etc.

Such principal discrepancies between two disciplines have been erased during the last two to three decades, when new synthetic and integral discipline arose. This discipline has been called as neuropsychiatry or behavioral neurology, and numerous handbooks and articles on these topics have appeared. The principal rules and canons of neuropsychiatry have been obtained on patients with epilepsy, and epileptology as a discipline is thought to be the principal part of neuropsychiatry.

From our point of view, neuropsychiatry cannot be simply reduced to the study of mental health and behavior in neurological patients. Moreover, neuropsychiatry is intended to search the neurological basis in all mental disorders. In other words, the principal aim of neuropsychiatry lies in the findings of the so-called cerebral substrate of different psychiatric disorders, and in this context, epilepsy represents the interesting useful model.

Besides neurology and psychiatry, other disciplines such as neurophysiology, biochemistry, genetics, and pharmacology have also caused impact on epileptology development, and now, it represents really multidisciplinary science.

The current book contains the chapters written by different specialists from many countries and may be helpful for neurologists, psychiatrists, and pharmacologists who are interested in multifarious epileptology problems.

Professor Vladimir V. Kalinin, MD, PhD
Department of Brain Organic Disorders and Epilepsy,
Moscow Research Institute of Psychiatry, Russia

Section 1

The Phenomenology, Neurophysiology and Pathogenesis of Epilepsy

Chapter 1

EEG Long-Term Dynamics to Measure Progress of Concurrent Patients in Drug-Resistant Childhood Syndromes

Ricardo Zavala Yoé and Ricardo Ramírez-Mendoza

Additional information is available at the end of the chapter

http://dx.doi.org/10.5772/64568

Abstract

It is well known that in order to study the evolution of a drug-resistant epilepsy, it is necessary to practice a lot of Electroencephalographic signals (EEG) studies during the child's life. The number of EEG collected by parents during the child's life might easily range between 10 and 20, depending of the severity of the affection, age and neurologist's requirements. With all these data, natural questions posed by parents and physicians are as follows: (a) Which zone of the brain has been the most affected so far? (b) On which year was the child better? Naturally, the neurologist would wish to correlate these answers with the prescribed drugs history but responding objectively those questions is certainly not easy (or even impossible). However, both questions were already answered quantitatively in [1] where a very difficult case of Doose syndrome (DS) was investigated. In this work, we propose to go further answering an additional question frequently posed by parents and physicians which is as follows: (c) How bad is our child with respect to other with similar affections? Note that replying this question results also very difficult because this would imply to compare *sets* of *multiple, massive* EEG (one for every kid involved in the study). In addition, the possibility of answering this question also implies to compare medications/results among all the children in the investigation. What we propose here is to answer *quantitatively* question (c) by using our complexity measures and indices introduced here and the experience obtained in [1] with all this linked to medications. The question arises as follows: Why to use complexity, that is, entropy to characterize EEG information? Because it would be formidable to determine a mathematical model which could represent *in general, each case of DS or LGS*. This is not yet possible but after analyzing a set of *nonlinear models*, we concluded that it is more reliable to work with *nonlinear statistics* (entropies) to extract information from EEG in children epilepsy [1]. As a result of this, we offer here the multiscale entropy (MSE) index and the bivariate multiscale (BMSE) index to evaluate all channels of multiple EEG.

Keywords: simultaneous EEG dynamics, time series entropy, drug-resistant children epilepsy, epileptic encephalopathies

1. Introduction

Epilepsy is defined as a disorder of the brain characterized by an enduring predisposition to generate epileptic seizures and by the neurobiological, cognitive, psychological and social consequences of this condition. The definition of epilepsy requires the occurrence of at least one epileptic seizure [3]. A syndrome is a group of signs and symptoms that, added together, suggest a particular medical condition. The International League Against Epilepsy (ILAE) defines an epileptic encephalopathy (EE) as the condition where the epileptic activity itself contributes to cognitive and behavioural impairments seen in severe epilepsy, beyond that expected from the underlying pathology alone [4, 5]. In addition, the ILAE Task Force has chosen the preferred term *drug resistant* to replace terms as *pharmacoresistant, intractable, refractory* because these would imply that there is no chance of remission, which is not necessarily the case [6–8]. Childhood epilepsy syndromes as Lennox-Gastaut (LGS) and Doose (DS) are typical examples of epileptic encephalopathies (EE). When these affections are drug resistant, finding reliable treatments becomes a challenge. Although some works in applied mathematics to epilepsy have been successfully conducted (see for instance [9] and references therein), papers which investigate quantitatively EEG in drug-resistant epileptic encephalopathies are practically null. Main attention has been devoted to adult affections as Alzheimer's disease, Creutzfeldt-Jakob disease, schizophrenia, Parkinson's disease and others [9–12]. About quantitative investigation of children epilepsy (see [1, 2]).

1.1. The Doose syndrome

Hermann Doose first described the features of a previously incompletely defined epilepsy syndrome characterized by very different seizures, consisting of jerks, drop attacks, or sometimes a jerk followed by a fall. Absence seizures can happen as well as the so-called generalized tonic-clonic seizures. The EEG may be initially normal, but development of the disease will exhibit patterns of generalized spike and wave activity, 4–7 rhythms/s and bursts. Photoparoxysmal reaction may be observed in the EEG as well. About 1–2% of all children epilepsy is confirmed by DS [7]. This illness affects children with an initial normal development which age ranges from 7 months to 6 years although early manifestations are typically exhibited from 2 to 5 years [13].

1.2. The Lennox-Gastaut syndrome (LGS)

Although precise definition of LGS is still controversial, it is accepted nowadays that three main features must be present in an LGS diagnosis: (a) slow spike wave activity in the EEG, (b) a wide variety of different kind of seizures (typically from sleep) and (c) intellectual

http://dx.doi.org/10.5772/64568

impairment. A very special feature in LGS is the presence of tonic seizures during sleep, which are often overlooked. Typically, onset is between 3 and 8 years of age and LGS shows up with drop or atonic seizures, but as mentioned, a lot of other phenomena may exist as tonic seizures and atypical absence seizures. As a result of this, providing a differential diagnosis can be quite difficult, particularly at the onset before the development of typical characteristics. Structural and brain damages are frequently reported as main causes of LGS [7, 8, 13].

Generalized epileptic seizures are conceptualized as originating at some point within, and rapidly engaging, bilaterally distributed networks. Focal epileptic seizures are conceptualized as originating within networks limited to one hemisphere. They may be discretely localized or more widely distributed [4]. In this work, we are interested in the preictal, ictal and postictal stages of a seizure.

1.3. Note about the subjects considered in this study

The present investigation is a pilot study of how mathematics can support neurologists in severe children epilepsy by means of entropy measures. We present a series of five cases of study; four patients with drug-resistant EE (one kid with a fuzzy transition from DS to LGS; two, confirmed LGS; and one with preponderant features of DS; see Section 2 for details). The fifth kid is neurologically normal, and his EEG collection was used merely as a comparison with the affected children. The EEG studies were recorded with sleep deprivation in the abnormal children, and the nonaffected one was awaken but relaxed developing several activities described in Section 2.5. We remark that finding a suitable (representative) population is quite difficult as a result of the rareness and conditions required in this research (see list below). All data were analyzed anonymously by paying attention only to the numerical information and medications. Artefacts were excluded by an expert neurophysiologist (**Figure 1**).

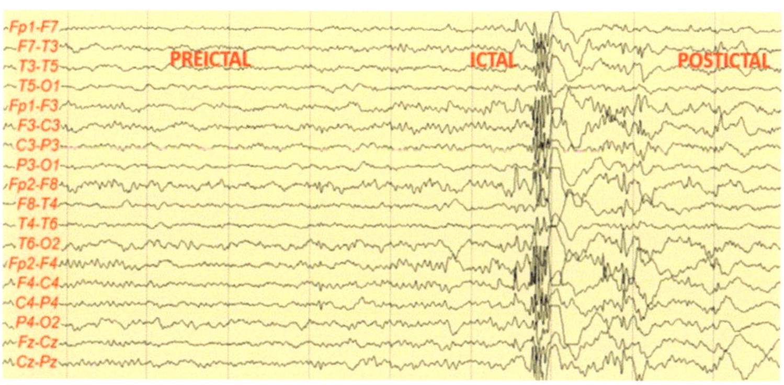

Figure 1. Stages of a seizure.

A question arises about EE: Why to work precisely with this type of affections? Because they have not been examined before (excluding [2] and [1]) and because this kind of epilepsy represents a challenge to deal with not only from a therapeutic viewpoint but also from a mathematical perspective. In addition, parents' observations are taken into account here when they described the type of seizures and improvement (or worsening) of them. Their remarks helped physicians to construct the tables and information about medications given in this work. Since our work is a pilot study, we do not offer, at this moment, neither hypothesis testing results nor power analysis;however, the conclusions shown here will guide the design and implementation of a larger scale study [14]. Such work is already being developed; nevertheless, we remark that a study as ours is still lacking. With the intention of giving examples of papers which considered just a few subjects in similar studies, we would like to cite [15] (one patient), [16] (three patients), [17] (seven patients), and [18] (15 patients). In those references, the investigation is conducted in absence of epilepsy and autistic children; more common affections than long term-drug-resistantepileptic encephalopathies.

The patients were selected in order to satisfy the following requirements; that is, they had to:

1. Be children (their epilepsy is more time-varying than adult's).

2. Suffer a drug-resistant EE of the type DS or a LGS since a long time ago, that is about 10 years.

3. Be adhered to medical treatments.

4. Continue such medical treatment in the same hospital (in order to follow their evolution continuously).

It was a challenge to find the subjects which could fulfil all the above-mentioned conditions. Note that as more we require, as less children we can collect. It is noteworthy mention that in developing countries complying with medical treatments in public hospitals may imply a lot of third party complications as lacking of beds, very long waiting lists to be attended, shortage of medicines, etc., just to mention a few [1, 19]. In addition, when parents cannot see a real improvement in short term, they change the physician or the hospital. The worst case is when parents do not understand the gravity of the illness and they do not comply the medical treatment [19–21]. These facts complicate even more to collect the required candidates for our investigation.

1.4. Main anticonvulsants prescribed for our subjects

A list of abbreviations for the anticonvulsants prescribed for the patients is given next. Details about action mechanism, dosages, etc., can be consulted in [22–24].

1. IMI = imipramine,

2. PA = piracetam,

3. VPA+ = valproate sodium,

4. TPM = topiramate,

5. CLB = clobazam,

6. VPA = valproic acid,

7. LTG = lamotrigina,
8. LEV = levetiracetam,
9. ATX = atomoxetine,
10. ESM = ethosuximide,
11. PSE = prednisone,
12. MDZ = midazolam,
13. CZP = clonazepam,
14. ZNS = zonisamide,
15. CZP = clorazepate dipotassium,
16. PB = phenobarbital,
17. LCM = lacosamide
18. PRM = primidone,
19. Q10 = co-enzyme Q10 (not an anticonvulsant),
20. Star (*) means that an EEG was recorded in a given year that such record was used in this work,
21. Letters *a* and *b* mean first and second semester of a year, respectively,
22. √ and × mean a relative good and poor control of seizures, respectively,
23. NA means not applicable.

2. Subjects, EEG description and medication

The set of subjects is composed by four children. Children A and B were born in 2002, child C in 2000,child D in 2003 and child E in 2000. Child A was diagnosed with DS, but it seemed to evolve to LGS, although not all physicians are agreed [1]. Kid B has been diagnosed as LGS; child C as DS and child D as LGS. Kid E is considered normal (no seizures). Children A-D suffer a multifocal effect, but child A has a main source in the frontal lobe while kid B present seizures which seem to originate from the frontal and temporal lobes. On the other hand, all records were sleep-deprived EEG for all non-normal subjects. The databases were retrieved from different children hospitals where the EEG was recorded from scalp in 32 channel-Grass Technologies Clinical Systems [25] according to the international 10–20 standards with 7 mm, 50 μv calibration [26]. In our work, the electrodes are as follows: Fp1, F3, F7, T3, C5, T5, P3, O1, Fp2, F4, F8, T4, C4, T6, P4, O2, Fz, Cz and Pz. The sample frequency was 200 Hz corresponding to 5 ms of sample time. The electrode Oz was not considered. In the case of the healthy subject, the equipment employed is produced by g.Tech and the model is g.Nautilus, a relatively new wireless biosignal acquisition system with possibility of having quality EEG recordings from 32/16/8 channels at 250–500 Hz of sampling frequency [27]. This device was very useful to record diverse activities in the normal kid. The version used is equipped with eight channels which are Fz, Cz, F3, Pz, P4, PO7, PO8 and Oz, and the sample frequency was 250 Hz, that is 4 ms of sample time. As known, these syndromes manifest very differently and that is why we offer our entropies perspective.

2.1. Patient A

A 12-year-old child was investigated in [1, 2], and her history is continued here. The onset of epilepsy in kid A was at 4 years with very short absence seizures. A few months later (when she became 5), seizures started as shivers and then they worsen as droop heads (See **Table 1**). A very wide spectrum of medications was tried without a clear success. Twenty anticonvulsants were used through all the child life and the worst season was at the beginning of 2014 when even 80 seizures a day were presented. The seizureslooked as shivers every 5 min and, as a consequence, the girl had to be admitted in the hospital emergency room but without any possibility of correcting this and deterioration started to be serious. The type of seizures was mainly drops, drop head and myoclonic. As a result of this, the child had to use a helmet and she had to interrupt her attendance to a special education school as well as psychomotor therapy. Some months were needed to admit this kid in the hospital in order to substitute clonazepam (CZP) byclobazam (CLB) because CZP had reached its highest dosage without positive results. This action ended up with about four months of relative success, but still several seizures were present. After many useless trials to improve her condition, parents took her child and left this hospital in order to let their kid to be treated in another institution where intravenous immune globulin (IVIG) was suggested as last resource (although with some doubts about success by some physicians).

Anticonvulsant	Year	Comments	Seizures	MSE	BMSE
IMI, PM	2006	First medicines consumed. Stopped suddenly	NA	NA	NA
VPA+, TPM, CLB, VPA	2007	Beginning of VPA+	NA	NA	NA
VPA, LTG, TPM, VPA+, CLB, LEV, ATX, ESM, PSE, MDZ	2008*	Pancreatitis. Beginning of ESM, LEV. ATX worsen seizures	√.	OK	OK
TPM, LEV, LTG, PSE, ESM, CZP, ZNS,	2009	ZNS useless. Retirement of ETS worsen seizures	NA	NA	NA
ZNS, ESM, CZP, LEV, CZP	2010*	CZP useless. Seizures worse	×	Bad	Bad
CZP, LEV, LTG, ESM, PB	2011*	PB useless	×	Bad	Bad
LCM, ESM, LEV, LTG, CZP	2012	LCM shows up.ETS retired again worsening seizures	NA	NA	NA
LCM, LEV, LTG, PRM, CZP, Q10, ESM	2013a*	Gastritis aggravate	√	OK	OK
LEV, ESM, LCM, LTG, CZP	2013b*	Idem.	√	OK	OK
LEV, ESM, LTG, CLB, *IVIG*	2014	LCM worsen seizures, CZP replaced by CLB	√	NA	NA
LEV, ESM, LTG, CLB, *IVIG*	2015	LCM retired, gastritis improved	√	NA	NA

Table 1. Anticonvulsants per year for patient A.

http://dx.doi.org/10.5772/64568

http://dx.doi.org/10.5772/64843

http://dx.doi.org/10.5772/64843

http://dx.doi.org/10.5772/64458

http://dx.doi.org/10.5772/64691

http://dx.doi.org/10.5772/64454

http://dx.doi.org/10.5772/63562

http://dx.doi.org/10.5772/63562

http://dx.doi.org/10.5772/64445

http://dx.doi.org/10.5772/64349

http://dx.doi.org/10.5772/64349

http://dx.doi.org/10.5772/64568

Nevertheless, it is remarkable how IVIG improved the life of this child which has received this treatment twice, one at the end of 2014 and another one by mid of 2015. She will repeat this by the end of 2015 (see [1] for disease details and its relation with other entropy measures). This information is an update of this case.

Although the disease process of this child starts in 2006, the EEG database encompasses only 2008, 2010, 2011, and 2013; missing years were not accessible for administrative purposes. The four EEG which compose the present database are referred to as EEG1, EEG2, EEG3, and EEG4, respectively. The entire set of the four EEG clearly shows typical features of DS although some clinical manifestations are not consistent with a typical DS (overlapping with LGS). This patient is a case of multifocal epilepsy which quickly spreads through all the brain. Apparently, the initial focus is the frontal lobe. Our results in [1] were in line with this.

Table 1 provides updated information about the main anticonvulsants prescribed for the kid during 2008–2015. In that table, the abbreviations used were already explained in Section 1.4. Details about those antiseizures can be reviewed in [8, 22–24, 28]. Note: The last two columns of **Tables 1** and **2** refer to the entropies described in this work which will be explained from Section 3 on.

Anticonvulsant	Year	Comments	Seizures	MSE	BMSE
VPA+	2007*	Onset of seizures, VPA+ prescribed	×	Bad	Bad
VPA+	2008	Seizures improve a bit	√	NA	NA
VPA+	2009	Seizures continue	×	NA	NA
VPA+	2010*	Seizures improve	√	OK	OK
VPA+	2011	VPA+ retired	√	NA	NA
VPA	2012*	Seizures starts to worsen	×	Bad	Bad
VPA, LTG	2013	Seizures improve, bad later	×	NA	NA
VPA, LTG	2014*	LTG prescribed, seizures improve	√	OK	OK

Table 2. Anticonvulsants per year for patient B.

2.2. Patient B

Kid B was diagnosed as LGS and started in 2007 with multifocal discharges with probable initial focus in the frontal and temporal lobes. The first medicine prescribed was VPA+ and continued until 2010. In 2011, this anticonvulsant was retired as a result of a relative improvement in his condition but seizures worsen and in 2012, and VPA was prescribed. LTG [28] was included to help in 2013 and 2014. More detailed information is missing (see **Table 2**). Notice the difference between the anticonvulsants needed by patient A and patient B. The available EEG was recorded in 2007, 2010, 2012 and 2014 and was named as EEG1-EEG4, respectively.

2.3. Patient C

This kid apparently suffers DS but (as in the case of child A) the border with LGS seems to be fuzzy. More information about child C is missing. We only could access the numerical database which corresponds to four records: 2005, 2008, 2012 and 2014. The main anticonvulsant was VPA, LTG, LEV and CLB. This disease is also multifocal.

2.4. Patient D

This kid is a case of LGS. The set of EEG was collected from 2005 to 2014. Here, we only could access the numerical databases of 2005, 2009 and 2014 as well. The main antiepileptic drugs consumed were VPA, ESM and LEV. This patient seems to be the less affected as a result of being DS. The level of consciousness seems to bebetter in this kid as a result of being DS.

2.5. Subject E

Kid D is healthy and his EEG was used to compare how entropy contrasts with epileptic affections versus normality. The EEG was recorded while the kid developed diverse activities (A1-A4) during a total of 5 min (M1=minute 1 to M5=minute 5), (1 min each). These actions are resumed below where the letters mean: R is the resting, MA is the muscle activity, HM is the hearing music (lying down), T is the talking (lying down), D is the drawing (sat down), LD is the lying down, SD is the singing/dancing (slowly) and W is the walking slowly (**Table 3**).

A/t	M1	M2	M3	M4	M5
A1	R	R	R	R	R
A2	R	MA	HM	R	T
A3	R	D	LD	SD	R
A4	R	W	W	W	R

Table 3. Activities in a normal kid.

3. Methods: nonlinear models or nonlinear statistics?

There are two main streams in modelling of EEG: (a) nonlinear dynamical systems (chaos-based theory) and (b) stochastic models [9–11, 29]. Although there have been interesting reports about this, they have been focused on adults epilepsy and literature about children epilepsy is rather scanty [1, 2]. But even considering their relative success, the models provided cannot be general as a result of the highly nonlinear, time-varying (and sometimes stochastic) nature of EEG in (children and adults) epilepsy. We sketch next our investigation about how we concluded to apply nonlinear parameters rather than nonlinear models to investigate EEG in children epilepsy.

As it was just mentioned, there have been good results in some adults epilepsy (Creutzfeldt-Jacob disease, schizophrenia, Alzheimer's disease, etc.) modelled by chaotic dynamical systems [9–11]. That is why we focused on time series (TS) characteristics considering TS as a particular case of a stochastic process. Those basic characteristics are as follows: normality (in distributional sense), stationarity and linearity of the TS.

http://dx.doi.org/10.5772/64568

3.1. Time series from EEG

A common consideration about EEG signals is that they are Gaussian and stationary. In this case, frequency analysis is a natural alternative [30]. If this were not the case, there also exists the possibility of dealing with nonstationary signals in frequency domain [31]. Some serious adult's brain disorders such as Alzheimer's disease (AD), Creutzfeldt-Jacob disease (CJD), schizophrenia obey neither stationary nor Gaussianity restrictions [10, 12]. Without being very formal, the following characteristics were explored in our databases.

3.1.1. Normality

In order to have an idea about the shape of the probability distributions of each channel in the patients' database, a very simple algorithm to test normality was used and it concerns the well-known Q-Q plot [32]. Using standard MATLAB commands, this test was run for all the databases resulting that all channels tends to present a non-normal (non-Gaussian) distribution. Providing a detailed statistical study for this is out of the scope of this work but for the time being it suffices to say that normality is not satisfied. The tails of the distributions are distorted in many channels of all patients.

3.1.2. Stationarity

It is well known that a process is called stationary in mean and stationary in variance if such quantities remain constant through time. From the amplitude vs. time plots, it can be seen by qualitative inspection that all patients' EEG signals have no trend, that is they are stationary in mean. In addition, in order to confirm absence of trend, two simple nonparametric tests were done; the Bendat-Piersol run and trend tests [33, 34] which agreedwith such observation. Later, the autocorrelation function was plotted showing that each channel of the whole database of the patients is not covariance stationary. A t test was also developed on all data, being in line with this. Correlograms of all EEG channels showed that they do not behave randomly (figures not shown).

3.1.3. Linearity

First, the notion of linearity has been established. Linearity with respect to what? It is known in our days that most of physiological signals represented by time series are nonstationary [35] and nonlinear in general. In the scope of this work, we will consider that an EEG signal is linear if its Q-Q plot is a straight line, that is, the distribution of a given EEG channel coincides almost perfectly with a normal distribution. However, as explained above, most of the EEG zones (channels) showed a non-normal distribution. In this sense, the meaning of statistical non-normality and medical non-normality coincides (see more details about this in [1, 36]).

As a result of all this, it was decided that working with nonlinear statistics (entropy of TS) was more reliable and useful because they can be computed for any TS (see next section).

3.2. Complexity of signals as time series

Time series complexity or entropy measures how regular a sampled signal is. For instance, a sine wave (or any periodic signal) will exhibit a low value of entropy because such signal is very predictable. As known, this signal is characterized only by its amplitude and frequency parameters. However, consider now a white noise variable. Since it is characterized by its random nature, its complexity value will be high (with respect to the sine wave). Broadly speaking, a signal will be complex if its entropy value is bigger (or equal to) than 1. Nevertheless, it is also important to determine *when* such value is reached. In order to explain deeper this important idea which supports our results, the basics of entropy are shown next. Immediately later, a workout example is provided.

3.2.1. What does entropy measure and how?

In time series context, entropy is the rate of information production [37]. Pincus [37] developed the theory for a measure of regularity, the rate of generation of new information that can be applied to clinical data. This statistic was called *approximate entropy, ApEn*. It had as a goal to measure systems complexity (the terms complexity and entropy are used interchangeably [37–39]). This statistic has been evolving, and it has taken new names depending of the improvements: *sample entropy* [40], *multiscale entropy, MSE* [39], our version of MSE and our proposed *bivariate MSE* (BMSE) and some others [1]. A collection of four entropy measures was evaluated in [1] showing that MSE was the more convenient to be used in our databases.

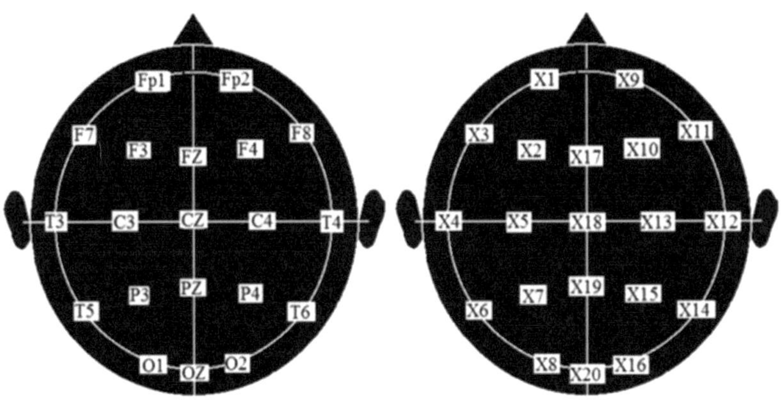

Figure 2. Schematic representation of the international standard 10–20 for electrodes placement and its corresponding nomenclature used in Algorithm 1 (see Section 3.2).

3.2.2. How to compute MSE?

Without loss of generality, before describing MSE, we would like to explain a generic algorithm to compute complexity, actually, ApEn. Later, we will comment how to modify this algorithm to determine MSE [1, 37, 39, 40]. For ease of exposition, this algorithm is explained for only one EEG channel:

http://dx.doi.org/10.5772/64568

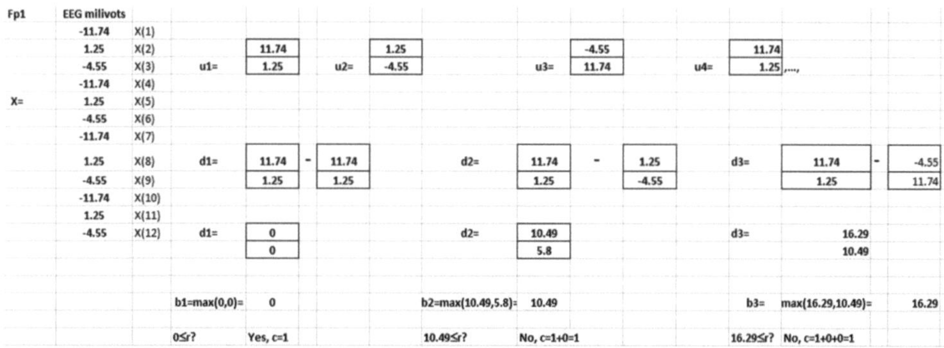

Figure 3. Basic steps to compute entropy generically in a hypothetical channel Fp1. In this example, $r = 3$ and the number of subvectors u whose distance is smaller or equal than r is 17 of a total of 50 samples (partially shown here). The value c means *count*. This figure encompasses Steps 1–7 from Algorithm 1. From Steps 8–10, the resultant entropy will be 0(see Section 3.2.3).

Algorithm 1. MSE

1. Define a time series for a chosen EEG channel, say X_1 (if we consider 19 EEG channels, we will have 19 numerical sets; one for each zone of the brain in the EEG). So, X_1 will correspond to Fp1, $X_2$to F3 and so on (see **Figure 2**). Recall that each vector $X = [X(1)\ X(2)\ X(3)\ldots]$ (the EEG channel) consists of voltage amplitudes, that is numerical values.

2. For the given EEG channel, X_1, that is, Fp1 do the following (see **Figure 3**):

3. Construct a set of test vectors (from X) called u of length m. Typically, $m = 2$. So, the test vectors will be formed taking sets of $m = 2$ elements from X. Hence, $u_1 =[X(1)\ X(2)]$. This means that the first vector $u_1$will be constructed with the first to components of X, the voltage amplitudes of the corresponding EEG channel. So, $u_2 =[X(2)\ X(3)]$, $u_3 =[X(3)\ X(4)]$, until finishing the elements of X. Recall that the length ℓ of X, the EEG channel is determined by the EEG time t_{EEG} (in seconds) and the sample time, T. So, $\ell = t_{EEG}/T$.

4. From vectors u, compute a set of *distances* called d as follows: $d_1 = [X(1) - X(2)]$, $d_2 = [X(2) - X(3)]$, $d_3 = [X(3) - X(4)]$, until exhaust all the elements of X.

5. From vectors u, compute a set of *distances* called d as follows: $d_1 = \underbrace{[X(1)-X(2)]}_{\text{From}\,u_1}$, $d_2 = \underbrace{[X(2)-X(3)]}_{\text{From}\,u_2}$, $d_3 = \underbrace{[X(3)-X(4)]}_{\text{From}\,u_3}$, until exhaust all the elements of X.

6. Choose the maximum value b between two consecutive elements of d (with no attention to its sign): $b_1 = max\ (d_1,d_2)$, $b_2 = max\ (d_3,d_3,d_4)$, etc.

7. Define $r = 0.2\sigma(X)$, where σ is the standard deviation. If $b_1 \geq r$ then count it as valid, else not. The same for b_2, b_3, etc. Add the total number of valid values of all b's in c_1. Take the natural logarithm of $c_1$as $ln(c_1)$.

8. Go to Step 3 and repeat it to 7 redefining $u_1 = [X(2)\ X(3)]$, $u_2 = [X(3)\ X(4)]$, $u_3 = [X(4)\ X(5)]$ etc., until exhausting all the values of the EEG channel, X.

9. Add all the natural logarithms computed in Step 7 and divide them by the total length (in time samples) of the EEG channel, A. Call this number F_1.

10. Go to Step 3 and use $m + 1$ instead of m and repeat all until Step 9 but name the result of all this F_2. Define the *entropy* of the EEG channel as F_1–F_2.

3.2.3. Worked out example

Assume that we want to analyze the complexity of a 50 samples long EEG signal given by X = …, 11.74,1.25, −4.55, 11.74, 1.25, −4.55, 11.74, 1.25, −4.55,…. (millivolts), $N = 51$. Assume that $m = 2$, $r = 3$. In this case, the sequence of subvectors u of length m (see Algorithm 1) is given by u_1 = [11.74 1.25], u_2 = [1.25 −4.55], u_3 = [−4.55 11.74], u_4 = [11.74 1.25]. Now, the distances are evaluated in such a way those vectors which satisfy the constraint $d = max(u_1,u_j) \leq r$ will be counted. Observe that $d_1 = (u_1,u_1) = 0$. (counted), $d_2(u_1,u_2) = max|11.74 - 1.25|, |1.25 - (-4.55)| = |11.74 - 1.25| = 10.49 > 3$ (not counted), where | | means absolute value (taking positive numerical value). Similarly, $d_3(u_1,u_3) = 16.29 > 3$ (not counted either) and $d_4\ (u_1,u_4) = 0 < 3$ (counted). Continuing this process, we realize that vectors which satisfy $d(u_1,u_j) \leq 3$ are the following: u_1, u_2, u_4, u_7, … u_{49} (seventeen elements). Next, b_1 will be given by 17/50. Continuing this way,F_1 will be 0.334. Analogously for F_2=0.334 and the resulting entropy will be F_1–F_2 = 0.

In this case, this periodic signal (or at least, the part considered here) is not complex. A complex signal has entropy values equal or above 1 [1]. In the case of Algorithm 1, we took continuous values of the EEG channel. If we repeat this process, downsampling a time series for τ = 2,3,4,

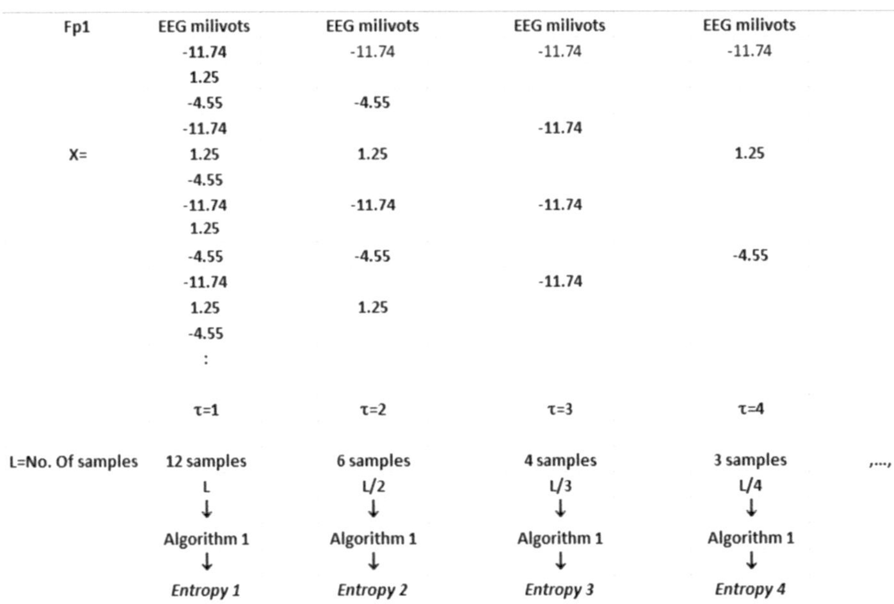

Figure 4. Algorithm 1 in Section 3.2.2 calculates a first value of entropy for the original time series (numerical values of a given EEG channel) taking contiguous elements (τ = 1). Forming subseries from the original one as shown above (i.e. by *downsampling*) and applying them again Algorithm 1 produce a collection of entropy *values* for each element of τ. Plotting τ vs. entropy produces an entropy plot (see Section 3.2.3 and **Figures 3**, **5**, and **6**).

τ_{max}, meaning that we take values of the EEG channel jumping in steps of 2,3,4… as just mentioned above, we will obtain a complexity plot in terms of τ the downsampling rate (see **Figure 4**).

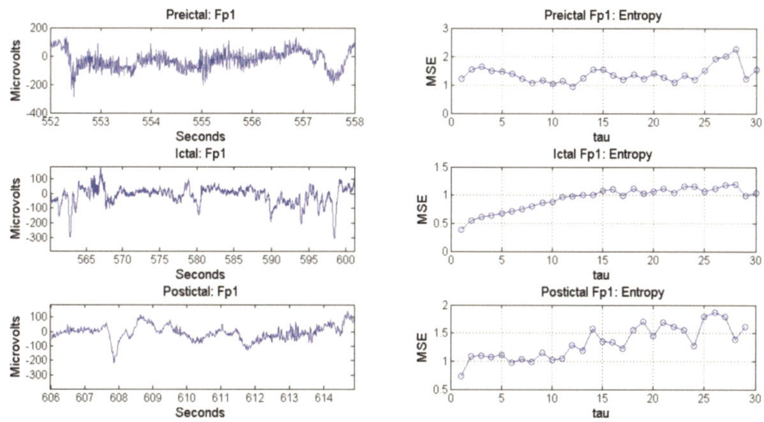

Figure 5. EEG stages and corresponding MSE plots for patient B. Note the entropy values above/below 1 (high/low complexity).

If we partition X in small subvectors and apply to them Algorithm 1, we obtain an entropy value referred to as *Multiscale Entropy* [1, 18, 39]. In this way, the latter algorithm permits to compute (and eventually) plot MSE curves for a time factor scale vector τ for a given period of time. This idea has been applied to a seizure in **Figure 5**, where each of its phases can be observed with their corresponding entropy (MSE) graphs.

3.2.4. *Why high complexity implies MSE ≥ 1?*

Consider a periodic (or quasi periodic) signal $y(t) = y(t + p)$, where p is the period. In this case, the number of elements which satisfy the distance threshold r is almost the same for vectors of length m and $m + 1$. This means that in Step 8 in Algorithm 1, the numerator and denominator of the logarithm of the ratio are almost equal to each other, and hence, we will take the logarithm of a quantity approximately equal to 1. Hence, its logarithm will be almost 0, a low value of complexity or entropy. In contrast, for an aperiodic signal, the result is the other way around and we will obtain high values of complexity(see [1] for details).

The ideas exposed above can be applied to a preictal-ictal-postictal event as shown in **Figure 5**. There, it is possible to compare the three stages of a seizure with respect to their complexity MSE curves. Such graphs were obtained by applying Algorithms 1 and 2 to patient B. Observe how during the preictal phase the complexity curve remains above MSE = 1 with some peaks; nevertheless, when the ictal stage comes, this complexity curvecomes down (below 1), and after some period, it improves finally by reaching values a little bit higher than 1. At the postictal phase, the complexity recovers going above 1 with some peaks which indicate no seizure activity.

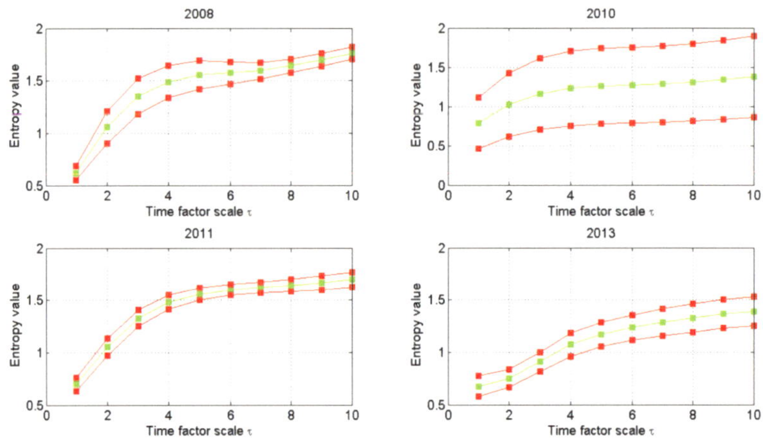

Figure 6. MSE plots averaging all channels per year for patient A. 2010 was the worst period. Observe the standard deviation curves especially wide with respect to the slightlybigger than one-average entropy plot (in the middle of the three curves). This indicates the presence of seizures as a preponderant behaviour in all channels in 2010 during a given period of EEG time (see also **Figure 4**).

This idea can be applied to all channels of a given EEG in order to obtain the average MSE plot for the year the EEG was recorded in. In **Figure 6**, the curves related to the average MSE (plus/minus one standard deviation) are shown for each year of the database of kid A. Notice how easy is to identify the worst year for this child (2010). This process was also applied to all years of the database to obtain an MSE average curve (plus/minus one standard deviation) for each *zone of the brain (channel)* allowing so to identify now the most affected zone (F3 in this patient). This process was applied to all our subjects' databases.

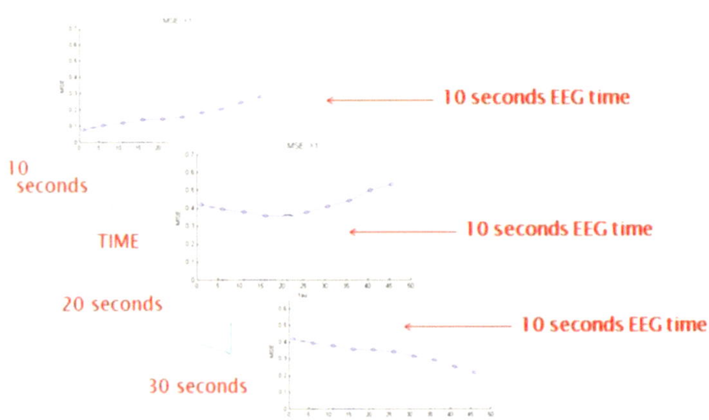

Figure 7. A single entropy plot is produced for a given period of EEG time. But partition this total EEG time in a collection of smaller periods would permit us to associate them a set of corresponding entropy plots (MSE) plots as shown here. Moreover, placing side-to-side dozens, hundreds or thousands of slices like these will form an entropy surface (see **Figure 8**).

http://dx.doi.org/10.5772/64568

It has been seen that we have obtained a single curve for a given period of EEG time. However, we can partition this EEG time in smaller periods in order to produce a single entropy plot for *each period*. So, we would obtain a collection of entropy plots as indicated in **Figure 7**.

Moreover, it is possible to put all these MSE curves together, side to side in order to construct an entropy *surface* (see **Figure 7**). This fact will define what we referred to as *Bivariate MSE*. These surfaces will allow us to make comparisons among several patients at the same time as it has been done in **Figure 9**. The surface can be formed with the following simplified version of an algorithm taken from [1]:

Algorithm 2. BMSE = MSE (t, τ)

1. Fix the EEG time to compute a set of MSE surfaces from.
2. Choose a number of MSE curves which will form BMSE (the complexity surface).
3. Divide the time given in Step 1 over the number of surfaces fixed in Step 2.
4. With Algorithm 1, compute a single MSE curve for each period of time defined in Step 3.
5. Plot all together the latter MSE curves. They will form a surface referred to as BMSE (bivariate MSE).

3.3. Complexity measures for MSE curves and BMSE surfaces

As mentioned above in Ref. [1], the complexity of signals was evaluated qualitatively, that is, those curves lying mainly above MSE = 1 or BMSE = 1 were classified as complex and those below 1 as noncomplex. A metric was missing, and we offer a simple one here. Such metric is referred to as *complexity index*, $\overline{MSE(\tau)}$, and is nothing but the mean of all the MSE values for each time factor scale τ in an MSE curve (see Algorithm 1), that is

$$\overline{MSE(\tau)} = \frac{1}{n}\sum_{i=1}^{n} MSE(\tau_i) \tag{1}$$

Moreover, the idea of a MSE curve (a bidimensional or 2D complexity plot) can be extended to a 3D one, a *complexity surface*. For this, we define $\overline{BMSE(t,\tau)}$ and compute a set of $n_s\overline{MSE(t,\tau)}$ curves (slices) which compound such surface (see Algorithm 2).

$$\overline{BMSE(t,\tau)} = \frac{1}{n_s}\sum_{i=1}^{n_s} \overline{MSE(\tau_i)} \tag{2}$$

A way to quantify the variation of MSE and BMSE is done via the standard deviation. Considering all the EEG database information about each patient, the algorithm, which permits to determine which kid was the most affected and on which zone of their brain, is (Algorithm 3) as follows:

Algorithm 3. $MSEZone_{Zone}$, $\sigma Zone_{Zone}$, MSE_{Year}, σ_{Year}

1. Define p, the number of patients, n_r the number of EEG for each patient and n_c the number of channels in each EEG record.

2. For all p, n_r and n_c, compute the average MSE, that is $\overline{MSE(t,i,j,k)}$

3. The most affected zone per patient will be determined by the *smallest MSE and its corresponding biggest standard deviation.*

In order to find *the year where the kids were most affected by their seizures*, we only need to change line 1 by n_y, where n_y is the year associated with each EEG. Hence, the new Step 3 follows. We remark that the EEG duration is implicit above. The number of samples per channel defines such time. As explained in Ref. [1] in order to extend the EEG time to much longer periods, we can use the BMSE and their surfaces. Fifteen minutes, half an hour or longer EEG durations can be compressed in BMSE surfaces. Once we have identified the worst zone/year of a patient, we plot its corresponding BMSE surface and obtain its BMSE index $\overline{BMSE(t,\tau)}$.

4. Results and discussion: which kid was healthier, when and on which region of the brain?

As an example, a period of 7 min was chosen as a duration of the EEG time to compute MSE and BMSE to know quantitatively which kid was healthiest and on which part of the brain. Notice that 7 min imply a lot of traditional EEG pages. Of course, this period can be much more longer. For all subjects, a set of entropy plots was generated. They are of two kinds: bidimensional (2D) MSE and three-dimensional (3D) MSE, that is BMSE [1]. MSE plots allowed us to determine the worst year/most affected area represented by a collection of EEG records. BMSE permits to create a 3D surface of the most affected channel in the worst year of the child.

4.1. Information from bidimensional MSE

4.1.1. Worst year/zone of brain for patient A

In [1] and [2], it was reported that 2010 was the worst year for this kid with F3 as the more discharging zone. This conclusion was obtained by scrutinizing the MSE mean and standard deviation curves (**Figure 6**). The MSE mean lies a little bit above 1, and the standard deviation curves are wider than in the other years. This means less complexity with higher variation in MSE as a result of more seizures with respect to the other years (**Figure 6**). The complexity indices were calculated for the four years to support the latter observations. In addition, the curves $\bar{\sigma}_+$ and $\bar{\sigma}_-$ were plotted for each EEGyear in **Figure 6**. There, the mean curve $\overline{BMSE(\tau)}$ lies between $\Delta = 2\bar{\sigma}(MSE(\tau)))$. So, the set of measures were as follows:

- $\overline{MSE}_{2008} = 1.8539, \bar{\sigma}_{2008} = 0.1481$

http://dx.doi.org/10.5772/64568

- $\overline{MSE}_{2010} = 1.3598, \bar{\sigma}_{2010} = 0.0185$(worst year)
- $\overline{MSE}_{2011} = 1.8329,\ \bar{\sigma}_{2011} = 0.2844$
- $\overline{MSE}_{2013} = 1.4802,\ \bar{\sigma}_{2013} = 0.4236$

The worst year combines the lowest value of MSE with the biggest variation $\bar{\sigma}$. More illustrations about the worst channel, years, zones of patient A can be found in [1, 2].

4.1.2. Worst year/zone of brain for patient B

Proceeding analogously as before, it was determined that 2007 was the worst year because the average MSE plot lies below 1 with wide standard deviation curves although 2014 showed a more complex mean curve with wider variation in the signals. This can be interpreted as having a relative good intellectual development, but accompanied of a continuous discharge state. See below the numerical values of the entropy index. It is remarkable how entropy makes comparable EEG studies per year/channel among several patients.

- $\overline{MSE}_{2007} = 0.7998, \bar{\sigma}_{2007} = 0.4993$ (worst year)
- $\overline{MSE}_{2010} = 1.1821, \bar{\sigma}_{2010} = 0.5658$
- $\overline{MSE}_{2012} = 0.8401, \bar{\sigma}_{2012} = 0.6392$
- $\overline{MSE}_{20147} = 1.2393, \bar{\sigma}_{2014} = 1.0104$

4.1.3. Worst year/zone of brain for patient C

Analogously as proceeded above, it was found that 2006 was the worst year and region T5 the one which suffers more discharges in this case. This kid is noteworthy as a result of his high average complexity. He was diagnosed with DS and recall that (in general) DS is less severe than LGS.

- $\overline{MSE}_{2005} = 1.4582, \bar{\sigma}_{2005} = 1.1140$
- $\overline{MSE}_{2008} = 1.1068, \bar{\sigma}_{2008} = 0.3415$ (worst year)
- $\overline{MSE}_{2012} = 1.3440, \bar{\sigma}_{2012} = 0.1153$
- $\overline{MSE}_{2014} = 1.7761, \bar{\sigma}_{2014} = 0.1447$

4.1.4. Worst year/zone of brain for patient D

Working as above, it was concluded that 2008 was the worst year with Fz the most affected area for this kid.

- $\overline{MSE}_{2005} = 1.1701, \bar{\sigma}_{2005} = 0.3131$

- $\overline{MSE}_{2009} = 1.0107, \bar{\sigma}_{2009} = 0.4101$ (worst year)
- $\overline{MSE}_{2014} = 1.3011,\ \bar{\sigma}_{2014} = 0.3805$

From the MSE indices, we conclude that the most affected patient among all was child B with the smallest $\overline{MSE(\tau)}$ and biggest $\sigma\left(\left(\overline{MSE(\tau)}\right)\right)$. Next, the MSE data will be used to generate the BMSE surfaces which will verify the latter conclusions for much longer EEG durations. See image 9.

4.2. Information from three-dimensional MSE: BMSE

A BMSE surface is illustrated in **Figure 8**, where 2.5 h (9000 s) have been compressed in a single image. The channel corresponds to Fp1, subject A, in 2013. Observe how the surface seems to be mounted on a constant plane equal to one. This means the main activity (red/orange tones) in child A tends to be normal. Notice also that there aretwo sinks (coloured in blue) at $t = 5500$ s and at $t = 6700$ s where episodes of seizures were present. Here, $\overline{BMSE} \approx 1.2$.

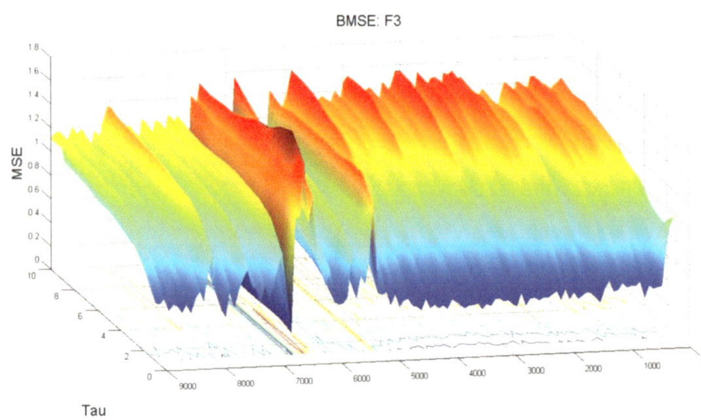

Figure 8. About 2.5Â h have been compressed in a single image for subject A, zone F3, in 2013. Blue sinks are seizures, and orange regions are high complexity regions. Note seizure/recovery times at t = 6000Â s and 7000Â s.

However, notice now that in **Figure 9**,we can compare the four patients' worst situation very easily instead of trying to compare among bunches of EEG. Moreover, the medication can be correlated with the MSE plots and BMSE surfaces as a useful support for the physician. Obviously, with all this, we do not try to replace the physician opinion, but to help it. In this sense, let us examine **Figure 9** where the BMSE surfaces have been plotted for the four subjects for the worst year and the most affected channel. Patient A exhibits a BMSE surface which lies mainly above 1 but with blue zones (low complexity) and a lot of ripples which are also coloured in orange/red meaning high complexity activity. This means that this patient suffers a constant discharging state but with a relative good consciousness and responsive state (note, however, the gash which appears at t≈ 125 s). Now, the BMSE of patient B tends to lies mainly below 1 (blue regions) with more pronounced peaks than patient A. This means that this subject suffer more acute seizures than patient A, and his consciousness is less active than patient's A. Subject's C BMSE surface lies mainly above 1 but observe the low and high complexity ripples during all the EEG record. Kids A and C are similar about consciousness state according to these graphs and to their affection. Now, let us examine child's D plot. This structure does not exhibit that many peaks as in cases A, B and C but rather tends to be flatter with low complexity. This means that the brain activity has slowed down (with respect to the other subjects) which could be the result of a relaxing mind state. Kid's E (normal one) graph lies mainly on 1 with a lot of high complexity ripples. Observe (and compare) child E with child A (which is closest to normality) and kids B, C and D where the lower part of the surfaces is quite close to small values of complexity.

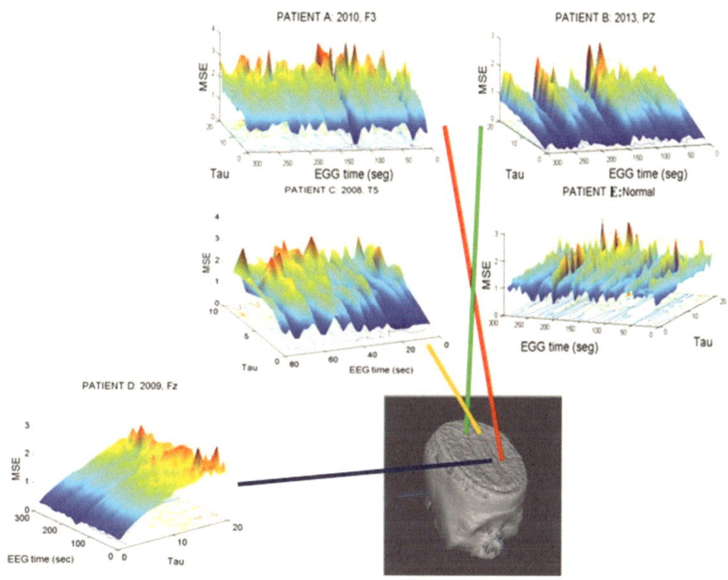

Figure 9. BMSE surfaces for the five subjects considering their worst year and zone of the brain. Note that it is easier to examine these surfaces than scrutinizing bunches of EEG in order to determine which subject was healthier and why. We remark that now all subjects are comparable to each other. Their corresponding BMSE indices are given in the text.

We remark that now all subjects are comparable to each other. Moreover, these facts are supported by the computation of $\overline{BMSE(t,\tau)}$ as follows:

- $\overline{BMSE(t,\tau)}_{A,F3,2010} = 1.6469, \bar{\sigma}_{A,F3,2010} = 0.3083$ (healthies patient)
- $\overline{BMSE(t,\tau)}_{B,PZ,2007} = 1.0469, \bar{\sigma}_{B,PZ,2013} = 0.5246$ (most affected kid)
- $\overline{BMSE(t,\tau)}_{C,T5,2008} = 1.2666, \bar{\sigma}_{C,T5,2008} = 0.0708$
- $\overline{BMSE(t,\tau)}_{D,Fz,2009} = 1.1140, \bar{\sigma}_{D,Fz,2009} = 0.0860$
- $\overline{BMSE(t,\tau)}_{E,C3,2015} = 1.7741, \bar{\sigma}_{D,C3,2015} = 0.3791$ (normal subject)

4.3. Conclusions: correlation with individual medication

Consider the medications of all the children in this study. Compare this resumed information with their corresponding complexity curves/indices. It is now visually easy to observe the effects of such drugs during treatments comparing all subjects at the same time. Our measures will allow neurologists to afford (objectively) the parents' questions established in the Abstract. We would like to recall that handling massive information to evaluate progress in a single patient is challenging, but objective comparisons among progress of different patients are practically impossible.

Declaration of conflicting interest

The authors declared no conflicts of interest with respect to the research, authorship and/or publication of this article.

Author details

Ricardo Zavala Yoé* and Ricardo Ramírez-Mendoza

*Address all correspondence to: rzavalay@itesm.mx

Tecnológico de Monterrey, Escuela de Ingeniería, Calzada del Puente, Ciudad de México, México

References

[1] Zavala-Yoé, R., Ramírez-Mendoza, R., Cordero, L.M.: Novel way to investigate evolution of children refractory epilepsy by complexity metrics in massive information. Springer Plus 4(437), 1–33 (2015).

[2] Zavala-Yoé, R., Ramirez-Mendoza, R., Jimenez-Botello, L.C.: Mathematical complexity as alternative to deal with multiple massive data EEG in children epilepsy. Journal of Epileptology 28(1), 12 (2015).

[3] Shorvon, D.S.: The etiologic classification of epilepsy. Epilepsy 52(6), 1052–1057 (2011).

[4] Berg, A.T., Berkovic, S.F., Brodie, M.J.: Revised terminology and concepts for organization of seizures and epilepsies: report of the ILAE Commission on Classification and Terminology, 2005–2009. Epilepsia 51(4), 676–685 (2010).

[5] Berg, A.T., Brodie, M.I., et al.: Revised terminology and concepts for organization of seizures and epilepsies: report of the ilae commission on classification and terminology. Epilepsia 51(4), 676–685 (2010).

[6] Kwan, P., Arimazinoglou, A., Berg, A.T., et al.: Definition of drug resistant epilepsy: consensus proposal by the ad hoc Task Force of the ILAE Commission on Therapeutic Strategies. Epilepsia 51(6), 1069–1077 (2010).

[7] Doege, C., Kleiss, R., Stephani, U., vonSpiczak, S.: Myoclonic-astatic epilepsy. Journal of Epileptology 2(27), 105–111 (2014).

[8] Stephani, U.: The natural history of myoclonic astatic epilepsy (Doosesyndrome) and Lennox Gastaut syndrome. Epilepsia 47(2), 53–55 (2006).

[9] Stam, C., vanStraaten, E.: Structure out of chaos: functional brain network analysis with EEG, MEG, and functional MRI. European Neuropsychopharmacology 23(1), 7–18 (2013).

[10] Stam, C.J., van Woerkom, T.C.A.M., Keunen, R.W.M.: Non-linear analysis of the electroencephalogram in Creutzfeldt-Jakob disease. Biological Cybernetics 77(4), 247–256 (1997).

[11] Stam, C.: Chaos, continuous EEG, and cognitive mechanisms: a future for clinical neurophysiology. American Journal of Electroneurodiagnostic Technology 43, 211–227 (2003).

[12] Abasolo, D., Escudero, J., Hornero, R., Gomez, C., Espino, P.: Approximate entropy and auto mutual information analysis of the electroencephalogram in Alzheimer's disease patients. Medical & Biological Engineering & Computing 46(10), 1019–1028 (2008).

[13] McTague, A., Cross, J.H.: Treatment of epileptic encephalopathies. CNS Drugs 27, 174–184 (2013).

[14] León, A.C., Davis, L.L., Kraemer, H.C.: Therole andinterpretation ofpilotstudies in clinical research. Journal of Psychiatric Research 45(5), 626–629 (2011).

[15] Reinicke, C., Muthuraman, M., Anwar, A.R., Mideska, K., Siniatchkin, M., Stephani, U., et al.: Neural networks in a patient with infantile epileptic encephalopathy. Clinical Neurophysiology 45, 179–182 (2014).

[16] Bruzzo, A.A., Gesierich, B., Santi, M., Tassinari, C.A., Birbaumer, N., Rubboli, G.: Permutation entropy to detect vigilance changes and preictal states from scalp EEG in epileptic patients. A preliminary study. Neurological Sciences 29(1), 3–9 (2008).

[17] Ouyang, G., Li, J., Liu, X., Li, X.: Dynamic characteristics of absence EEG recordings with multiscale permutation entropy analysis. Epilepsy Research 104(3), 246–252 (2013).

[18] Catarino, A., Churches, O., Baron-Cohen, S., Andrade, A., Ring, H.: Atypical EEG complexity in autism spectrum conditions: a multiscale entropy analysis. Clinical Neurophysiology 122(12), 2375–2383 (2011).

[19] Mbuba, C.K., Ngugi, A.K., Newton, C.R., Carter, J.A.: The epilepsy treatment gap in developing countries: a systematic review of the magnitude, causes, and intervention strategies. Epilepsia 49, 1491–1503 (2008).

[20] Nogués-Solán, X., Sorli-Redó, M.L., Villar-García, J.: Measuring instruments of adherence to treatment. Annals of Internal Medicine 24(3), 138–141 (2007).

[21] Morisky, D.E., Green, L.W., Levine, D.M.: Concurrent and predictive validity of a self reported measure of medication adherence. Medical Care 24, 67–74 (1986).

[22] WHO: WHO Model List of Essential Medicines for Children. 4th List, 2013. WHO, World Health Organization, Geneva, Italy (2013).

[23] WHO: WHO Model List of Essential Medicines. 18th List, 2013. WHO, World Health Organization, Geneva, Italy (2013).

[24] Steinhoff, B., Bast, T.: Compendium Antiepileptic Drugs, 2012–2013. German Society of Epileptology, Berlin, Germany (2013).

[25] Natus Technology. Grass Comet Plus EEG: Lab-Based Portable EEG Systems. Natus Technology, Natus Neurology Incorporated, Middleton, WI (2015).

[26] Gil-Nagel, A.: Manual de Electroencefalografia. McGraw-Hill-Interamericana, Mexico City, Mexico (2001).

[27] g.tec medical engineering Gmbh. Advanced Biosignal Acquisition Processing and Analysis, Products 2013/2014. g.tec medical engineering Gmbh, Schiedlberg, Austria (2014).

[28] Doege, C., May, T., Michael, S., von Spiczak, S., Stephani, U., Boor, R.: Myoclonic astatic epilepsy (Doose syndrome) – a lamotrigine responsive epilepsy? European Journal of Paediatric Neurology 2013(17), 29–35 (2013).

[29] Nakamura, T., Small, M., Hirata, Y.: Testing for nonlinearity in irregular fluctuations with long-term trends. Physical Review E74(026205), 026205–10262058 (2006).

[30] Barnett, A.G., Wolff, R.C.: A time domain test for some types of nonlinearity. IEEE Transactions on Signal Processing 53(1), 26–33 (2005).

[31] Sandsten, M.: Time Frequency Analysis of Non-Stationary Processes. PhD Thesis, Center for Mathematical Sciences (2013).

[32] Garcia Ben, M., Yohai, J.V.: Quantile-quantile plot for deviance residuals in the generalized linear model. Journal of Computational and Graphical Statistics 13(1), 36–47 (2004).

[33] Kipinski, L., Konig, R., Sieluzycki, C., Kordecki, W.: Application of modern tests for stationarity to single trial MEG data. In: Biological Cybernetics, pp. 183–195. Publisher Springer Berlin Heidelberg (2011).

http://dx.doi.org/10.5772/64568

[34] Bendat, J.S., Piersol, A.G.: Measurement and Analysis of Random Data. John Wiley and Sons, NY, USA (1966).

[35] Guarin, D., Delgado, E., Orozco, A.: Testing for nonlinearity in non-stationary physiological time series. In: 33rd Annual International Conference of IEEE-EMBS, pp. 2671–2674 (2011), Boston, Massachusetts USA, August 30–September 3, 2011. IEEE(The Institute of Electrical and Electronics Engineers).

[36] Nachane, D.M.: Selected problems in the analysis of non-stationary and nonlinear time series. In: IGIDR Proceedings/Project Report Series, pp. 1–17 (2009). Quantitative Approaches to Public Policy –Conference in Honour of Professor T. Krishna Kumar Held in conjunction with the Fourth Annual International Conference on Public Policy and Management Indian Institute of Management Bangalore (IIMB) 9–12 August 2009.

[37] Pincus, S.M.: Approximate entropy as a measure of system complexity. Proceedings of the National Academy of Sciences of the United States of America. 88(1), 2297–2301 (1991).

[38] Chon, K.H., Scully, C.G., Lu, S.: Approximate entropy for all signals. IEEE Engineering in Medicine and Biology Magazine 0739–5175, 18–23 (2009).

[39] Costa, M., Goldberger, A., Peng, C.K.: Multiscale entropy analysis of complex physiologic time series. Physical Review 89(6), 068102–10681024 (2002).

[40] Richman, J., Moorman, J.R.: Physiological time series analysis using approximate entropy and sample entropy. American Journal of Physiology – Heart and Circulatory Physiology 278(H2039), 2039–2049 (2000).

Chapter 2

Benign Childhood Epilepsy Syndromes

Tamer Rizk

Additional information is available at the end of the chapter

http://dx.doi.org/10.5772/64843

Abstract

Epileptic syndromes usually carry a devastating outcome and poor prognosis; patients usually present with epileptic encephalopathy, delayed milestones, multiple comorbidities and refractory seizures, although not all epileptic syndromes behave the same, among the big group of children with epilepsy who do not fit within any of the currently recognized syndromes, epilepsy in many children follows a benign course.

Keywords: benign, epilepsy, syndromes, Rolandic, Panayiotopoulos, Gastaut

1. Introduction

International League Against Epilepsy (ILAE)'s definition of a benign epilepsy syndrome is "a syndrome characterized by epileptic seizures that are easily treated, or require no treatment and remit without sequelae". Many children who have epilepsy syndromes that are not usually considered benign, nevertheless, have a good outcome. Many children with congenital hemiplegia who develop focal seizures have only a few seizures, respond well to medication, and eventually successfully discontinue treatment [1].

Benign epilepsy syndromes have been classified according to age of onset into three types: benign neonatal epilepsy syndromes with onset during early neonatal period; benign infantile epilepsy syndromes with onset outside the neonatal period and before first birthday; and benign childhood epilepsy syndromes with its subclassification; these usually occur in children older than 1 year [2].

1.1. Benign neonatal epilepsy syndromes

Most of early-onset neonatal convulsions are characterized by their poor prognosis, except for fifth-day seizures, which carry an excellent outcome. Exclusion of toxic, metabolic, hypoxic-ischemic insult and structural abnormalities is a must prior to diagnosis of benign familial neonatal convulsions. Benign epilepsies in the neonatal period are generally characterized by good prognosis and long-term favorable outcome.

1.2. Benign infantile epilepsy syndromes

Benign infantile epilepsies, with presumed genetic origin, with an increased risk of epileptic seizure disorders are present in children with positive family history of benign focal epilepsies [3].

1.3. Benign childhood epilepsy syndromes

Benign childhood epilepsies are present in about one fourth of children with afebrile seizures. They are also called benign childhood focal seizures and related idiopathic epilepsies, which are subclassified into three types: epilepsy with centrotemporal spikes (CTSs) or "Rolandic" epilepsy, Panayiotopoulos syndrome with its two forms, namely early-onset benign childhood occipital epilepsy and late-onset idiopathic childhood occipital epilepsy (Gastaut type), and idiopathic photosensitive occipital lobe epilepsy of childhood [2].

2. Epilepsy with centrotemporal spikes "Rolandic epilepsy" versus "benign childhood epilepsy with centrotemporal spikes (BECTS)"

2.1. Definition

In 1958, Beaussart was the first to recognize benign focal epilepsies. Lombroso established its recognition in the United States later on. It is now considered the single most common epilepsy syndrome after febrile seizures [4].

The term "Rolandic Epilepsy" is widely used by pediatricians; BECTS was so labeled as centrotemporal spikes (CTSs), which are more predominantly seen in the central (rolandic) fissure; nevertheless, infrequent or even rare spikes may be located in the temporal electrodes bilaterally [5].

The presence of CTS remained a prerequisite for diagnosis of BECTS, though many studies showed that BECTS may take place without CTS and on the contrary some children may show CTS with no history of seizures and it may be encountered in children with other benign focal epilepsies. The word "temporal" may be mistakenly linked to manifestations similar to those taking place in temporal lobe seizures, though this has not been suggested as a characteristic feature of BECTS [5].

2.2. Epidemiology

Age of onset ranges between 1 and 15 years. Up to 75% of cases have onset of seizure between 7 and 10 years. There is marked male predominance with boys being more often affected than girls, with a ratio of 3:2.

2.3. Clinical manifestations

Rolandic epilepsy, being idiopathic, is expected to occur in children who are otherwise normal, though recent studies showed that the presence of excessive spike and wave epileptiform discharges has been linked to learning difficulties and lower school performance.

They are characterized by hemifacial sensorimotor symptoms, oro-pharyngo-laryngeal manifestations, speech arrest and hypersalivation. Secondary generalization is frequent. From all these multiple seizure types, the most recognizable form remains facial symptoms in the form of oro-pharyngo-laryngeal symptoms in addition to hemifacial motor, sensory or more frequently combination of sensorimotor symptoms which is encountered in more than 30% of patients usually in the form of unilateral funny feeling with paresthesia and numbness associated with hemifacial twitches involving tongue, inner cheeks, teeth, gums, pharynx and larynx.

Sensory manifestations of the hemifacial seizures are usually described as numbness or tingling sensations in the corner of the mouth. Speech arrest is very common in Rolandic seizures. The child with speech arrest will often try to communicate using other means, such as gestures. Aphemia (motor aphasia) and aphonia (inability to produce sound as a consequence of laryngeal dysfunction) have been reported. Hypersalivation is reported in around one-third of cases. Ictal syncope has also been recently reported as a rare feature of Rolandic seizures. Panayiotopoulos has argued that it is an anarthria or dysarthria (implying an articulatory disturbance). In support of this, it appears to occur equally in left and right-sided seizures.

Motor manifestations start with abrupt, sustained or episodes of focal clonic contractions involving the lower limb, with deviation of the ipsilateral angle of the mouth, and less frequently, widespread motor components to involve the ipsilateral upper limb. These motor manifestations are responsible for gurgling, grunting and guttural noises, sometimes producing a so-called death rattle.

In more than one-half of Rolandic seizures, consciousness is retained throughout the seizure, such that the child can often give a vivid description of his or her experiences after the seizure. Spread and secondary generalization (generalized tonic clonic seizures [GTCSs]) is much more likely with seizures occurring in sleep; Rolandic epilepsy is one of the commonest causes of nocturnal GTCS in children, exceptionally associated with GTCS when awake.

Seizures are usually brief, mostly lasting 1–2 minutes and may be longer if they progress to GTCS. Focal motor and hemiconvulsive status epilepticus (SE) are well described. Hemiconvulsive SE is more common in younger children, may be followed by Todd's paresis, usually sparing the face. Opercular status is encountered as part of the atypical evolution sometimes encountered in the syndrome. Convulsive SE is exceptional.

2.4. Diagnostic evaluation and differential diagnosis

There is controversy regarding the need of investigations for cases with BECTS. Most investigations, other than EEG, are expected to be normal. Neuroimaging is not required if the clinical presentation, taking into account age, the absence of any comorbidities, seizure semiology and EEG features, is typical.

Neuroimaging, preferably MRI is considered a necessity in the presence of atypical features, abnormal neurological exam, developmental regression or abnormal disease course. MRI brain may show structural brain lesions involving the rolandic regions, coincidental finding of other abnormalities, especially white matter changes and hippocampal abnormalities have been reported, though their significance remains an area for further studies.

2.4.1. EEG

Interictal EEG shows high amplitude sharp and slow wave foci, which are usually localized to the central or centrotemporal electrodes. Three-quarters of seizures occur in non-rapid-eye movement (non-REM) sleep, usually shortly after sleep commences or before wakening [6].

The EEG trait characteristic of Rolandic epilepsy is considered to be inherited in an autosomal dominant manner. The interictal EEG in children with Rolandic epilepsy usually shows a normal background but with the hallmark centrotemporal/Rolandic spikes, complexes of high amplitude epileptiform sharp and slow waves are mainly seen in the central electrodes (C3/C4) or in between central and temporal electrodes (C5/C6). EEG findings can be seen unilateral or bilateral with or without secondary generalization; synchronous as well as asynchronous reports have been delineated [7].

Various studies of CTS utilizing EEG single- or multiple-dipole modeling computerized techniques showed that modeling of the negative spike component can be done by a single and stable tangential dipole source along the central (rolandic) region, the negative pole is maximally delineated in the centrotemporal region while the positive pole is maximally delineated in the frontal regions.

CTSs are highly activated by sleep with preservation of normal sleep architecture. The interictal EEG be normal in rare settings. Trivial findings in the form of subtle background slowing most likely considered as a postictal effect, antiepileptic medication effect, or may be seen if CTSs are particularly abundant. Extracentral sharp and slow wave complexes such as occipital, parietal, frontal and midline regions may occur concurrently with CTS. They are of similar morphology to CTS. Rarely, generalized discharges occur. An unusual feature of the EEG apparent in some children with rolandic epilepsy is the provocation of extreme somatosensory evoked spikes (giant somatosensory evoked potentials) in the contralateral hemisphere by tapping of the fingers or toes [6].

CTS maximally seen at the age of 8–9 years, incidence of 2–3% in normal children and even in children with neurological deficits without history of seizures or epilepsy. There is no link between CTS' frequency, location, persistence and clinical scenario, manifestation, progression of seizures or long-term prognosis. Before the onset of the ictal discharge, CTSs become sparse. There are very few ictal EEG recordings of Rolandic seizures. The ictal discharge consists of unilateral slow waves intermixed with fast rhythms and spikes located in the central regions [6].

Marked EEG abnormalities over many years may not correlate with the clinical condition; some patients will be entirely normal with markedly abnormal EEG abnormalities without any linguistic or neuropsychological deficits and good school achievement.

2.4.2. Magnetoencephalography (MEG)

MEG shows that the dipoles of the prominent negative sharp waves of rolandic discharges appear as tangential dipoles in the central (rolandic) region, with positive poles being situated anteriorly. In rolandic epilepsy, equivalent current dipoles of spikes are located and concentrated in the rolandic regions and have regular directions [6].

2.5. Treatment

Prognosis is not influenced by regular AED treatment. Frequent or diurnal seizures are considered a reasonable indication to start regular antiepileptic medications. Sudden unexplained death in epilepsy (SUDEP) will remain a worry for many parents who will consider regular medications.

Seizure control is easily reached with monotherapy in most of the cases, though recent studies had raised the possibility that it is the secondary generalized tonic clonic seizure (GTCS) that is controlled not the focal ones as previously assumed. There is a lack of strong evidence-based protocol for choosing a first or second line antiepileptic, though the most commonly used medication is still carbamazepine, with oxcarbazepine, valproate and levetiracetam considered as second line choices [8].

2.6. Course and prognosis

Most cases with rolandic epilepsy will have less than ten seizures, single seizures are common. Up to 20% will have frequent seizures, especially at the start of the disorder. The prognosis, however, remains excellent, with remission within 1–2 years of onset and certainly before late adolescence. Incidence of occurrence of GTCS is more or less comparable to normal population (<2%). Patients with rolandic epilepsy are still at higher risk of developing absence seizures later on. Despite being labeled as benign seizures, rolandic epilepsy has been associated with multiple neurodevelopmental effects, cognitive impairment and learning difficulties mainly demonstrated as a consequence of CTS; this has been an area of research and studies focusing on the difference between ictal and interictal EEG abnormalities and their overall effect on the patient even in the absence of clinical seizures. Some patients with BECTS will suffer from multiple speech, reading, behavioral and sleep problems, it is controversial if regular antiepileptic medications should be used in such scenarios and their usefulness to control or even reverse these conditions keeping in mind the side effects of AEDs themselves should be taken in consideration when deciding to start regular antiepileptic medications.

Less than 1% of children with rolandic epilepsy have the so-called atypical evolutions. These include the development of severe linguistic, cognitive or behavioral problems. If such problems develop in a child with rolandic epilepsy, a sleep EEG should be obtained, because continuous spike-and-wave during slow-wave sleep (CSWS) may be present. Landau-Kleffner syndrome is sometimes said to develop from rolandic epilepsy. Atypical focal epilepsy of childhood in which other seizure types, including tonic and atypical absence seizures, may also develop in children with otherwise typical rolandic epilepsy. CSWS may also be seen in children with opercular status characterized by continuous positive or negative myoclonias around the mouth or elsewhere in the face and pseudobulbar problems [9, 10].

3. "Panayiotopoulos syndrome" or "early-onset benign childhood occipital epilepsy (Panayiotopoulos type)"

3.1. Introduction and definition

In 1973, this syndrome was first described by Panayiotopoulos in a 30-year prospective study. After rolandic epilepsy, it is the most common of the benign focal epilepsy syndromes of childhood, which is manifested with autonomic seizures (epileptic seizures characterized by altered autonomic function occurring at the onset of the seizure or as the sole manifestation of the seizure). It is likely to be misdiagnosed as a nonepileptic disorder [11].

Panayiotopoulos syndrome seizures manifest with emesis-like symptoms with retching, nausea, with or without other autonomic symptoms. Episodes of syncope-like behavior have been frequently reported. Seizures are usually long lasting. Interictal EEG usually showed focal high amplitude sharp and slow epileptiform discharges with shifting predominance throughout various cortical areas.

3.2. Epidemiology

Panayiotopoulos syndrome cases vary between late infancy where cases present in the late infancy period and the age of early adolescence at the age of 14 years. However, most cases lie between preschool age (3–6 years) with peak onset age (4–5 years). Boys and girls are equally affected. Prevalence is 6% (1–15 years) and 13% in those (3–6 years). Therefore, a clinician might expect to see at least one case of Panayiotopoulos syndrome for every three cases of rolandic epilepsy [12].

3.3. Clinical manifestations

Panayiotopoulos syndrome is an idiopathic epilepsy syndrome; it occurs in children who are otherwise normal. No specific precipitants can be identified.

http://dx.doi.org/10.5772/64843

Two-thirds of seizures occur during sleep, including daytime naps, and they usually begin with emetic symptoms (nausea, retching with or without vomiting). Some mothers will find their children retching or even vomiting in bed, if seizures start during night sleep, though most of the kids will wake up complaining of nausea and tendency to vomit.

During wakefulness, seizures usually commence with feeling of nausea, mostly associated with behavioral changes, irritability and agitation. Repetitive vomiting is less frequently encountered throughout the seizure onset, usually over many hours. In rare occasions, seizures in Panayiotopoulos syndrome can happen without any feature of the classic "emetic triad". Pallor as well as various autonomic manifestations can concomitantly take place; pupillary abnormalities (mydriasis usually more frequently encountered than miosis), cyanosis and flushing are less common. Urinary and occasionally fecal incontinence may occur [11].

Hyperthermia may be encountered during or immediately after a seizure and may represent a true ictal symptom, rather than being a precipitant of the seizure. Tachycardia is certainly a feature of seizures recorded on EEG with simultaneous ECG recording. Cardiorespiratory arrest during a typical seizure of Panayiotopoulos syndrome has been reported in few case reports. Rarer ictal symptoms that have been reported include headache and other "cephalic sensations," hypersalivation and coughing. Breathing changes are sometimes reported, particularly before convulsions. Episodes of ictal syncopal-like attacks infrequently occur, which have been assumed to result from brief cortical hypoperfusion.

Seizures usually commence during full wakefulness, they start as simple partial seizure, shortly after that, consciousness will be impaired with emergence of a complex partial seizure with some preservation of ability to respond to external stimuli. Behavioral changes in the form of restlessness, agitation and terror, being apparently reported in full consciousness. The occurrence of autonomic manifestations like pallor, while the kid is atonic and unresponsive, raises the possibility of syncope. Seizures often end in hemiconvulsions (in about 20% seizures) or GTCS (also in about 20% seizures). 44% seizures that lasted for 30 minutes or more (maximum is 7 hours) represent a form of nonconvulsive status epilepticus and might reasonably be classified as autonomic status epilepticus, may end spontaneously or as short hemiconvulsions/GTCS and returned to normal within a few hours of such episodes. Convulsive status epilepticus is exceptional. The mean duration is around 9 minutes.

Initial reports of Panayiotopoulos syndrome described lateralizing manifestations such as aversive movement of the head and, as an initial manifestation, eyes to one side; although this feature is not consistent over subsequent reports, data re-evaluation confirmed that is a common featurethatoccurs when consciousness is impaired, which usually takes place sometime after seizure starts.

3.4. Diagnostic evaluation and differential diagnosis

Panayiotopoulos syndrome is frequently mistaken for paroxysmal nonepileptic disorders and occasionally for other types of epilepsy; this is mainly due to its peculiar ictal clinical features and the presence of abnormal interictal EEG changes associated with Panayiotopoulos syndrome.

Seizures in Panayiotopoulos syndrome are usually prolonged and it is not uncommon that many patients will present to emergency room during a clear ictal state; it is sometimes confusing for the attendant physician especially if the presentation is with impaired level of consciousness and vomiting to consider epileptic seizure in the differential diagnosis. Top differential diagnoses will be encephalitis, meningitis and herpetic meningoencephalitis; this will lead the patient to the intensive care unit with broad spectrum antibiotics and antiviral management.

Long-lasting seizures may also be confused with acute confusional migraine and, if vomiting is particularly prominent, with cyclical vomiting syndrome or gastroenteritis. Some seizures may simply be dismissed as travel sickness.

Children with Panayiotopoulos syndrome commonly present to emergency departments while still seizing or in the immediate postictal period.

Panayiotopoulos syndrome should be considered in the differential diagnosis of all previously well young children, (3–6) years, who have rapid onset of emetic symptoms followed by impaired (often fluctuating) consciousness. Eye or head deviation may be a useful finding. However, it may still be appropriate to manage the child for a suspected encephalopathy.

If Panayiotopoulos syndrome is suspected from the history, the most useful investigation is likely to be the EEG (including sleep study if necessary). Symptomatic epilepsies may mimic Panayiotopoulos syndrome, so even if the history is typical, most authorities recommend neuroimaging.

3.4.1. EEG

Interictal EEG usually shows normal background with high-amplitude sharp, sharp and slow-wave foci (sometimes labeled as functional spikes), which is similar, in morphology; but not in location, to those seen in rolandic epilepsy. The EEG abnormalities in Panayiotopoulos syndrome are accentuated in sleep. Cloned-like, repetitive and multifocal spike wave complexes in which repetitive spike or sharp and slow wave complexes appear concurrently in different brain locations of one or both hemispheres.

Previously the occipital location of these changes was emphasized, along with their occurrence in long trains (occipital paroxysms) and abolition by central fixation (fixation-off sensitivity). Although fixation-off sensitivity is common, photosensitivity is exceptional. It now appears that these features were overemphasized, and in Panayiotopoulos syndrome the characteristic functional spikes can occur in multiple locations, albeit with a posterior predominance. Focal or diffuse slowing may be seen postictal. However, spikes' frequency, distribution and persistence are not time-locked to clinical manifestations, progression, seizures' frequency or intensity and are not consistent with prognosis of Panayiotopoulos syndrome.

Various ictal EEG changes have been reported; trains of focal rhythmic delta or theta activity associated with the presence of epileptic spikes. These changes used to be delineated mainly in the posterior areas, but may be anterior. Rarer EEG findings: small, spikes, slow waves intermixed with small spikes and brief generalized discharges. Occasionally, repeated EEGs can all be normal.

In some cases, EEG findings of patients with Panayiotopoulos syndrome may be misleading and may lead to wrong diagnosis. EEG findings may look similar or even identical to those of other benign epilepsies such as BECTS or Gastaut idiopathic childhood occipital epilepsy, which is highly possibile is higher if proper clinical history is not obtained. Multifocal spike discharges and bursts of repetitive multifocal spike wave complexes within the delta range may look similar to EEG findings associated with some malignant epilepsies such as the Lennox-Gastaut syndrome, though they run a totally different clinical course.

3.4.2. MEG

MEG study for patients with Panayiotopoulos syndrome usually shows equivalent current dipoles of spikes concentrated in the rolandic regions and occipital areas. In MEG combined with MRI, equivalent current dipoles cluster preferentially in cortical locations along the parietal-occipital, the calcarine or the central fissure. The equivalent current dipole clustering may be unilateral or bilateral, monofocal or multifocal. These findings are in keeping with the condition being a multifocal rather than a purely occipital epilepsy. The directions of each equivalent current dipole in each area are quite regular as if three small round toothbrushes are placed in each of the three areas.

3.4.3. MRI

MRI is considered a better modality than CT scan. However, if MRI will require sedation or general anesthesia, CT may be appropriate.

3.5. Treatment

Regular prophylactic AED medication is usually reserved for patients with frequent seizures, which distressed them and their families or even interfere with their daily living activities and regular life style. There is a lack of well-structured study to suggest the first line AED to be used. Carbamazepine and sodium valproate are considered equally efficacious, though carbamazepine was found to exaggerate seizures in a minority of children with PS [13].

Panayiotopoulos syndrome is considered a benign syndrome, so it is important to try to avoid side effects of various AEDs. It is considered a good practice to try to wean AED after 2 years if the child remained seizure-free throughout this period; it is still controversial whether or not to have a normal EEG prior to that as clinical improvement may be reached prior to electrographical one. I think that the emergence of association between Panayiotopoulos syndrome and cardiorespiratory arrest will be a valid indication to continue AED for longer duration; this area still needs further studies.

3.6. Course and prognosis

Seizures in Panayiotopoulos syndrome are considered infrequent. 30% of cases with Panayiotopoulos syndrome will encounter only one seizure and only 5–10% will have more frequent seizures reaching more than 10, though sometimes seizures are very frequent. One-fifth will have one or more seizures typical of one of the other benign focal epilepsies of childhood, especially rolandic epilepsy [14].

The duration of active seizures is short; remission usually occurring within 1–2 years from onset. Seizures in adult life are no greater than in the general population [14, 15].

There are few case reports of atypical evolutions in Panayiotopoulos syndrome, including the development of absences and drop attacks [1, 14].

4. Idiopathic childhood occipital epilepsy (late-onset childhood occipital epilepsy, "Gastaut type", and idiopathic photosensitive occipital lobe epilepsy)

4.1. Introduction and definition

"Idiopathic childhood occipital epilepsy" includes both late-onset childhood occipital epilepsy —Gastaut type and idiopathic photosensitive occipital lobe epilepsy. This is because both conditions share many common features and it is not clear that they merit separation into two distinct syndromes [1, 16].

Idiopathic childhood occipital epilepsy with and without photosensitivity was first established as an epileptic syndrome by Gastaut. Recently, it has been classified separately by the ILAE Task Force as late-onset childhood occipital epilepsy (Gastaut type) and idiopathic photosensitive occipital lobe epilepsy. Idiopathic childhood occipital epilepsy can be defined as an idiopathic focal seizure disorder of childhood manifested mainly by elementary visual seizures and ictal blindness, which are often frequent and usually occur without impairment of consciousness [1, 16].

Idiopathic photosensitive occipital epilepsy is an idiopathic focal seizure disorder mainly of childhood manifested mainly by elementary visual seizures provoked by various forms of environmental light stimulation [1, 16].

The likelihood of remission in these syndromes is considerably less than rolandic epilepsy and Panayiotopoulos syndrome. Some children with these conditions remit completely [1, 16].

4.2. Epidemiology

Idiopathic childhood occipital epilepsy usually starts at toddler age group in children as young as 3 years and extends to involve adolescents as old as 15 years of age. Peak age of onset is around 8 years. Boys and girls are equally affected. Furthermore, idiopathic photosensitive occipital epilepsy may start as early as the second year of life or as late as young adult life.

http://dx.doi.org/10.5772/64843

However, it peaks at around 12 years of age. There is probably a slight female preponderance, but nowhere near as great as for photosensitivity alone [16].

Panayiotopoulos estimated that idiopathic childhood occipital epilepsy accounted for about 2–7% of all benign focal epilepsies of childhood.

4.3. Clinical manifestations

Idiopathic childhood occipital epilepsy hallmark is visual hallucinations which the patient described as small multicolored patterns that run in circles, most commonly occurring unilaterally in the peripheral visual field; they increase in size and number with seizure progression, sometimes moving horizontally across the visual field, with or without other more complex movements. Normal vision may be hindered by these hallucinations, but in others it may not. Visual illusions as shape and distance distortions have been reported; even more complex visual hallucinations as formed shapes and faces may be encountered, though they are less frequent [12, 16].

Ictal blindness is considered the second most common complaint reported by patients with idiopathic childhood occipital epilepsy after visual hallucinations. Ictal blindness is usually bilateral, but may be unilateral or even partial involving less than one half of a visual field. It usually occurs in the form of sudden black outs, though others will describe that everything goes white. Ictal blindness is usually an initial seizure manifestation but sometimes follows visual hallucinations. Other ictal ocular symptoms are relatively common, e.g., ocular pain and ictal eye deviation, often with simultaneous head deviation in about 70% of cases. Forced eye closure and eyelid blinking are other reported phenomena [12, 16].

Seizures are usually brief, lasting for few seconds, though prolonged seizures lasting for few minutes have been described, mainly those seizures with ictal blindness which may last for even hours; this has been described as "status amauroticus" [12, 16].

Headache has been described as a common manifestation in idiopathic childhood occipital epileptic seizures (post ictal > ictal). It often has a migrainous character. Autonomic manifestations have been reported in idiopathic photosensitive occipital lobe epilepsy, e.g., vomiting which characterizes Panayiotopoulos syndrome [12, 16, 17].

Patients with idiopathic childhood occipital epilepsy usually maintain their consciousness during most seizures, though occasionally impaired level of consciousness will be reported in cases of secondarily generalization with occurrence of generalized tonic clonic seizures. Occurrence of temporal lobe symptoms has been reported and is considered to result from local spreading of epileptiform discharges.

Seizures usually occur in day time with high frequency; multiple seizures take place on a daily or sometimes weekly basis. Nocturnal seizures with hemiconvulsions or even generalized tonic clonic seizures are not uncommon [12, 16].

Photosensitivity in idiopathic photosensitive occipital lobe epilepsy is significant, as seizures may be provoked by variable light sources, e.g., video-games, watching television. Photosensitivity ranges between different subjects; some will have high photosensitivity resulting in high seizure frequency while others with less photosensitivity will have few seizures. Nevertheless, spontaneous seizures without photosensitivity have also been reported. Some cases with idiopathic childhood occipital epilepsy have developed absences and myoclonic jerks provoked by photic stimulation [12, 16].

4.4. Diagnostic evaluation and differential diagnosis

These syndromes, like all occipital epilepsies, are very prone to misdiagnosis as migraine. However, the elementary visual hallucinations are unlike those of migraine. In the latter they tend to be black and white, rather than colored, and have jagged or sharp contours rather than being predominantly rounded. They may mimic symptomatic occipital lobe epilepsies, and neuroimaging, preferably MRI, is indicated [12, 16].

4.4.1. EEG

In late-onset childhood occipital epilepsy 'Gastaut type', interictal background is normal, occipital paroxysms are characteristic and isolated occipital spikes may be seen. Extraoccipital paroxysmal abnormalities may occur, but are much less common than in Panayiotopoulos syndrome [12, 16].

The ictal EEG is expected to show attenuation of occipital paroxysms followed by appearance of an occipital discharge of fast rhythms, fast spikes or both.

In some subjects, EEG abnormalities may only be seen in sleep; occasionally both awake and sleep EEGs may be consistently normal [12, 16].

In idiopathic photosensitive occipital lobe epilepsy, interictal EEG is expected to have a normal background. No spontaneous epileptiform abnormalities or else there may be occipital spikes or paroxysms. Extraoccipital epileptiform abnormalities may also be seen. Intermittent photic stimulation will, in all subjects, show occipital or generalized photoparoxysmal responses [12, 16].

4.5. Treatment

Given the frequency of seizures in idiopathic childhood occipital epilepsy, including the likelihood of occasional GTCS, regular AED treatment is considered necessary in most if not all subjects. There are no controlled studies comparing alternatives, although carbamazepine appears to be most often used in subjects who are not photosensitive. Broad spectrum agents such as sodium valproate and levetiracetam, active against focal and generalized seizures and photosensitivity, would appear to be reasonable choices. However, it appears that carbamazepine, not usually considered a useful drug for photosensitivity, may sometimes be effective [12, 16].

Attempt withdrawal after two seizure-free years is associated with significant risk of relapse. Some subjects with idiopathic photosensitive occipital lobe epilepsy who are only mildly photosensitive and who do not have spontaneous seizures can remain seizure-free by avoiding precipitants. Others will require AED treatment.

http://dx.doi.org/10.5772/64843

4.6. Course and prognosis

Prognosis for both idiopathic childhood occipital epilepsy and idiopathic photosensitive occipital lobe epilepsy is variable. About 50–60% of Gastaut type have remission of seizures within 2–4 years of them starting. However, in a significant minority, seizures will continue into adulthood [18].

In children with idiopathic photosensitive occipital lobe epilepsy who are only mildly photosensitive and can control their exposure to relevant provoking factors, freedom from seizures may be easily achieved. For others, particularly those who are highly photosensitive, the likelihood of seizures continuing into adult life is high [18].

Atypical evolutions in idiopathic childhood occipital epilepsy with cognitive deterioration and CSWS. Carbamazepine is sometimes implicated in precipitating such atypical evolutions [18].

5. Other described benign focal epilepsies of childhood

The syndromes discussed previously are the only benign focal epilepsies of childhood currently recognized by the ILAE. However, others have been proposed and are more or less well characterized: benign childhood seizures with affective symptoms, benign childhood focal seizures associated with frontal or midline spikes, benign focal epilepsy in infants with central and vertex spikes and waves during sleep and Benign childhood seizures with affective symptoms are associated by and frequent extreme somatosensory-evoked spikes [19, 20].

5.1. Benign childhood seizures with affective symptoms

The onset is between 2 and 9 years of age. They are characterized by multiple, usually short, daytime and nighttime seizures in which the predominant symptom appears to be fear or terror, accompanied by autonomic disturbances (pallor, sweating, abdominal pain and salivation), arrest of speech and mild impairment of consciousness with automatisms [21].

Interictal EEG shows sharp and slow wave complexes similar to those in rolandic epilepsy but located in the frontotemporal and parietotemporal electrodes [21].

This is likely to be an intermediate phenotype between Panayiotopoulos syndrome and rolandic epilepsy. Benign childhood seizures with affective symptoms are associated by and frequent giant somatosensory evoked potentials. Remission in 1–2 years from onset is expected [21].

This putative disorder is mainly defined by its interictal EEG features reflected in its name. These features are, however, said to often be associated with a phenotype characterized by mainly daytime versive seizures, which are infrequent and have an excellent prognosis [21].

5.2. Benign childhood focal seizures associated with frontal or midline spikes

This putative disorder is mainly defined by its interictal EEG features. These EEG features can be seen in children with febrile seizures, rolandic epilepsy, Panayiotopoulos syndrome and idiopathic childhood occipital epilepsy.

5.3. Benign focal epilepsy in infants with central and vertex spikes and waves during sleep

Benign focal epilepsy in infants with central and vertex spikes and waves during sleep has been recently described as a new benign syndrome [22].

It lies in the transition zone between benign infantile seizures and Panayiotopoulos syndrome with age of onset usually in the first two years of life. Males and females are equally affected. Clinical examination, including developmental assessment, should be normal; investigations and imaging are always normal [3].

Benign focal epilepsy in infants with central and vertex spikes and waves during sleep usually starts with staring, arrest of activity, autonomic features with facial cyanosis, loss of consciousness and tonic contractions of both upper limbs; rarely clonic movements and automatisms may be encountered. Seizures usually last for less than 5 minutes, most of the time they occur during daytime, though nocturnal seizures have been described. They are usually infrequent with less than four seizures annually, but they may occur in clusters [3, 22].

Interictal EEG changes mainly encountered in non-REM sleep stages, consist of central spike and wave epileptiform discharges of low amplitude, localized to the vertex [3, 22].

Benign focal epilepsy in infants with central and vertex spikes and waves during sleep carries a favorable prognosis in families with strong history of benign epilepsies. Prognosis is excellent with more or less complete seizures remission, normal neurodevelopment and even EEG normalization before the fourth year of life [3, 22].

6. Genetics

Benign focal epilepsies of childhood do not follow simple Mendelian inheritance, which has strong concordance for idiopathic generalized epilepsies in monozygotic twins, but not for rolandic epilepsy. Autosomal dominant genetic linkage has been reported to 15q14 for BECTS [23].

Researchers found that EEG traits characterizing these disorders may surprisingly show Mendelian inheritance even if the seizure phenotype did not; this is still an area of debate and needs further studies [24].

Vadlamudi et al. found strong concordance for idiopathic generalized epilepsies in 26 monozygotic twins, but no concordance for Rolandic epilepsy in six monozygotic twins [25].

http://dx.doi.org/10.5772/64843

Mendelian inheritance in individual families with forms of benign focal epilepsy has been established. EEG trait characterizing these disorders may show Mendelian inheritance, even if the seizure phenotype does not [23].

Author details

Tamer Rizk

Address all correspondence to: drtamergaber@gmail.com

1 Al-Takhassusi Hospital, Riyadh, Saudi Arabia

2 Habib Medical Group Holding Company, Riyadh, Saudi Arabia

References

[1] Engel J Jr. A proposed diagnostic scheme for people with epileptic seizures and with epilepsy: report of the ILAE Task Force on Classification and Terminology. Epilepsia 2001; 42:796–803.

[2] Panayiotopoulos CP. Benign childhood partial epilepsies: benign childhood seizure susceptibility syndromes [editorial]. J Neurol Neurosurg Psychiatry 1993; 56:2–5.

[3] Capovilla G, Beccaria F, Montagnini A. "Benign focal epilepsy in infancy with vertex spikes and waves during sleep." Delineation of the syndrome and recalling as "benign infantile focal epilepsy with midline spikes and waves during sleep" (BIMSE). Brain Dev 2006; 28:85–91.

[4] Beaussart M, Loiseau P, Roger H. The discovery of "benign rolandic epilepsy." In: Berkovic SF, Genton P, Hirsch E, Picard F, Eds. Genetics of Focal Epilepsies. London: John Libbey & Company, 1999:3–6.

[5] Lombroso CT. Sylvian seizures and midtemporal spike foci in children. Arch Neurol 1967; 17:52–59.

[6] Kanazawa O. Benign rolandic epilepsy and related epileptic syndromes: electrophysiological studies including magnetoencephalography in ictal and interictal phenomena. In: Benjamin SM, Ed. Trends in Epilepsy Research. New York: Nova Science Publishers, Inc., 2005: 19–54.

[7] Heijbel J, Blom S, Rasmuson M. Benign epilepsy of childhood with centrotemporal EEG foci: a genetic study. Epilepsia 1975; 16:285–293.

[8] Corda D, Gelisse P, Genton P, Dravet C, et al. Incidence of drug-induced aggravation in benign epilepsy with centrotemporal spikes. Epilepsia 2001; 42:754–759.

[9] Fejerman N, Caraballo R, Tenembaum SN. Atypical evolutions of benign localization-related epilepsies in children: are they predictable? Epilepsia 2000; 41:380–390.

[10] Fejerman N. Atypical evolutions of benign partial epilepsies in children. Int Pediatr 1996; 11:351–356.

[11] Panayiotopoulos CP. Benign childhood focal seizures and related epileptic syndromes. In: Panayiotopoulos CP, Ed. The Epilepsies: Seizures, Syndromes and Management. Oxford: Bladon Medical Publishing, 2005:223–269.

[12] Panayiotopoulos CP. Occipital seizures and related epileptic syndromes. In: Panayiotopoulos CP, Ed. Benign Childhood Partial Seizures and Related Epileptic Syndromes. London: John Libbey & Company, 1999:101–228.

[13] Kikumoto K, Yoshinaga H, Oka M, Ito M, et al. EEG and seizure exacerbation induced by carbamazepine in Panayiotopoulos syndrome. Epileptic Disord 2006; 8:53–56.

[14] Caraballo RH, Astorino F, Cersosimo R, Soprano AM, et al. Atypical evolution in childhood epilepsy with occipital paroxysms (Panayiotopoulos type). Epileptic Disord 2001; 3:157–162.

[15] Ferrie CD, Koutroumanidis M, Rowlinson S, Sanders S, et al. Atypical evolution of Panayiotopoulos syndrome: a case report [published with video sequences]. Epileptic Disord 2002; 4:35–42.

[16] Gastaut H. A new type of epilepsy: benign partial epilepsy of childhood with occipital spike-waves. Clin Electroencephalogr 1982; 13:13–22.

[17] Panayiotopoulos CP. Elementary visual hallucinations, blindness, and headache in idiopathic occipital epilepsy: differentiation from migraine. J Neurol Neurosurg Psychiatry 1999; 66:536–540.

[18] Tenembaum S, Deonna T, Fejerman N, Medina C, et al. Continuous spike-waves and dementia in childhood epilepsy with occipital paroxysms. J Epilepsy 1997; 10:139–145.

[19] Fonseca LC, Tedrus GM. Somatosensory evoked spikes and epileptic seizures: a study of 385 cases. Clin Electroencephalogr 2000; 31:71–75.

[20] Tassinari CA, De Marco P. Benign partial epilepsy with extreme somato-sensory evoked potentials. In: Roger J, Bureau M, Dravet C, Dreifuss FE, et al, Eds. Epileptic Syndromes in Infancy, Childhood and Adolescence. London: John Libbey & Company, 1992:225–229.

[21] Dalla Bernardina B, Colamaria V, Chiamenti C, Capovilla G, et al. Benign partial epilepsy with affective symptoms ("benign psychomotor epilepsy"). In: Roger J, Bureau M, Dravet C, Dreifuss FE, et al, Eds. Epileptic Syndromes in Infancy, Childhood and Adolescence. London: John Libbey & Company, 1992:219–223.

[22] Bureau M, Cokar O, Maton B, Genton P, Dravet C. Sleep-related, low voltage Rolandic and vertex spikes: an EEG marker of benignity in infancy-onset focal epilepsies. Epileptic Disord 2002; 4:15–22.

[23] Bray PF, Wiser WC. Evidence for a genetic etiology of temporal-central abnormalities in focal epilepsy. N Engl J Med 1964; 271:926–933.

[24] Neubauer BA, Hahn A, Stephani U, Doose H. Clinical spectrum and genetics of Rolandic epilepsy. Adv Neurol 2002; 89:475–479.

[25] Vadlamudi L, Harvey AS, Connellan MM, Milne RL, et al. Is benign rolandic epilepsy genetically determined? Ann Neurol 2004; 56:129–132.

Chapter 3

GABAergic Interneurons in Severe Early Epileptic Encephalopathy with a Suppression-Burst Pattern: A Continuum of Pathology

María Carmen Carrascosa-Romero and
Carlos De Cabo De La Vega

Additional information is available at the end of the chapter

http://dx.doi.org/10.5772/64458

Abstract

Early infantile epileptic encephalopathy (EIEE) and early myoclonic encephalopathy (EME) are catastrophic epilepsies starting in the neonatal period. The International League Against Epilepsy classifies both of them as generalized symptomatic epilepsies of nonspecific etiology, characterized by early onset, presence of burst-suppression EEG pattern and serious prognosis. The critical difference lies in their presumed etiologies and the prevailing clinical seizure type at onset: EIEE (known as Ohtahara syndrome) usually manifests with tonic seizures, while EME is mainly associated with myoclonic seizures. However, the distinction between those two pathologies is not always easy due to clinical and etiological overlap. Both mutations in the ARX gene for EIEE (OMIM 308350) and disruption in the neuregulin receptor ErbB4 for EME (OMIM 609304) impair interneuron migration and alter the number of GABAergic interneurons in the postnatal cortex. These findings could explain the occurrence of severe epileptic encephalopathy with a burst-suppression pattern and represent a continuum of progressive pathology. In the present chapter we review the genes involved in EIEE and EME including their possible mechanisms of action, particularly via GABAegic interneurons. Their clinical manifestations are myoclonic or tonic seizures, which represent the expression of the underlying pathology and correlate with degree of brain damage.

Keywords: ARX gene, burst-suppression EEG pattern, early infantile epileptic encephalopathy, early myoclonic encephalopathy, early-onset epileptic encephalopathy, encephalopathy, epilepsy, ErbB4, GABA, interneurons, genetics, development, children, neonatal epilepsies, newborn, Ohtahara syndrome, seizures

1. Introduction

Neonatal seizures are the most characteristic sign of neurological disease and the most frequent neurological events during the neonatal period (babies less than 28 days old), often reflecting a variety of different pre-, peri-, or postnatal disorders of the central nervous system (CNS). The incidence of seizures is highest during the neonatal period. The overall risk of neonatal seizures in the United States was 2.84 per 1000 live births, and risk estimates were consistently higher in low-birth-weight infants (relative risk of 3.9) [1]. We have found an absolute incidence of neonatal convulsions in newborns (NBs) infants of 2‰ in live births (in full term of 1.4‰, in preterm of 13.4‰, and in immature NBs (with a gestational age of <29 weeks) of 27.8‰) [2]. Besides, higher incidence and prevalence rates of epilepsy have been found in developing countries [3]. They may be symptomatic or cryptogenic, precursory or subsequent epilepsies, and acquired causes are the most frequent. Thus, in our study the etiology was distributed as follows: hypoxic-ischemic encephalopathy (HIE, 32%), brain malformations or cerebral dysgenesis (24%), intracranial hemorrhage (16%), and, less frequently, infections, metabolic disorders and pharmacological changes (8%), and epileptogenic diagnosis (4%). Notwithstanding, we are currently observing a decrease down to 7.9% in brain malformations as a cause of neonatal seizures due to the impact of the implementation of the legal termination of pregnancy due to congenital anomalies or birth defects.

The neonatal period is the most vulnerable time for the occurrence of seizures. Overall, neonatal seizures are the expression of a serious neurological condition that requires urgently both etiological and symptomatic treatment, because by themselves can aggravate brain damage. The study of neonatal seizures also allows us to better understand the mechanisms that affect the developing brain [4]. The burden of acute recurrent seizures in neonates may also impact chronic outcomes independently from the etiology [5].

The developing brain has a higher incidence of seizures in both animal and human models. These neonatal seizures can produce long-lasting consequences that are stage-dependent [6]. The nervous system (NS) of the newborn presents singularities related to the lower maturation of its structures. The neonatal brain has an increased neuronal metabolism, and, therefore, a high rate of oxygen consumption. Such energetic costs seem also to exert a selective pressure toward a metabolically efficient neural morphology, leading to a metabolically efficient patterning of dendritic arborizations, neural codes, and brain-wiring patterns [7]. However, the theory of energy failure has largely been disproved. Brains of immature animals have been shown to be capable of using anaerobic metabolism and require less adenosine triphosphate (ATP) when aerobic energy production ceases, even during status convulsive. Recent explanations for the injurious consequences of prolonged convulsions postulate that neuronal damage occurs from excessive release of excitatory amino acids (EAA) which, by binding to their ligand-gated ionic receptors, cause a large influx of Ca^{2+}, resulting in acute excitotoxic cell death and neuronal apoptosis [8].

On the other hand, neurotransmitters (NTs)—especially γ-aminobutyric acid (GABA) and glutamate—as well as N-methyl-D-aspartate receptors (NMDARs) play key roles in successive steps of brain development, including the proliferation, migration, survival, and differentiation of neurons. Cerebral cortical circuits are composed of both excitatory (glutamatergic) projection and local inhibitory (GABAergic) neurons. The NMDA receptor subunits in the developing brain are more permeable and less susceptible to block than mature forms, with the result that immature brains are far more excitable and epileptogenic than the adult brain (9). Although in general the neonatal brain is more resistant to hypoxia than the adult brain, the former seems to be more vulnerable to the neurotoxic amino acids that occur during seizures [9].

Although early-onset epileptic syndromes are a rare and not a common cause for neonatal seizures, they have aroused increasing interest since they generally involve genetic diseases. Thus, it is very important to establish the diagnosis in order to allow adequate genetic counseling. The study of these syndromes has also helped to clarify the role of NTs and receptors, signal transduction, intracellular transporters, and enzymes in the origin of seizures. More accurate molecular genetics diagnostic tools will allow diagnosing a larger number of cases previously considered of unknown etiology and open the door to pharmacogenomics.

2. Neonatal epileptic encephalopathy (EE) with suppression-burst EEG pattern

2.1. Concept of epileptic encephalopathies

The International League Against Epilepsy (ILAE) defines epileptic encephalopathies (EEs) as follows: they "are a group of diseases in which epileptic activity itself contributes to severe cognitive and behavioral impairments above and beyond what might be expected from the underlying pathology alone. These impairments can worsen over time" [10]. This means that not only refractory seizures but also that serious epileptiform discharges observed in the electroencephalogram (EEG) background contribute to the progressive decline in brain function. The three main features of EEs are refractory seizures, severe EEG abnormalities, developmental delay, and/or intellectual disability. Around 40% of seizures that occur during the first 3 years of life are due to EEs. A few syndromes are considered epileptic encephalopathies, also known as early-onset epileptic encephalopathies (EOEEs) (for a review, see [11, 12]):

- Early myoclonic encephalopathy (EME) and Ohtahara syndrome (OS) in the neonatal period;
- West syndrome (WS), epilepsy of infancy with migrating focal seizures (EIMFS), and Dravet's syndrome (DS) during infancy;
- Lennox-Gastaut syndrome (LGS), epileptic encephalopathy with continuous spikes and waves during sleep (CSWS), and Landau-Kleffner syndrome (LKS) during childhood.

2.2. Classification epilepsy syndromes

In the last International Classification of the Epilepsies (ILAE classification), the epilepsy syndromes are classified by reliably identified common clinical and electrical characteristics. Such "electro-clinical" syndromes have a typical age of seizure onset, specific seizure types, and EEG characteristics, and often other features, which when taken together allow the diagnosis of every specific epilepsy syndrome [13]. The classification, which has been updated on an ongoing basis by the ILAE Commission on Classification and Terminology in Epilepsy Diagnosis [14] (a cutting-edge online diagnostic manual of the epilepsies), includes within the *electro-clinical syndromes* of neonatal/infantile onset the following syndromes (arranged by age at onset):

2.2.1. Neonatal period

- Self-limited neonatal seizures and self-limited familial neonatal epilepsy
- Early myoclonic encephalopathy (EME)
- Ohtahara syndrome (OS) or early infantile epileptic encephalopathy (EIEE)

2.2.2. Infancy

- Self-limited familial and nonfamilial infantile epilepsy
- West syndrome (WS)
- Dravet's syndrome (DS)
- Myoclonic epilepsy in infancy (MEI)
- Epilepsy of infancy with migrating focal seizures (EIMFS)
- Myoclonic encephalopathy in nonprogressive disorders
- Febrile seizures plus, genetic epilepsy with febrile seizures plus

"Early myoclonic encephalopathy" (EME) and "Ohtahara syndrome" (OS), are listed as two separate syndromes in the classification of epilepsies. Both are characterized by early onset (EIEE may also occur later), presence of "burst-suppression" (BS) EEG pattern, seizures that do not respond to anti-seizure medication, and serious prognosis. EEG pattern is the most important diagnostic feature for both clinical entities. BS means that the EEG tends to display periods of very little electrical brain activity or flattening of the brain waves, followed by a burst of high spiky activity before returning to very low activity again. The BS is characterized by high-voltage bursts (multifocal spikes of 150–350 mV, and 1–3-s duration) alternating regular rate with almost flat suppression phases (2–5 s). These changes can be seen both during sleep and when the child is awake [15]. The differential diagnosis is based mainly on the different types of seizures: fragmentary myoclonus, erratic focal seizures, and massive myoclonias for EME, and tonic seizures and predominantly tonic spasms (flexor or extensor/ stiffening of arms or legs, uni-, or bilateral) for EIEE [16, 17] (see **Table 1**).

http://dx.doi.org/10.5772/64458

	Early myoclonic encephalopathy (EME)	Early infantile epileptic encephalopathy (EIEE) Ohtahara syndrome
General description	• Both entities are syndromes consisting of frequent intractable seizures and severe early encephalopathy resulting in limited development and reduced life expectancy. • They are considered "epileptic encephalopathies". This term implies that the epileptic activity itself might be directly implicated in additional neurodevelopmental impairments besides those expected from the underlying etiology alone, and that suppression of epileptic activity might minimize this additional disability. • Treatable ***metabolic etiologies*** (especially pyridoxine and pyridoxal-5-phosphate disorders) should be excluded early. • Both sexes are affected equally.	
Age of occurrence	Onset of seizures in the first 2 months of life (during the first week in 76% of the cases, with 96% occurring by the first month)	The onset of seizures is in the first month of life (range 1–3 months).
Different seizure types	**Myoclonic seizures are frequent:** fragmentary myoclonus, erratic focal seizures, and massive myoclonias. Tonic seizures are observed later, usually around 3–4 months of age.	**Tonic seizures predomínate**. Many seizure types may occur, but myoclonic seizures are rare.
Electroencephalograph	**Suppression-burst pattern:** ***Consisting of alternating periods of slow waves of high amplitude (the burst) and periods of so-called flat EEGs (the suppression)***	
Clinical course	Severe developmental delay is seen, with or without regression.	
		Children with this syndrome may evolve to West or Lennox Gastaut syndrome.
Antecedent and birth history	Typically normal	
Neurological examination	Abnormal neurological behavior may be present prior to onset of seizures.	
	Abnormal in keeping with the presence of severe neurological impairment. ***Head size is typically normal at onset; microcephaly may develop over time.***	Abnormal in keeping with underlying brain structure abnormalities and the presence of severe neurological impairment. Head size is typically normal; however, microcephaly may occur.
Causes: There is overlap in the etiologies that cause Ohtahara syndrome and early myoclonic encephalopathy.	Metabolic etiologies are common (nonketotic hyperglycinemia is the commonest cause, amino and organic acidopathies, urea cycle disorders, mitochondrial disorders, pyridoxine and pyridoxal-5-phosphate disorders, molybdenum cofactor deficiency,	**Structural brain etiologies** are common Metabolic etiologies (mitochondrial disorders, nonketotic hyperglycinemia, pyridoxine/pyridoxal-5-phosphate disorders, carnitine palmitoyl transferase deficiency, and others).

	Early myoclonic encephalopathy (EME)	Early infantile epileptic encephalopathy (EIEE) Ohtahara syndrome
	sulfite oxidase deficiency, Menke syndrome, Zellweger syndrome, and other disorders are also seen). Structural brain abnormalities are rare.	
Genetic causes	**SLC25A22, ErbB4, etc.**	**ARX, STXBP1, KCNQ2, SCN2A, GNAO1, etc.**

Table 1. Epilepsy syndromes with debut neonatal/infantile and suppression-burst EEG pattern.

2.3. Early myoclonic encephalopathy (EME)

EME was first reported in 1978 by Aicardi and Goutieres [18], as "Encephalopathie myoclonique neonatale". It is characterized by early-onset fragmentary myoclonus, erratic focal seizures, and massive myoclonias during the neonatal period (before the first week 76% of the cases, and 96% occurring within the first month). Tonic seizures are observed later, generally around 3–4 months of age [16, 19]. Suppression-burst pattern (SBP) becomes more apparent in sleep in EME. The prognosis is grave [20] and evolves into hypsarrhythmia in 41% of patients [21].

2.4. Early infantile epileptic encephalopathy (EIEE), and Ohtahara syndrome (OS)

OS is also known as "early infantile epileptic encephalopathy" (EIEE) or "early infantile epileptic encephalopathy with burst-suppression pattern". EIEE was first described by Ohtahara and contributors in 1976 [22], mainly characterized by tonic spasms that start during the first month of life (range of 1–3 months, but may occur within the first 10 days of life or during the first hour after delivery). The epileptic spasms may be either generalized and symmetrical or lateralized, and may occur in clusters or singly, while awake and during sleep alike. The duration of tonic spasms is up to 10 s, and the interval between spasms within cluster ranges from 9 to 15 s. In one-third of cases, other seizure types include partial motor seizures or hemiconvulsions, but myoclonic seizures are rare [23]. Interictal EEG shows a BS with high-voltage paroxysmal discharges separated by prolonged periods of nearly flat tracing that last for up to 18 s. OS is considered to be the result of developmental static structural brain damage. Patients show a poor outcome with severe psychomotor retardation or death. In the majority of patients (76%), EIEE evolves to infantile spasms (ISS) [21].

2.5. Severe early-onset epileptic encephalopathy (EOEEs) with a suppression-burst pattern: a continuum of pathology

Ohtahara and Yamatogi in 2006 [24] explain the differential diagnosis of EME versus EIEE/OS. Etiologically, structural brain lesions are most likely in OS, and nonstructural/metabolic disorders in EME. Clinically, tonic spasms are the main seizures in OS, while myoclonia and frequent partial motor seizures in EME. Another difference is noted in th EEG findings: SBP is consistently observed in both waking and sleeping states in OS, but SBP becomes more apparent during sleep in EME. In OS, the SBP evolves to hypsarrhythmia around 3–4 months of age, and sometimes it progresses further to diffuse slow spike waves; by contrast, in EME the SBP may persist up to late childhood after a transient evolution to hypsarrythmia in the middle to late infancy. The evolution of the two syndromes is also different: OS evolves to West syndrome (WS), and further to Lennox-Gastaut syndrome (LGS) with age, but EME persists long without such an evolution except a transient phase of West syndrome.

Nevertheless, the border between the two syndromes unfortunately is not always clear since they share many common features (age of onset, BS-EEG pattern, grave prognosis), but also each of them can evolve from one to the other. Due to this overlap, the classification is sometimes questionable even among the published cases. Thus, they have also been generally referred to as "neonatal epileptic encephalopathy" [25]. To the point that Aicardi and Ohtahara finally recognized that they may be one single epileptic syndrome, and they proposed the designation of "severe neonatal epilepsies with suppression-burst pattern" [16]. Various authors have also suggested that both entities constitute a single syndrome that has a predictable age-related evolution and its clinical manifestations express a continuum of the progressive brainstem dysfunction, with frequent evolution toward West and Lennox-Gastaut syndromes [21, 26, 27].

The severe epileptic encephalopathies (EIEE, WS, late infantile epileptic encephalopathy, and LGS) share many common clinical features and in certain individuals there is a progression from one syndrome to the next. Ohtahara proposed that these epilepsies occur on an electroclinical spectrum and that the clinical and EEG features depend on the maturity of the NS [28]. However, there are differences between the disorders that may not be explained by the concept of "age-dependent encephalopathy" [29]. Other authors such as Lombroso [30] conclude that there is some justification to provisionally support a nosological place for the EME syndrome, whereas a nosologically separate position for the EIEE syndrome seems to be less justified, and it would be safer to consider it for now as an early variant of the West syndrome (WS).

Most of the cases of EIEE are associated with structural brain anomalies while the better part of EME with metabolic disorders (including nonketotic hyperglycinemia) [16, 20, 30–33]. Nevertheless, the etiology of EIEE is heterogeneous, and patients with EIEE often have acquired causes (e.g., HIE), structural brain defects (e.g., cortical brain malformations), or metabolic disorders [34, 35]. Thereby, the recognition is that multiple etiologies can produce under certain circumstances either syndrome, and there is an overlap in both severe early-onset epileptic encephalopathies (EOEEs) that may share a common mechanism. On the other hand, recent molecular genetics studies have shown that these encephalopathies are genetically heterogeneous and phenotypically diverse disorders, such that similar gene mutations have been found in several different epileptic encephalopathies syndromes, reinforcing the notion that these epilepsies are unlikely to be distinguished on the basis of cause alone. Thus, the ILAE emphasizes in its classification the symptomatic nature and nonspecific etiology of these syndromes.

Lombroso et al. found that asphyxiated babies meeting EME criteria exhibited both erratic myoclonia and BS, while presenting clinical and EEG parameters and evolutions differing from others who had homogeneous enough profiles to justify their inclusion in a provisional EME syndrome [8]. However, since HIE can be the common cause of neonatal seizures, brain damage, and BS pattern (BS is caused in 44.1% of cases by HIE) [36], it may serve as a model to study the correlation of progressive brain damage and evolution of the crisis. In our clinical experience, we have observed that the two entities (EME and EIEE) may be present in the evolutionary course of an epileptogenic encephalopathy neonatal secondary to HIE. As an illustrative example, we report the case of a newborn infant admitted to the Pediatrics Department at the Albacete General Hospital (Spain), who initially presented early neonatal seizures as tonic extension of the limbs, eye deviation, as well as sucking, pedaling, and swimming movements. Their initial EEG showed severe depression of brain bioelectrical activity, which progressed into EME at 15 days, with myoclonic convulsions and a BS-EEG pattern. Neuroimaging studies objectified a deep ischemia with the involvement of basal ganglia. Within 2 months of life, the clinical picture changed and it was suggestive of EIEE: flexion spasms appeared together with radiological progression toward a "multicystic encephalomalacia". In our patient, the presence of myoclonic seizures with subsequent flexion spasms associated with the appearance of brain structural abnormalities and the persistence of a BS-EEG pattern also support the notion of one epileptic syndrome with different clinical manifestations depending on age at presentation and brain damage/maturational status of the patient.

We have also observed the clinical course and EEG evolution of an extreme low-birth-weight preterm neonate with glycine encephalopathy (already published [37]), in which the BS pattern and seizures did not appear until the third month after birth (40 weeks corrected gestational age). An immature brain could have been responsible, at least in part, for the long asymptomatic period before the onset of convulsions in our patient. This suggests that an adequate maturation and organization of the brain development—particularly regarding GABAergic interneurons—is required for the onset of EME.

The most prominent distinctive points between both epilepsy syndromes are the observation that patients with OS exhibit predominantly tonic seizures, their crises evolve to ISS, and the outlook is often worse than in patients with EME. Although both syndromes may have different courses, the differentiation at the beginning may be impossible, since both myoclonus and tonic convulsions may coexist and present the same electrical pattern, although some specialists report to be able to find distinctive features between the EEG patterns. Tonic seizures are considered to be a manifestation of brainstem dysfunction and it is possible that this is more prominent in OS. Thereby, in a review article Djukic and collaborators [21] analyze preliminary studies that would suggest the following:

- Evidence that the brainstem is involved in the expression of tonic seizures;
- Evidence of increased excitability/epileptogenicity in the immature brainstem;
- Evidence of decreased seizure-controlling substrate in the immature brainstem;
- Clinical evidence supporting the notion that tonic seizures are associated with the severity of brainstem dysfunction in EIEE and EME;

- For the Ohtahara syndrome, some mothers retrospectively reported movements consistent with seizures in utero [38]. Unable to rule out that the myoclonic component had occurred in utero.

The standard notion is that when the brain is intact and a strong harmful event happens leading to acute excitotoxic cell death and neuronal apoptosis (e.g., acute cerebral injury in HIE and metabolic disorders), a BS-EEG pattern is acutely developed. However, the newborn shows a first stage of frequent and diverse seizure types: fragmentary myoclonus, erratic focal seizures, and massive myoclonias compatible with the specific epilepsy syndrome EME. Conversely, when there is brain damage established—nonprogressive static structural developing brain damage (e.g., brain injury such as as multicystic encephalomalacia in HIE, cortical brain malformations, brainstem dysfunction, and metabolic disorders with intrauterine brain damage, among others)—also a BS-EEG pattern may occur that can be demonstrated, but the infant is more likely to show tonic intractable seizures that are typical of EIEE. In view of these evidences, we believe that these syndromes do not correspond so much to an "age-dependent encephalopathy" but rather to a "damage-dependent encephalopathy". Thereby, it is possible that these syndromes represent successive stages of "a continuum and progressive neuronal injury" from an epileptic process.

3. Genetic factors in severe early-onset epileptic encephalopathy

3.1. Genome instability and neurotransmitter signaling

The genetic factors are thought to play a role in at least 70% of patients with epilepsy [39]. Genetic analysis for copy number variants (CNVs) and single EOEEs candidate genes have become increasingly important investigations in clinical practice. Data suggest that mutations causing EE are often sporadic, mostly due from de novo dominant mutations in a single autosomal gene, although inherited autosomal recessive and X-linked forms also exist [40].

Over recent years, huge steps have been made to clarify the genetics of epilepsy, and the amount of reports on novel genetic causes of EOEEs has increased due to fast developments and dramatically reduced costs in molecular genetic techniques, especially the "next-generation sequencing" (NGS) technologies (for a review, see [41–43]).

Mutations have been identified in several genes in infants with severe EOEEs, clustering in several biological pathways that are often shared by patients with similar mutations. But the complexity of phenotype/genotype correlations—one syndrome having multiple genetic causes (genetic heterogeneity) and one gene being associated with different phenotypes (pleiotropy)—has been progressively unraveled for both EIEE and EME. To date, the genetic origin of up to 36 genetic phenotypes (EIEE 1 to EIEE36), as referred in the Online Catalog of Human Genes and Genetic Disorders "Online Mendelian Inheritance in Man" (OMIM), has been identified [44]. Many of them are related to mutations in NT receptors, transporters, or associated proteins.

Title (OMIM)	Gene	Phenotype Clinical	Age	Seizures predominate	EEG
EIEE1 (308350)	ARX	Ohtahara syndrome	1–3 months	Tonic seizures	SBP
EIEE2 (300672)	CDKL5	X-linked dominant infantile spasm syndrome-2 (ISSX2). Dysmorphic.	1–10 weeks	Infantile spasms. Atypical Rett syndrome	H
EIEE3 (609304)	SLC25A22	Early myoclonic encephalopathy (EME)	Neonatal period	Myoclonic seizures	SBP
EIEE4 (612164)	STXBP1	Ohtahara and West syndrome with cerebral hypomyelination	3 days to 4.5 months	Tonic seizures	SBP/H
EIEE5 (613477)	SPTAN1	West syndrome with pontocerebellar atrophy and hypomyelination	3 months	Infantile spasms.	H
EIEE6 (607208)	SCN1A	Dravet S. and FEB3A, MHP3	Mean 6 months	Multiple types.	GSWD
EIEE7 (613720)	KCNQ2	Ohtahara Syndrome and BFNS1	Neonatal period	Tonic seizures	SBP
EIEE8 (300607)	ARHGEF9	Hyperekplexia and epilepsy	Neonatal period	Tonic seizures provoked by tactile stimulation	Varies
EIEE9 (300088)	PCDH19	EFMR. Juberg-Hellman syndrome	6–36 months	Multiple types	Varies
EIEE10 (613402)	PNKP	Microcephaly, seizures, and developmental delay (MCSZ)	<6 months	Complex partial type	Varies
EIEE11 (613721)	SCN2A	EIEE and benign familial infantile seizures-3 (BFIS3)	Neonatal period	Tonic-clonic seizures. Infantile spasms	SBP GSWD
EIEE12 (613722)	PLCB1	West Syndrome and MMPSI	10 weeks to 6 months	Tonic seizures/infantile spasms	MF/H
EIEE13 (614558)	SCN8A	Intractable seizures	First days to 6 months	Multiple types	Varies/H
EIEE14 (614959)	KCNT1	Refractory focal seizures. MMPSI	<6 months	Multiple types	MF
EIEE15 (615006)	ST3GAL3	West syndrome	3–7 months	Infantile spasms	H
EIEE16 (615338)	TBC1D24	Familial infantile myoclonic epilepsy (FIME) and MMPSI	First weeks or months	Myoclonic seizures. Multiple types	Varies
EIEE17 (615473)	GNAO1	Intractable seizures	First weeks or months	Tonic seizures	SBP

http://dx.doi.org/10.5772/64458

Title (OMIM)	Gene	Phenotype Clinical	Age	Seizures predominate	EEG
EIEE18 (615463)	SZT2	Dysmorphic feature and thick corpus callosum	First months or years	Tonic-clonic seizures	Varies
EIEE19 (615744)	GABRA1	Dravet syndrome	8–11 months	Multiple types	GSWD
EIEE20 (300868)	PIGA	Multiple congenital anomalies—hypotonia-seizures, Syndrome 2	First days to 9 months	Myoclonic seizures	SBP/H
EIEE21 (615833)	NECAP1	Intractable seizures	First years	Multiple types	Varies
EIEE22 (300896)	SLC35A2	Congenital disorder of glycosylation type IIm (CDG2M)	First days to 3 months	Tonic seizures. Infantile spasms	Varies/H
EIEE23 (615859)	DOCK7	Intractable seizures. Dysmorphic feature and cortical blindness	2–6 months	Tonic seizures. Multiple types	MF/H
EIEE24 (615871)	HCN1	Resembling Dravet syndrome with pharmacoresistant febrile seizures	4–13 months	Tonic-clonic, progress to atypical absences	Varies
EIEE25 (615905)	SLC13A5	Developmental delay and tooth hypoplasia	First 7 days	Focal clonic seizures. Status epilepticus	Focal MF
EIEE26 (616056)	KCNB1	Intractable seizures	First years	Multiple types	H/MF
EIEE27 (616139)	GRIN2B	West syndrome	First months	Infantile spasms	H
EIEE28 (616211)	WWOX	Lethal microcephaly syndrome. Simplified gyral pattern	Mean 2 months	Multiple types	Varies
EIEE29 (616339)	AARS	Hypomyelination. Charcot-Marie-Tooth disease, axonal, type 2N	3–6 months	Myoclonic seizures	MF
EIEE30 (616341)	SIK1	Intractable seizures	Neonatal period	Myoclonic. Tonic and infantile spasms	SBPMF H
EIEE31 (616346)	DNM1	Intractable seizures. West syndrome	2–13 months	Multiple types. Infantile spasms	Varies/H
EIEE32 (616366)	KCNA2	Ataxia and myoclonic epilepsy	5–17 months	Myoclonic seizures. Multiple types	Varies
EIEE33 (616409)	EEF1A2	West syndrome	First week or month	Myoclonic seizures. Infantile spasms	MF/H
EIEE34 (616645)	SLC12A5	Refractory migrating focal seizures	First weeks or months	Focal seizures	Varies

Title (OMIM)	Gene	Phenotype Clinical	Age	Seizures predominate	EEG
EIEE35 (616647)	ITPA	Lack of myelination of early structures	Neonatal period	Multiple types	Varies
EIEE36 (300884)	ALG13	Congenital disorder of glycosylation Is	First week or month	Infantile spasms	MF/H

SBP: suppression-burst pattern on EEG. **H:** hypsarrhythmia. **GSWD:** generalized spike-wave discharges. **MF:** multifocal epileptogenic foci. **MMPSI**: malignant migrating partial seizures of infancy. **FEB3A:** febrile seizures, familial, 3A. **MHP3:** migraine, familial hemiplegic, 3. **BFNS1:** benign familial neonatal seizure 1. **EFMR:** epilepsy, female-restricted, with mental retardation.

Table 2. EIEE following the classification of OMIM.

Despite these evidences, in the last International Classification of epilepsies these entities are included as epilepsy syndromes and they are classified according to the age of onset and their electro-clinical features, for example, Ohtahara and West syndromes. However, in OMIM these syndromes are included in the so-called "epileptic encephalopathy, early infantile", or "early infantile epileptic encephalopathy" (EIEE), paying great attention to their genetic origin and less so to their phenotype. Thus, epileptic encephalopathy, early infantile 1 (EIEE1) is Ohtahara syndrome (OMIN 308350) caused by a mutation in the "aristaless-related homeobox gene" (ARX; 300382) on chromosome Xp22. Whereas early myoclonic encephalopathy (EME; OMIM 609304) caused by mutation in the "solute carrier family 25 (mitochondrial carrier, glutamate), member 22 gene" (SLC25A22; 609302), is named EIEE3 (609304) Dravet's syndrome, caused by mutation in SCN1A gene (182389), is named EIEE6 (6070208) (see **Table 2**).

Nevertheless, the heterogeneity of the epileptic features is often the rule for most of the reported genes, and, inversely, the same gene mutation can cause several seizure types, even in the same patient across ages. Therefore, in many cases, clinical prediction of causative genes is challenging for some patients, since the association between phenotypic pleiotropy and genetic heterogeneity phenotype is not sufficiently distinctive. Sequential single-gene analysis (by direct Sanger sequencing) is costly, time consuming, and often unsuccessful. With the current development of the NGS technologies—via gene panel analysis—diagnostic rates improve. NGS can also help to clarify and broaden the phenotypic spectrum of the genes involved. In a recent study, Trump et al. [45], in a 400 series of patients with early-onset seizure disorders and/or severe developmental delay, identified causative mutations in 18% of the individuals with seizures. The diagnostic rate was highest among those with seizure onset within the first 2 months of life (39%). The most frequently mutated gene was SCN2A (11 patients). Other recurrently mutated genes included CDKL5, KCNQ2, SCN8A (six patients each), FOXG1, MECP2, SCN1A, STXBP1 (five patients each), KCNT1, PCDH19, TCF4 (three patients each), and ATP1A3, PRRT2, and SLC9A6 (two patients each). Mutations in EHMT1, GABRB3, LGI1, MBD5, PIGA, UBE3A, and ZEB2 were each found in single patients. These authors also pointed out that only in 15% of them, the clinician had sufficient clinical certainty for a specific mutated gene as the probable cause prior to genetic testing. Neurometabolic disorders and frequent major structural brain anomalies were not included in the panel, which may explain the absence of the ARX gene.

3.2. Genetic mutations in Ohtahara syndrome

A phenotype relatively similar to that of Ohtahara syndrome can be a consequence of various mutations on a single gene, with special mention to the ARX gene, but also to KCNQ2, SCN2A, STXBP1, and GNAO1 among other genes.

3.2.1. The homeobox gene ARX (MIM 300382)

One of the most important and well studied is the mutation in the ARX gene, which is the one responsible for OS named EIEE1 (OMIM 308350) that causes severe disorganization of forebrain with aberrant migration and differentiation of interneurons containing gamma-aminobutyric acid (GABAergic interneurons) [46–49] via the Dlx pathway [50]. Additionally, the ARX gene modifies glutamatergic neurons excitability and morphology. Pyramidal neurons show a dramatic rise in the frequency of excitatory inputs associated with a redevelopment of their axonal arborization resulting from glutamate network remodeling. Thus, secondary alterations are instrumental for the development of disease-specific phenotypes and should be regarded to explain the "phenotypic pleiotropy" associated with epileptogenic mutations [51].

The homeobox gene ARX is one of the most frequently mutated genes in "phenotypic spectrum of disorders", comprising a nearly continuous series of X-linked developmental disorders with intellectual disability (ID), ranging from syndromic (S-XLMR) and nonsyndromic X-linked mental retardation (XLMR), to lissencephaly and infantile spasms without brain malformations. At least seven well-defined clinical entities have been described including [47, 52, 53].

- Ohtahara syndrome (308350),
- Nonsyndromic X-linked mental retardation with or without seizures, ARX-related (OMIM 300419),
- Partington syndrome, characterized by the association of mild to moderate intellectual deficit, dysarthria, and variable movement disturbances—dystonic hand movements—(OMIM 309510),
- Proud syndrome or microcephaly—corpus callosum agenesis—abnormal genitalia syndrome (OMIM 300004),
- X-linked lissencephaly with ambiguous genitalia (LISX2, XLAG), as well as hydranencephaly and abnormal genitalia (OMIM 300215).

The genetic heterogeneity (same clinical entities being associated with several mutations in ARX) together with intra- and interfamilial pleiotropy is becoming a hallmark of ARX mutations [53]. It appears to be a consistent genotype-phenotype correlation and both intra- and interfamilial variability of expression of some of the mutations, particularly the common 428-451dup (24 bp) mutation [54]. On the other hand, brain-imaging abnormalities can also be highly variable, ranging from lissencephaly/hydranencephaly and cortical dysplasia (among others) to normal brain. Microarray analysis has identified a total of 1006 gene promoters bound by ARX, and around 24% of Arx-bound genes were found to show expression changes following ARX overexpression or knock-down. Several of the ARX target genes are known to be important for a variety of functions in brain development and some of them suggest new functions for ARX [55]. Phenotype/genotype studies in humans suggest that truncating mutations cause X-linked lissencephaly, and insertion/missense mutations result in epilepsy and intellectual deficit without cortical dysplasia [56].

3.2.2. Dysfunctions of potassium (K+) channels

Several epileptic phenotypes have been associated to dysfunctions of potassium (K+) channels, and it has been recently proposed to name such epilepsies as "K+ channelepsies" [57]. Based on their structures, biophysical characteristics, pharmacological sensitivities, and physiology, these channels are classified as (for a review, see [58]) follows:

- Voltage-gated (Kv 1-12): Regulation of outward K+ currents and action potentials, modulation of NT release, control of both excitability and electrical properties of neurons.
- Inwardly rectifying (Kir1-7): Maintenance of the resting membrane potentials and regulation of the cell excitability.
- Sodium-activated channels (K_{Na}): Regulation of delayed outward currents IKNa and contribution to adaptation of firing rate.
- Ca^{2+}-activated channels (K_{Ca}): Regulation of neuronal firing properties and circuit excitability.

3.2.2.1. KCNQ2 (# 602235)

As an example of phenotypic diversity, reference is made to mutation in the KCNQ2 gene on chromosome 20q13.3 (encoding the Kv7.2 channel), characterized by benign familial neonatal seizures-1 (BFNS1) that can also cause early infantile epileptic encephalopathy-7 (EIEE7, OMIM 613720). Reported genotype-phenotype observations for KCNQ2 with truncating mutations are associated with the benign, inherited phenotype and missense mutations affecting key residues with the severe, sporadic phenotype [45]. Cellular experiments indicate that these latter mutations may have a dominant negative effect on cellular function [59].

The EIEE7 is an atypical severe early-onset epilepsy with refractory seizures and prominent tonic component. Most patients showed a BS-EEG pattern and were diagnosed clinically with Ohtahara syndrome (but with an earlier start during the neonatal period), infrequent evolution to West syndrome, and good response to sodium channel blockers (phenytoin, carbamazepine, zonisamide,…), topiramate (TPM), or valproic acid, but poor developmental prognosis [60]. Weckhuysen et al. in 2012 [61] reported eight unrelated patients with EIEE7 confirmed by genetic analysis. All patients had the onset of seizures during the first week of life, and two mothers retrospectively noted intrauterine jerking during the last 2 months of pregnancy. Early magnetic resonance imaging (MRI) of the brain showed characteristic hyperintensities in the basal ganglia and thalamus. These evidence supports (as we mentioned above) that the myoclonic component had occurred in utero while tonic crises may be a manifestation of brainstem dysfunction [21].

3.2.2.2. KCNT1

The KCNT1 gene encodes the K_{Na} channel subunit KCNT1, called Slack (sequence such as a calcium-activated potassium channel). Mutations in KCNT1 gene have been found in different epilepsy syndromes (EIEE 14): autosomal dominant nocturnal frontal lobe epilepsy (ADN-FLE), epilepsy of infancy with migrating focal seizures (EIMFS), and other types of EOEEs, including OS [62]. Patients displaying KCNT1 mutations have a very high occurrence of severe mental and intellectual disability.

3.2.3. SCN2A (MIM 182390)

The three isoforms of the brain sodium channel alpha subunit are encoded by three distinct sodium channel, voltage-gated genes (SCN1A, SCN2A, and SCN3A) that share a common ancestral origin [63].

De novo mutations in SCN2A are increasingly recognized as a cause of an early-onset seizure and developmental delay. The clinical spectrum named EIEE11 (MIM 613721) includes OS and benign familial infantile seizures-3 (BFIS3) [64]. While inherited SCN2A mutations have been identified in multiple mild epilepsy cases, by contrast in cases with EIEE and severe or profound developmental delay, the majority of mutations were de novo missense variants, similarly to the abovementioned findings for KCNQ2 [45, 65].

3.2.4. STXBP1 (MIM 602926)

STXBP1 (mapping to 9q34.1) encodes the n-Sec1 (neural-specific, syntaxin-binding protein), which participates in the constitutive secretory pathway between the Golgi apparatus and the plasma membrane, and implicated in vesicle trafficking and NT release [66]. The mutation in STXBP1 (named EIEE4, MIM 612164) shows a relatively similar phenotype to OS but with frequent evolution to West syndrome [67] and cerebral hypomyelination in MRI brain imaging. Mutations in STXBP1 are not limited to patients with Ohtahara or West syndrome, but are also present in about 10% of patients with an EOEE without a specific recognized epilepsy syndrome [68].

A *de novo* heterozygous missense mutation in the STXBP1 gene was found for the severe phenotype of early infantile epileptic encephalopathy with suppression burst (EIEE4) [69, 70]. By contrast, a *de novo* truncating mutation in STXBP1 was identified in nonsyndromic intellectual disability (NSID) with/without history of epilepsy [71, 72].

3.2.5. GNAO1 (139311)

The GNAO1 gene encodes an alpha subunit (Go, alpha subunit) of the heterotrimeric guanine nucleotide-binding proteins (G proteins), a large family of signal-transducing molecules. Go-alpha has been implicated in ion channel regulation. Most of the reported cases present EIEE17 (OMIM 615473), characterized by OS with intractable tonic seizures in the first weeks of life associated with BS pattern on EEG, involuntary movements, and progressive cerebral atrophy. Delayed myelination and thin corpus callosum were common features in brain images [73].

A novel heterozygous missense pathogenic GNAO1 variant is report in an EIEE presented at birth with twitching movements and convulsions, with nonspecific electro-clinical signs, and no radiological abnormalities [74]. Other reports demonstrated that GNAO1 variants can cause involuntary movements and severe developmental delay with/without seizures, suggesting that GNAO1 variants can cause various neurological phenotypes [75].

3.3. Genetic mutations in EME

On a genetic point of view, several genes have been associated with EME.

3.3.1. SLC25A22 gene

As referred to above, the SLC25A22 gene is most often associated with EME (or EIEE 3) and encodes mitochondrial carriers that transport a variety of metabolites across the inner mitochondrial membrane (it is one of the two mitochondrial glutamate/H+ symporters), with strong expression in the developing brain. Mutated SLC25A22 expression in areas of the brain decreased glutamate transport activity and contributed to the genesis and control of myoclonic seizures [76]. Malignant migrating partial seizures in infancy (MMPSI, or EIEE14, OMIM 614959) that may occur as a result of heterozygous mutation in the KCNT1 gene (608167) on chromosome 9q34 can also be caused by a SLC25A22 gene mutation, expanded the phenotypic spectrum associated with this gene [77].

3.3.2. PIGA

Phosphatidylinositol glycan class A (PIGA, OMIM 311770) is involved in the first step of glycosylphosphatidylinositol (GPI) biosynthesis, a glycolipid that attaches dozens of different proteins to the cell surface. Many proteins, including CD55 and CD59, are anchored to the cell by GPI. The loss of CD55 and CD59 on erythrocytes causes complement-mediated lysis in paroxysmal nocturnal hemoglobinuria (PNH).

Multiple congenital anomalies-hypotonia-seizures syndrome-2 (MCAHS2, or EIEE20, OMIM 300868) is an X-linked recessive neurodevelopmental disorder characterized by neonatal hypotonia, myoclonic seizures, dysmorphic features, and variable congenital anomalies involving the central nervous, cardiac, and urinary systems. EEG, in the most severe cases, showed hypsarrhythmia or BS pattern. Some affected individuals die in infancy [78].

3.3.3. SIK1

SIK1 (OMIM 605705) is a member of the AMP kinase subfamily with several roles in the CNS and is involved in the regulation of corticotropin-releasing hormone in the hypothalamus. SIK1 abundance and activity are also increased by stimulation with ACTH (adrenocorticotrophic hormone), which is a first-line treatment for ISS [79].

The mutations in SIK1 gene have been associated with a spectrum of developmental epilepsies [80], mainly EME (EIEE30, 616341), and also with OS and ISS. Brain was either normal, mild hypoplasia of the frontal lobes. Interestingly, one of the patients described in this work that developed intermittent myoclonic jerking movements did not respond to anticonvulsants. Their EEG on day 14 of life showed BS pattern, and at 8 months of age the EEG had not improved, with continued BS associated with both myoclonic and tonic seizures. Brain MRI showed no structural malformations. In another OS patient with tonic seizures, the brain exhibited "a simplification of the gyral pattern", and asymmetric thinning of the WM. This evidence also supports the idea that tonic seizures in OS are associated with structural and static brain damage, while the EME requires a good cerebral cortical development.

3.3.4. Neuregulin-1 receptor ErbB4

The neuregulins (NRGs) are cell-cell signaling proteins that are ligands for receptor tyrosine kinases of the ErbB family. Recently, it has been known also that disruption in the neuregulin-1 receptor ErbB4 (family members of tyrosine kinase receptors, OMIM 600543) also contributes to EME (OMIM 609304) [81] by impairing interneuron migration [82] and altering the number of GABAergic interneurons in the postnatal cortex [83]. NRG1 is crucial for maintaining a normal radial glial scaffold and signals allowing neuronal migration. It also induces the expression of brain lipid-binding protein (BLBP), a well-known marker of radial glia [84]. NRGs also regulate the timing of astrogenesis in the developing brain [85], as well as in the myelination of Schwann cells [86].

3.4. Genetic analysis for copy number variants (CNVs)

Advances in molecular genetic testing have greatly improved diagnostic rates in EIEE, with an important role of array-comparative genomic hybridization (array-CGH) investigation in this group of disorders. Array CGH can readily detect micro-chromosomal aberrations at a much finer resolution than the 5-Mb limit of the conventional karyotype. There are over 200 disorders where epilepsy is or can be part of the clinical condition, but not the primary feature (Online Mendelian Inheritance in Man, OMIM). Many of these can be associated with various micro-chromosomal anomalies; therefore, the array CGH is more widely applied as a frontline diagnostic tool, especially for children with syndromic epilepsy.

CNVs can be recurrent due to non-allelic homologous recombination (NAHR) in *"hotspots"* regions of segmental duplication (SD) or low-copy repeats (LCRs). The most common of the recurrent microdeletions associated with generalized epilepsy are typically seen at a frequency close to 1% at 15q13.3, 16p13.11, and 15q11.2. These loci also confer susceptibility to ID, autism spectrum disorders (ASDs), and schizophrenia (for a review, see [87]). Rare copy number variants—deletions and duplications—have recently been established as important cause of epileptic encephalopathies. Pathogenic CNVs play an important role in the genetic etiology of unknown cause EOEEs: 7.9% of affected individuals carried at least one rare CNV [88], and in at least 3.4% [89] to 4.1% [88] of patients, CNVs were clearly pathogenic.

4. GABAergic neurons in the developing brain

To accomplish stability, neurons must maintain a homeostatic balance between adjustment output (to meet new requirements) and preservation output within a satisfactory performance range. This balancing act is performed through the combination of synaptic plasticity and changes in intrinsic neuronal excitability. The neuronal components of brain circuitry are generally considered to be "stable" across an animal's life, excepting the growth and degeneration phases that happen during development, aging, or pathology. The periods of greatest neuronal instability occur during the early ontogenesis and CNS development. The EEA (glutamate and especially GABA acting like an excitatory) plays a fundamental role in the developing brain. The hypothesis of a "homeostatic-like" regulation [90] (by NT and receptors) of neuronal migration that controls final position, timing, and number of cells at destination depends on the following:

- the type of migration: radial, tangential, or chain migration;
- the type of cells: principal glutamatergic neurons versus GABAergic interneurons; and
- the brain area: neocortex, cerebellum, rostral migratory stream.

4.1. Distinct modes of migration in the developing cortex

The newly specified neurons migrate long distances before they differentiate and form synapses. Neuron migration routes in the developing mammalian brain are generally a long and complex process, but it can be summarized in the following: (for a review, see [91, 92])

a. Radial-type migration: postmitotic neurons migrate away from the germinal ventricular zone to their positions in the developing cortex, using two forms of radial movement: somal translocation, which is adopted by the early-generated neurons, and glia-guided locomotion, which is used predominantly by pyramidal cells.

b. Tangential-type migration: cortical interneurons migrate tangentially into the cortex and then seek the ventricular zone before moving radially to take up their positions in the cortical anlage.

4.2. Transient and permanent circuitry elements

In lower mammals, all hippocampal and almost all neocortical neurons are born in a specific region named ganglionic eminence in the ventral (basal) part of the telencephalon. The glutamatergic principal cells (i.e., projection neurons) migrate from the proliferative layer to their target region following a radial orientation. Meanwhile, GABAergic interneurons via long-distance tangential migration (parallel to pial surface) move from the ganglionic eminence to their target layer in the cerebral cortex. A substantial body of evidence indicates that in humans neocortical GABAergic interneurons of local cortical circuitry are likely to originate in two different areas: 65% are born in the ventricular/subventricular zone of the dorsal telencephalon, and 35% originate from the ganglionic eminences (proliferative zones of the subpallium) [93].

http://dx.doi.org/10.5772/64458

The subplate zone (SPZ) is a transient cytoarchitectonic compartment of the fetal telencephalic wall, situated between the fetal white matter (WM) (i.e., intermediate zone) and the cortical plate, and it is the crucial laminar compartment for the development of the human cerebral cortex. The subplate contains numerous neurons of various morphological types and molecular phenotypes, including differentiated projection (glutamatergic) neurons and local (GABA and peptidergic) interneurons [94]. The developing human cortex goes through three major early stages of functional development: (1) between 13 and 15 postconceptional weeks (PCW): initial-transient fetal circuitry, centered at the SPZ, which is endogeneously (spontaneously) driven; (2) 15 and 30 PCW: perinatal dual circuitry (coexistence of endogeneously driven subplate-centered transient circuitry with developing cortical plate-centered permanent circuitry) that slowly disappears toward the end of gestation and during the early postnatal period; and (3) postnatally established permanent (externally driven) cortical circuitry, centered at the cortical plate (i.e., developing cortical layers I–VI). While the SPZ disappears during the perinatal and early postnatal period, numerous subplate neurons survive and remain embedded in the superficial (gyral) WM of adolescent and adult brain as the so-called *interstitial neurons* [95]. There is also a prolonged coexistence of transient and permanent circuitry elements in the developing cerebral cortex. Therefore, the neuronal elements in transient fetal zones form a developmental potential for plasticity after perinatal cerebral lesions [96].

The subpallium also generates oligodendrocytes (OLs) that migrate in a similarly tangential path to the cortex. These are the cells that give rise to myelin, a major component of WM, and play an important role in assuring fast neuronal signaling in the CNS [97]. The proliferation and differentiation of developing oligodendroglial cells and their myelination of axons are partly controlled by NT (glutamate, GABA, glycine, etc.) (for a review, see [98]). Numerous studies refer connections among this OLs and the GABAergic system [99, 100]. The growth of the axonal pathways in preterm newborn explains their vulnerability and plasticity, while conversely in neonates the vulnerability is related to the intracortical circuitry. In addition to OLs loss, axonal disruption, and excess apoptosis, a significant loss of telencephalon GABAergic subplate neurons expression was found in neonatal brains with WM lesions, compared with neonatal brains without WM lesions, which could contribute to the pathogenesis of neurological deficits in children [101]. On the other hand, innate immunity mediated by microglia plays a crucial role in initiating and propagating seizure-induced inflammatory responses, as long-term epileptogenic effects of early-life seizure, such that seizure-induced microglia activation primes the central immune response to overreact and to increase the susceptibility to a second seizure later in life [102].

4.3. GABAergic interneurons

GABAergic neurons in cerebral cortex mostly correspond to local circuit neurons (interneurons), which release GABA as their output, and are the major inhibitory cells of the mature CNS. Despite including only 20–30% of the cerebral cortical neuronal population, these cells play an essential part and mighty role in modulating the electrical activity in the synapse of the excitatory pyramidal cells. In the epileptogenic neocortex, there is preferential loss of GA-

BAergic neurons, namely "basket cells" (BCs) and chandelier cells (ChCs) (for a review, see [103, 104]).

The interest in developing human cortex and GABAergic neurons has increased in the past decade. GABAergic interneurons develop early in the cortical anlage during embryonic development, whereas glutamatergic activity arises later. Although interneurons are present in all regions of the mature telencephalon, many studies have shown that during embryogenesis these cells are generated in specific compartments of the subcortical telencephalon and migrate across WM to reach their final destinations in the mature brain. Studies of histological sections of progressively more developed embryonic brains revealed that GABAergic cells were firstly present in the preplate, subventricular, and ventricular proliferative zones, migrated later to the subplate, marginal zone, and intermediate zones and finally reached the cortical plate (for a review, see [93, 105]).

Despite progress toward understanding the genetic determinants that specify the fate of neural progenitors, much remains unknown about the complex molecular machinery that directs the migration of immature neurons to specific regions of the cerebrum. Interestingly, in addition to its function in synaptic transmission, NTs have been shown to promote several developmental processes that contribute to the creation and maintenance of the CNS. In this regard, a growing body of literature has highlighted a role for NT through the activation of its receptors in the regulation of cell migration in the telencephalon during development and in adulthood [106, 107]. Thus, it seems that the activation of $GABA_AR$ regulates neuronal proliferation, migration, and differentiation of GABAergic interneurons in the developing cerebral cortex [108]. Most interestingly, GABAergic interneuron dysfunction may contribute to a subset of genetic developmental epilepsies [104]. It is also worth noting that, in experimental animals, it has been shown that status epilepticus altered neurogenesis and decreased the number of GABAergic neurons in the septal dentate gyrus at the early phase of epileptogenesis. This could modify the connectivity between these cells and disturb the maturation of the GABAergic neurotransmission in the immature brain [109].

Lévesque et al. [110] described the interneurons spark seizure-like activity in the cortex in an in vitro model of epileptiform synchronization:

- Interneurons (66.7%) are more likely to fire in association with interictal discharges than principal cells (35.3%).
- The pre-ictal period is characterized by increased interneuron firing that reaches its peak at ictal onset, while the activity of principal cells does not change.
- The tonic phase of the ictal discharges is associated with high firing from interneurons that fire in a phase-locking relationship with low-voltage fast (LVF) oscillations.
- Interneurons continue to generate action potentials in association with the interictal discharges occurring during blockade of ionotropic glutamatergic transmission.

Their results illustrate the major role of interneurons in interictal discharge generation and in the transition to ictal activity.

http://dx.doi.org/10.5772/64458

5. Excitotoxicity in developing brain

Amino acids are among the most abundant NTs in the CNS, and most neurons use GABA and glutamate, both primary regulators of the excitability of most neurons in the brain (glutamate is an excitatory NT, while GABA is an inhibitory NT in the adult mammalian brain), and are therefore involved in important physiological processes and in pathophysiologic events.

Receptor families of EAA are overexpressed in the immature brain. Due to the abundance of EAA receptors in early ontogenesis and age-dependent changes in intrinsic neuronal excitability, an excitotoxic hypothesis as the source of neonatal seizures seems plausible, even though some observations do not support this theory [8]. Many reports reviewed here aimed to demonstrate that both NTs (GABA and glutamate) modulate neuronal migration and brain maturation in humans by early paracrine actions, and cytoskeletal dynamic changes are regulated by intracellular calcium. Thus, there is evidence that the activation of specific GABA and glutamate receptors is instrumental in cell migration by promoting motility and acting as an acceleratory or stop signal. Therefore, the modification of glutamate and GABAergic systems, among other mechanisms, can trigger disorders in cortical migration of neurons, the most common CNS developmental alteration observed in human patients and a significant cause of seizures [9].

5.1. The amino acid glutamate

Glutamate is the major excitatory NT in the CNS, released from both neurons and glial cells. During neurotransmission, glutamate is released from presynaptic neurons by means of depolarization of the presynaptic neuronal end plate and then diffuses across the synaptic cleft to activate postsynaptic glutamatergic receptors.

The mammalian genome contains five glutamate transporter genes—"solute carrier family" —(EAAT1, slc1a3; EAAT2, slc1a2; EAAT3, slc1a1; EAAT4, slc1a6; EAAT5, slc1a7). The most important and most abundant transporters for the removal of transmitter glutamate in the brain are EAAT2 (GLT-1) and EAAT1 (GLAST). These transporters keep the extracellular level excitatory amino acids low and provide amino acids for metabolic purposes (for a review, see [111]).

Glutamate is one of the NTs with the most receptors; therefore, its classification is complex. There are two known groups of glutamate receptors: ionotropic (iGluRs, ligand-gated ion channels) and metabotropic (G-protein-coupled) receptors. IGluRs are further divided into the following subgroups with respect to their pharmacological properties: GluN (the N-methyl-D-aspartic acid), GluA (AMPA, the alpha-amino-3-hydroxy-5-methyl-4-isoxazole propionic acid), GluK (kainate), and GluD (δ) receptors [112]. NMDA receptors are named "slow" (slow transmission, synaptic currents are typically very slow) and non-NMDAs "fast" (fast transmission, synaptic currents are typically very fast) [113].

Metabotropic glutamate (mGlu) receptors are further subdivided into three groups of eight subtypes: group I with components mGlu1 and mGlu5 (coupled to Gq/G11), group II consisting of mGlu2 and mGlu3; and group III composed of mGlu4, mGlu6, mGlu7, and mGlu8 (members of both latter groups are coupled to Gi/Go) [114].

Glutamate receptors are regulated in both neuronal and glial cells within the developing brain. Rapid synaptic excitation in the CNS is mediated primarily by the activation of postsynaptic ionotropic (AMPA and NMDA) glutamate receptors. Both of these receptors play different, well-defined roles in excitation: AMPA receptors (AMPARs) are considered to be the primary mediators of fast neurotransmission under resting conditions, whereas NMDA receptors, based on their unique properties, detect the coincidence of glutamate release and postsynaptic depolarization and are involved in the induction of long-term synaptic changes [115, 116]. Several studies indicate that glutamate receptor-mediated excitotoxicity is a key player in neuronal and glial cell death and that its involvement in the developing brain is more critical than in the adult brain [117, 118]. Other studies have shown a dual effect of glutamate on GABAergic interneuron survival during cerebral cortex development, expressed as either excitotoxicity lesions or antiapoptotic effects depending on the cortical layers. In layer VI, NMDA led to excitotoxicity, sustained calcium mobilization and necrosis; conversely, in the immature layers II–IV, NMDA decreased apoptosis and induced transient calcium mobilization [119].

5.1.1. NMDA receptors

The NMDA receptor is an essential executive and integrative element of the glutamatergic system and crucial for proper functioning of neuronal circuits. NMDA receptors have received a great deal of attention over the last few decades, due to their key role in neuronal excitotoxicity (their hypofunction or overactivation can result in neuronal disturbances and neurotoxicity) and their involvement in many types of neural plasticity (for a review, see [120, 121]).

The NMDA receptor subunits in the developing brain create populations of receptors that flux more calcium, open more easily, and block less frequently than mature forms, allowing these receptors to fulfill their special role in development. However, this makes the immature brain more susceptible to excitotoxic injury if energy levels are compromised. For instance, neurotoxicity mediated by NMDA is more enhanced in the neonatal brain than in the adult brain. Therefore, development-dependent changes in the expression of NMDA receptor subunits and their composition are, at least, partially responsible for the fact that immature brains are far more excitable and epileptogenic than the adult brain. Nevertheless, the important role that NMDA receptors play in activity-dependent neuronal plasticity during development contraindicates treatments that block NMDA receptors at specific neurodevelopmental stages due to their potential adverse effects on brain development [122].

5.1.2. AMPA receptors

AMPA receptors are Na^+ and K^+ (in some cases Ca^{2+}) permeable ion channels constituted by four subunits (GluA1-GluA4), playing the major determinants of the rapid component of excitatory synaptic currents in the brain. They exhibit fast activation and deactivation kinetics aside from rapid desensitization. The receptor subunits interact with transmembrane AMPA regulatory proteins (TARPs), exerting its influence on the synthesis, trafficking and localization of AMPA receptors at the cell surface, aside from their functional properties such as open probability, channel conductance, activation, deactivation, and desensitization [121].

In the developing brain, early alterations of the AMPA receptors (AMPARs) play a significant role in epileptogenesis, seizure susceptibility, and seizure-induced neuronal injury, and mediate synaptic potentiation induced by neonatal seizures [123]. Changes in AMPA receptor number are of great significance for CNS function, for instance, in shaping mechanisms underlying synaptic plasticity in cognitive aging [124]. Several studies have thrown light on the role of AMPA receptor maturation in perinatal seizures and brain injury. In immature subjects, AMPA receptors are relatively overexpressed in WM OLs, while after maturation those receptors predominate in neurons of cortex and hippocampus. Besides, in rodent models, it has been observed that hypoxia/ischemia causes neuronal damage at postnatal day 7 and seizures at postnatal days 10–12, but not at younger or older ages. These effects were found to be reversible by the administration of an AMPA receptor antagonist [125].

5.2. The amino acid GABA

GABA is a major NT expressed from the embryonic phase and throughout life. GABA is a versatile molecule with multiple functions during neocortical development and plays an important role in the developing brain even prior to synaptogenesis: stem cell proliferation, migration, synaptogenesis, and circuit formation. These diverse roles of GABA seem to depend both on cell-intrinsic properties (particularly high intracellular Cl^- gradient in immature neurons) and on extrinsic factors [126]. By changing the excitatory/inhibitory balance, GABAergic plasticity can regulate excitability, neural circuit function, and contribute to learning and memory [127]. GABA exerts depolarizing effects mostly contributing to the expression of spontaneous activities that are instructive for the construction of neural networks but GABA also acts as a potent trophic factor (for a review of metabolism and transport, see [128, 129]). The mammalian genome contains four genes encoding GABA transporters—"solute carrier family"—(GAT1, slc6a1; GAT2, slc6a13; GAT3, slc6a11; and the Betain/GABA transporter type 1 (BGT-1), slc6a12). GABA transporter types 1 and 3 (GAT-1 and GAT-3, respectively) are the two main subtypes of GATs responsible for the regulation of extracellular GABA levels in the central nervous system [111, 130]. GABA is actively taken up by neuron and astrocyte carrier proteins and broken down into succinic acid semialdehyde by glutamic acid decarboxylase (GAD) or repackaged into a vesicle that is released again at the next synaptic transmission [131].

There are two main types of GABA receptors: the ionotropic GABAsubtype A receptor and the metabotropic GABAsubtype B receptor [93]. The GABA receptor type A ($GABA_A$ receptor) is a ligand-gated chloride channel that mediates major inhibitory functions in the adult CNS. $GABA_A$ receptors function mainly as pentamers containing α, β, and either γ or δ subunits. At an early developmental stage, GABA, acting at $GABA_A$ receptors, produces a rapid synaptic excitatory response and is implicated in most processes of neurogenesis, including neuronal migration, proliferation, differentiation, and preliminary circuit building. In the mature CNS, GABA acts in an inhibitory manner, a switch mediated by chloride/cation transporter expression. In contrast to the ionotropic $GABA_A$ receptors, GABAB receptors are responsible for the latter and slower component of inhibitory transmission [132]. The composition of $GABA_A$ receptors is different in newborns, with less $\alpha1$ and more $\alpha2/3$ subunits, rendering them less responsive to benzodiazepines [133].

In the adult NS, due to low intracellular levels of neuronal chloride [Cl^-] gradients, GABA inhibits most neurons by the activation of GABA subtype A receptor channel chloride currents ($GABA_A$Rs), causing Cl^- influx, membrane hyperpolarization, and inhibition. During development, GABAergic neurotransmission undergoes a switch from excitatory to inhibitory due to a reversal of [Cl^-] gradients [134]. In immature neurons, high levels of expression and robust activity of the chloride-importing Na-K-2Cl cotransporter NKCC1 cause the accumulation of intracellular [Cl^-] and, therefore, a depolarized Cl^- equilibrium potential, responsible for an excitatory effect in the developing brain; besides the Cl^- exporting activity of KCC2 is lower than in mature neurons, and in the context of NKCC1 expression, neuronal [Cl^-] is higher and $GABA_A$ reversal potential (EGABA) is more depolarized, such that the binding of GABA to ligand-gated $GABA_A$ receptor-associated Cl^- channels triggers Cl^- efflux and depolarizing excitation. This results in the outward flux of [Cl^-] through $GABA_A$ channels, the opposite direction compared with mature neurons. In adults, NKCC1 expression decreases and the expression of the genetically related chloride-extruding K-Cl cotransporter KCC2 increases, which turns $GABA_A$ receptor activation inhibitory because Cl^- flows into the cell (for a review, see [135]).

6. GABAergic system in early-life epilepsies

The incidence of seizures classified as reactive, symptomatic, or idiopathic is particularly high in the early ages of life. The most common reactive seizures in early life are febrile convulsions, although they must be differentiated from symptomatic seizures precipitated by fever. Symptomatic seizures are often associated with different levels of CNS insults, including HIE, metabolic storage diseases gray matter, and brain congenital malformations. In the neuronal migration disorders and idiopathic seizures, increasingly a genetic defect can be identified (e.g., LIS1 mutations for lissencephaly). In all these instances, the GABAergic system has been proposed as a key player in "age-dependent vulnerability to seizures" [136, 137].

During seizures, the release of GABA occurs, and this outward flow of Cl^- in neonatal neurons is excitatory. The immaturity of GABAergic inhibitory systems has been implicated in the heightened susceptibility of neonates to seizures in early-life epilepsies, and contributes to a greater seizure propensity and poor electroencephalographic response to GABAergic anticonvulsants such as phenobarbital (PB) and benzodiazepine [133]. This is thought to be due to shunting inhibition or inhibition via excitatory effects upon inhibitory interneurons [138]. During seizures, the excessive GABAergic stimulation of the substantia nigra reticulata that is believed to occur has been reported to be proconvulsant in neonatal animals while it would be anticonvulsant at older ages [139]. This developmental switch seems to occur earlier in female rats [140]. But in addition to GABA synapses, also the intact glutamatergic transmission

http://dx.doi.org/10.5772/64458

has been linked to the appearance of a BS pattern [141]. Therefore, certain neocortical cell types may act as EEG burst-suppression pacemakers, in particular the "fast-rhythmic-bursting" neurons described in neocortex [142].

Gene symbol	Titles	Locus	OMIM	EIEE
Genes impair interneuron migration				
ARX	Aristaless-related homeobox, X-linked	Xp21.3	300382	EIEE 1/LISX2
HER4/ERBB4	Tyrosine kinase–type cell surface receptor HER4 (Neuregulin-1receptor ErbB4)	2q34	600543	EIEE 3 (EME)
Genes encoding ion channels				
SCN1A	Sodium channel, neuronal type 1a subunit;	2q24.3	182389	EIEE 6 or Dravet Synd. GEFSP2/FEB3A/MHP3
SCN2A	Sodium channel neuronal type 2a subunit	2q24.3	182390	EIEE 11/BFIS3
SCN8A	Sodium channel neuronal type 8a subunit	12q13	600702	EIEE 13
KCNA2	Potassium channel, voltage-gated, shaker-related subfamily, member 2	1p13.3	176262	EIEE 32
KCNQ2	Potassium channel, voltage-gated, KQT-like subfamily, member 2	20q13.3	602235	EIEE 7/BFNS1
KCNB1	Potassium channel, voltage-gated, Shab-related subfamily, member 1	20q13.13	600397	EIEE 26
KCNT1	Potassium channel, subfamily t, member 1	9q34.3	608167	EIEE 14
CACNA2D2	Calcium channel, voltage-dependent, alpha 2/delta subunit 2	3p21.31	607082	VUS
HCN1	Hyperpolarization-activated cyclic nucleotide–gated potassium channel 1	5p12	602780	EIEE 24
Genes encoding regulators of synaptic vesicles release				
DNM1	Dynamin-1	9q34.11	602377	EIEE 31
NECAP1	Necap endocytosis–associated protein 1	12p13.31	611623	EIEE 21
TBC1D24	Tbc1 domain family, member 24	16p13.3	613577	EIEE 16
STXBP1	Syntaxin-binding protein 1	9q34.1	602926	EIEE 4
Genes encoding regulators of intracellular/intercellular signal transduction				
DOCK7	Dedicator of cytokinesis 7	1p31.1	615730	EIEE 23
GNAO1	Guanine nucleotide–binding protein, alpha-activating activity polypeptide 1	16q13	139311	EIEE 17
ARHGEF9	Rho guanine nucleotide exchange factor 9	Xq11.1	300429	EIEE 8/hyperekplexia
ST3Gal III	St3 beta-galactoside alpha-2,3-sialyltransferase 3	1p34.1	606494	EIEE 15

Gene symbol	Titles	Locus	OMIM	EIEE
WWOX	Ww domain-containing oxidoreductase	16q23	605131	EIEE 28
SPTAN1	Spectrin, alpha, nonerythrocytic 1	9q34.11	182810	EIEE 5
PCDH19	Protocadherin 19	Xq22.1	300460	EIEE 9
PLCB1	Phospholipase c, beta-1	20p12.3	607120	EIEE 12
PIGA	Phosphatidylinositol glycan, class A	Xp22.2	311770	EIEE 20
AARS	Alanyl-tRNA synthetase	16q22.1	601065	EIEE 29
SIK1	Salt-inducible kinase 1	21q22.3	605705	EIEE 30
ALG13	Asparagine-linked glycosylation 13	Xq23	300776	EIEE 36
Genes encoding neurotransmitters membrane receptors				
GRIN 2A	Glutamate receptor, ionotropic, N-methyl-D-aspartate, subunit 2[a]	16p13.2	138253	FESD
GRIN2 B	Glutamate receptor, ionotropic, *N*-methyl-*D*-aspartate, subunit 2b	12p13.1	138252	EIEE 27
GABRA 1	Gamma-aminobutyric acid receptor, alpha-1	5q34	137160	EIEE 19
Genes encoding intracellular transporters				
SLC12A5	Solute carrier family 12 (potassium/chloride transporter), member 5	20q13.12	606726	EIEE 34
SLC13A5	Solute carrier family 13 (sodium-dependent citrate transporter	17p13.1	137160	EIEE 25
SLC25A22	Solute carrier family 25 (mitochondrial carrier, glutamate) member 22	11p15.5	609302	EIEE 3 (EME)
SLC35A2	Solute carrier family 35 (UDP-galactose transporter), member 2	Xp11.23	314375	EIEE 22
EEF1A2	Eukaryotic translation elongation factor 1, alpha-2	20q13.33	602959	EIEE 33
Genes encoding enzymes				
SZT2	Seizure threshold 2	1p34.2	615463	EIEE 18
CDKL5	Cyclin-dependent kinase–like 5	Xp22.13	300203	EIEE 2
PNKP	Polynucleotide kinase 3-prime phosphatase	19q13.4	605610	EIEE 10
ITPA	Inosine triphosphate pyrophosphohydrolase	20p13	147520	EIEE 35

EIEE: early infantile epileptic encephalopathy. LISX2: lissencephaly, X-linked 2. EME: early myoclonic encephalopathy. GEFSP2: epilepsy, generalized, febrile plus, type 2. FEB3A: febrile seizures, familial, 3A. MHP3: migraine, familial hemiplegic, 3. BFIS3: benign familial infantile seizures-3. BFNS1: benign familial neonatal seizures. VUS: variant of uncertain significance because its contribution to EIEE has not been confirmed. FESD: focal epilepsy and speech disorder.

Table 3. Genes of early-onset epileptic encephalopathies.

Mutations or genetic variations of the genes encoding the $\alpha1$, $\alpha6$, $\beta2$, $\beta3$, $\gamma2$, or δ subunits (GABRA1, GABRA6, GABRB2, GABRB3, GABRG2, and GABRD, respectively) of the $GABA_A$ receptor have been associated with the pathomechanisms of human epilepsy and genetic epilepsy syndromes, both with and without febrile seizures syndromes, including pure febrile seizures (FSs), generalized epilepsy with febrile seizures plus (GEFS+), Dravet's syndrome (DS, also known as severe myoclonic epilepsy in infancy, SMEI), childhood absence epilepsy (CAE), and juvenile myoclonic epilepsy (JME). Related genotypic and phenotypic spectra of mutations of $GABA_A$ receptor are changeful, thus, mutations of GABRA1 (137160) in 5q34 were associated with EIEE19 or DS. Recently, mutations of GABRA1, GABRB2, and GABRB3 were associated with ISS and Lennox-Gastaut syndrome, and also GABRB3-related EOEE [143]. These mutations that compromise hyperpolarization through $GABA_A$ receptors are found in both translated and untranslated gene regions. Interestingly, most of the insufficiencies are not caused by receptor-gating abnormalities, but by multiple mechanisms, including (I) endoplasmic reticulum (ER)-associated degradation; (II) reducing subunit mRNA transcription or stability, impairing subunit folding, stability, or oligomerization; (III) intracellular-trafficking defects; and (IV) ER stress [144, 145].

While ion channel genes were considered for a long time as the only major group of genes involved in genetic epilepsies, at present, an increasing number of non-ion-channel genes and new pathways have been identified and it is difficult to find a common mechanism to explain EOEE. In 2015, Mario Mastrangelo [43] summarized clinical presentations, genotype-phenotype relationships, and genes involved in the pathogenesis of EOEE comprising genes encoding ion channels, regulators of synaptic vesicles release, regulators of intracellular/intercellular signal transduction, NT, membrane receptors, intracellular transporters, and enzymes (see **Table 3**).

The study of epilepsy due to single gene defects has helped to clarify certain seizure mechanisms. The role of ARX mutations is well defined on downstream targets of this interneuron-expressed transcription factor as well as their effects on cell migration and maturation of GABAergic interneurons, which can help to explain the phenotype of ISS and electrographic seizures [146]. During the early stages of development, ARX is expressed in a significant proportion of neurons in the cortex, striatum, ganglionic eminences, and the spinal cord. In the adult, the expression of ARX is still present but restricted to regions that are known to be rich in GABAergic neurons, such as the amygdala and olfactory bulb [47]. SCN1A mutations also implicate a predominant role for GABA interneurons due to disturbed GABAergic function [147].

A variety of the named "epilepsy-age-dependent epileptic encephalopathies" is considered to share a common pathological mechanism connected with the structural and functional disturbance of interneurons, and therefore they have been designated with a new term "interneuronopathies" [55, 148, 149, 150]. However, not only interneurons but also pyramidal neurons could be at the origin of these encephalopathies. Therefore, those genes that disrupt the glutamate metabolism via mitochondrial respiratory chain damage (i.e., mitochondrial glutamate carrier SLC25A22) should also be considered as an important cause of the neonatal epileptic encephalopathy (EME, EIEE3) [151].

Another example of a gene that presents mutations related to EIEE23 is DOCK7 (Dedicator of cytokinesis 7, locus 1p31.3). Overexpression of human DOCK7 in transfected embryonic rat hippocampal neurons induced the formation of multiple axons, whereas knockdown of Dock7 inhibited axon formation. DOCK7 is an important regulator of microtubule assembly both in the context of neurogenesis and in the establishment of neuronal polarity in newborn pyramidal neurons. It also promotes the development of nascent axons by activating Rac1 (a Rac guanine nucleotide exchange factor). In addition, DOCK7 controls the development and the morphological differentiation of GABAergic interneurons in the developing cortex. In human, the loss of DOCK7 function causes a syndromic form of epileptic encephalopathy and cortical blindness (EIEE23) by affecting multiple neuronal processes, with different types of seizures, including tonic seizures, infantile spasms myoclonus, partial complex seizures with rotation of the head, drop attacks, and tonic seizures among other crises [152]. Thus, some genes may be involved in several pathways of cortical development.

Quoting the words of Connie Wu [93], "the so called "GABA shift" is a fascinating change in the effect of GABA from depolarizing action in the developing brain to hyperpolarizing action in the adult brain". The depolarizing action of the GABAergic system would be governed by glutamate with an inhibitory effect on this early excitatory activity of the GABA in the early neocortex [153], and by $GABA_B$ receptors-mediated inhibition of $GABA_A$ receptor calcium elevations in the developing hypothalamus, providing a mechanism for excitatory-inhibitory balance during development [154].

Additionally, the full maturation of the GABAergic system in humans occurs after the neonatal period. In the human cerebral cortex and WM, there is evidence that an important part of the development of the GABAergic system takes place during the latter half of gestation and into the first few years of infancy [155]. In point of fact, it is possible that the human GABAergic system does not completely mature until adolescence [156]. The interruption of any aspect of this sequence of events during development, due to either an environmental insult or genetic mutations, could have devastating consequences on normal brain function [157], and may interfere neuronal morphology, differentiation, and connectivity, manifesting as cognitive or neurodevelopmental deficits. In the same vein, further dysregulation of inhibitory GABA systems has been shown to play a major role in facilitating seizures, particularly marked in the early neonatal ages [158].

One hypothesis that has been presented is that the normal variability in the number of interneurons could explain the propensity of some individuals to develop epilepsy more than others as a result of an injury or any other trigger that could lead to neuron loss. Particularly, if chandelier cells (which are considered to be the most powerful cortical GABAergic inhibitory interneuron) were affected, it would have serious consequences for the inhibitory control of the pyramidal cells [159]. Recent data have shown that early postnatal transplantation of interneuronal precursor cells increased GABAergic inhibition in the host brain and dramatically suppressed seizure activity in epileptic mice [160]. These data create future expectations for "the Promise of an Interneuron-based Cell Therapy for patients with intractable forms of epilepsy" [161].

http://dx.doi.org/10.5772/64458

7. Antiepileptic drugs (AEDs) in EIEE

As we mentioned previously, epilepsy in children represents a symptom of complex brain diseases, presenting with a variety of syndromes, with many treatment options and disparing results. The prognosis is generally good, with a large proportion responding well to the first treatment given. But a substantial share (particularly children with epileptogenic encephalopathies), however, will not respond well to AEDs, despite aggressive and often off-label use of a variety of drugs. For these patients, the clinical goal is to find an optimal balance between the benefits and side effects of a particular medication.

Before 1993, the management of epilepsy was limited to six major AEDs consisting of phenobarbital, primidone, phenytoin, valproate, carbamazepine, and ethosuximide (ESM). These were referred to as the "first-generation AEDs" or traditional AEDs. Since the 1990s new drugs were introduced and called "second-generation" antiepileptic drugs, including felbamate, gabapentin (GBP), lamotrigine, topiramate, tiagabine (TGB), levetiracetam (LEV), oxcarbazepine, zonisamide, vigabatrin (VGB), and pregabalin [162]. Newly published evidence-based treatment guidelines have helped physicians to choose the most effective AED in pediatric epilepsy, although data do not always fully support new antiepileptic drugs due to lack of well-designed, randomized controlled trials [163].

At present, there are about 20 novel antiepileptic drugs, categorized as "third generation". Some of these drugs are derived from others that can be found in today's market place. Among the most representative include brivaracetam and seletracetam (analogs of levetiracetam), pregabalin, ganaxolone (GNX) (belong to neurosteroids), carisbamate and fluorofelbamate (analog of felbamate), rufinamide, safinamide (inhibit the release of glutamate), lacosamide, eslicarbazepine (analog of the antiepileptic drug oxcarbazepine), and talampanel (glutamate antagonist). Some of these drugs are recommended only in adults, but it is expected that they would also be included for therapy in children in the future, as it happened with the second-generation AEDs (see **Table 4**).

The second-generation AEDs have less effect on hepatic metabolism and cytochrome P450 induction, fewer drug interactions, and lower protein binding. Their off-label use in pediatric patients is fairly widespread and has given new options for the treatment of patients with epileptic encephalopathy and refractory epilepsy, despite most of these agents not having US Food and Drug Administration (FDA) indications for use [164, 165]. However, the newer AEDs are not more efficacious than the older-generation AEDs. In particular, there is no clinical evidence to suggest that the newer agents should be considered as a first-choice treatment in any form of epilepsy in children [166].

The Task Force Report for the ILAE Commission of Pediatrics, in a recent report [167], summarizes the recommendations for the management of infantile seizures. For focal seizures, levetiracetam is effective (strong evidence); for generalized seizures, weak evidence supports levetiracetam, valproate, lamotrigine, topiramate, and clobazam (CLB); for Dravet's syndrome, strong evidence supports that stiripentol is effective (in combination with valproate and clobazam), whereas weak evidence supports that topiramate, zonisamide, valproate, bromide, and the ketogenic diet are possibly effective; and for Ohtahara syndrome, there is weak evidence that most antiepileptic drugs are poorly effective.

Main mechanism of action		Main groups		AEDs
Factors that influence excitatory postsynaptic potential (EPSP): - Na^{+} influx - Ca^{++} currents - Paroxysmal Depolarization	**Sodium Influx**	**Sodium channel blockers**		Phenytoin (PHT) Carbamazepine(CBZ) Oxcarbazepine (OXC) Eslicarbazepine Zonisamide (ZNS) Lamotrigine(LTG) Lacosemide
	Calcium Channel	**Calcium current inhibitors**		Ethosuximide(ESM)
Factors that influence inhibitory postsynaptic potential (IPSP). - K^{+} efflux - Cl^{-} influx - Pumps - Low pH	**GABA-A receptor by Cl influx.**	**GABA enhancers**	**GABA A agonist** (enhanced by binding directly to GABA-A receptors)	Barbiturates Primidone Benzodiazepines Progesterone Ganaloxone
			Uptake inhibitor (by blocking presynaptic GABA uptake)	Tiagabine(TGB)
			GABA-transaminase inhibitor (by inhibiting the metabolism)	Vigabatrine (VGB)
			GAD modulation (increasing the synthesis of GABA)	Gabapentin(GBP) Valproate (VPA) Pregabalin Progabide(Prodrug)
	GABA-B receptor by K efflux		**GABA-B receptors antagonist**	CGP35348
	Glutamate receptors facilitate the flow of both Na and Ca ions into the cell, while K ions flow out of the cell, resulting in excitation	Glutamate blockers	NMDA	Felbamate
			AMPA/KAINATE	Topiramate (TPM) Parampanel
	Neuronal Potassium Channel Openers			Ezogabine (known as retigabine)
	Carbonic anhydrase inhibitors (decreases the pH)			Acetazolamide
Unknow	Binds the Synaptic vesicle protein 2A (SV2A) (function has not been clearly defined; by Ca^{++}?)			Levetiracetam (LEV) (Glycine?) Brivaracetam Rufinamide

AEDs Main Group Classification, basis in main mechanism of action: excitatory postsynaptic potential (EPSP) and inhibitory postsynaptic potential (IPSP). Several mechanisms of action are indicated by arrows

Table 4. Mechanism of action of antiepileptic drugs (AEDs).

Research on the molecular basis and pathways of some epilepsy syndromes has become practical clinical task and has a clear value for both the patient and his family. It is now possible for some cases to make therapeutic decisions made based on genetic findings of EIEE. This capacity for precision therapy is expected to become more usual in the near future [168].

An extensive knowledge of the genes involved in EIEE may allow a more appropriate use of AEDs based on their mechanism of action. The AEDs can also be grouped according to their primary mechanism of action, although many of them have various actions and others have unknown mechanisms of action. The main groups include (1) GABA enhancers and (2) non-GABAergic antiepileptic drugs: sodium channel blockers, calcium current inhibitors, glutamate blockers, neuronal potassium channel openers, carbonic anhydrase (CA) inhibitors, and drugs with unknown mechanisms of action (see **Table 4**).

7.1. AEDs and GABAergic system

The current GABAergic antiepileptic drugs (especially GABA receptor agonists), while often effective for adults, are not always capable of stopping seizures and preventing their sequelae in neonates. The GABAergic drugs mainly include phenobarbital, benzodiazepines, tiagabine, vigabatrin, gabapentin, valproate, and pregabalin.

7.1.1. GABA receptor agonists: drugs that enhance the actions of the neurotransmitter GABA

A number of antiepileptic drugs (AEDs) have agonistic effects on GABA subtype A ($GABA_A$) receptors. Currently, the first-line medical treatment for neonatal seizures is composed of drugs that increase $GABA_A$Rs, such as phenobarbital and benzodiazepines (clobazam, clonazepam); another treatment strategy is the indirect manipulation of the GABAergic system, via the modulation of neuronal Cl(−) gradients, by targeting the cation-Cl(−) cotransporters (NKCC1 and KCC2) or their regulatory signaling molecules [169].

- **Phenobarbital (PB)** increases $GABA_A$Rs. PB has been the gold standard and remains the preferred drug for the management of neonatal seizures for the treatment of seizures in neonates [170]; however, PB controls seizures in less than half of newborns [171]. This reduced efficacy of GABA-enhancing AEDs has been linked to neuronal chloride transport in the developing brain. It is also intriguing to consider that recent insights regarding the impact of maturational changes in neuronal chloride transporter expression on GABA receptor function may provide strategies for adjunctive therapies of neonatal seizures, and could improve the neuroprotective efficacy of PB in the neonate.

Specifically, blocking the neonatal neuronal chloride transporter with **bumetanide** (a specific inhibitor of the NaC-KC- $2Cl^-$ cotransporter NKCC1) can augment the inhibitory activity of GABA agonists such as PB [172, 173]. Low concentrations of the diuretic bumetanide have been shown to alter the ion gradient that underlies the excitatory effects of GABA. Blocking the NKCC1 transporter with bumetanide prevents outward Cl- flux and causes a more negative GABA equilibrium potential in immature neurons. While several studies have reported anticonvulsant effects of bumetanide [174], others have found no significant anticonvulsant effect. The alteration of Cl- transport by bumetanide reduces electrographic seizures, and the combination of bumetanide and PB is significantly more effective than PB alone on seizure occurrence, frequency, and duration [172].

- **Stiripentol (STP):** STP enhances central GABA transmission through a barbiturate-like effect, since it increases the duration of opening of GABA-A receptor channels, and also may increase the GABA levels by interfering with its uptake and its metabolism. In 2007, the European Medicines Agency granted STP a marketing authorization for Dravet's syndrome whose seizures are not adequately controlled with clobazam and valproate. The combination of STP with clobazam (CLB) and valproate seems promising for therapy of severe myoclonic epilepsy in infancy (SMEN) with a responder rate of 54% [175], as well as to suppress convulsive status epilepticus [176].

- **Benzodiazepines:** The benzodiazepines most often used for the treatment of epilepsy are diazepam, midazolam, lorazepam, clonazepam, and clobazam. The first three drugs are used primarily in protocols for emergency treatment of seizures and status epilepticus due to their rapid onset of action, the availability of intravenous (IV) forms, and anticonvulsant effects. Its use for long-term treatment is limited due to the development of tolerance. Benzodiazepines are used in (phenobarbital) refractory cases of neonatal seizures [177].

– **Clonazepam** has higher affinity for the $GABA_A$ receptor site than diazepam and binds to $GABA_A$ receptors that do not bind other benzodiazepines. Clonazepam is the drug of choice for myoclonic seizures and subcortical myoclonus.

– **Clobazam (CLB):** In addition to its agonist action at the $GABA_A$ receptor, clobazam may affect voltage-sensitive conductance of calcium ions and the function of sodium channels, which makes CLB a potent anticonvulsant for partial epilepsy.

7.1.2. Uptake inhibitor (by blocking presynaptic GABA uptake)

Tiagabine (TGB) represents a new generation of AEDs. It is a derivative of nipecotic acid, with a unique mechanism of action: uptake inhibitor, by blocking presynaptic GABA uptake. TGB was approved for use by the FDA in 1997 as an adjunct agent for adults and children past 12 years of age with epilepsy, suffering from partial seizures, with and without secondary generalization. Following a period of great enthusiasm for the use of TGB, it was put aside. The FDA on 18 February 2005 issued a warning about the possible occurrence of nonconvulsive as well as convulsive status epilepticus in a subset of nonepileptic and epileptic patients treated with TGB [178], and should be under surveillance of frequency and severity of TGB overdoses and reported to the American Association of Poison Control Centers (AAPCC).

There are very little data on TGB use in children, but this agent appears to be effective and have a good tolerability profile and it still has its place in the treatment of drug-resistant epilepsy.

7.1.3. GABA transaminase inhibitors (inhibition of the GABA-degrading enzyme)

- **The Vigabatrin (VGB)** has been widely used for the treatment of refractory epilepsies in epileptic encephalopathies. The anti-seizure effect of VGB is a result of enhanced brain

http://dx.doi.org/10.5772/64458

extracellular GABA levels by irreversible inhibition of the GABA-degrading enzyme GABA aminotransferase (GABA-T) [179]. VGB inhibits GABA-T and elevates GABA in the subthalamic nucleus (STN) [180].

ACTH, corticosteroids, and VGB are the first-line drugs for the treatment of ISS. However, the detection of an irreversible visual field defect observed in as high as 30–50% of children treated with VGB has contraindicated its use as first-line drug. Regarding West syndrome, there is some evidence for the preference of hormonal treatments over VGB, except for children under 3 months. In children with tuberous sclerosis complex (TSC), VGB is the treatment of first choice. Around 30% of patients who present with ISS respond well to treatment with VGB. VGB should be considered as an early treatment option in early-onset epileptic encephalopathies (EIEE and EME) [181]. Patients with mutation in STXBP1 gene could especially benefit from treatment with VGB [182]. Interestingly, VGB can cause swelling and loss of myelin, suggesting that excessive activation of $GABA_A$ receptors while oligodendrocytes are undergoing myelinization may be deleterious for that process [183].

7.1.4. GAD modulation

GAD modulation increases GABA turnover/synthesis of GABA.

- **Gabapentin (GBP)** was approved on January 1994 as an adjunctive treatment in patients 12 years or older with partial seizures, with or devoid of secondary generalization, which were resistant to the traditional AEDs. GBP is an anticonvulsant GABA-mimetic and considered as a structural analog of the inhibitory NT GABA. However, preliminary studies proposed that GBP did not bind to either $GABA_A$ or $GABA_B$ receptors, nor was it transformed metabolically into GABA. GBP prevents voltage-dependent sodium currents, and it is also claimed to reduce presynaptic glutamate release and binding to postsynaptic calcium channels and prevent central desensitization due to glutamate neurotransmission in the dorsal horn of the spinal canal [184].

GBP has been used in both adults and children for numerous neurologic conditions, including management of epilepsy, neuropathic pain (control of pain and irritability attributed to neurologic impairment), refractory insomnia, and occasionally movement disorders (e.g., restless legs syndrome, dystonia, and nystagmus) [185]. GBP use for seizure has been limited as a result of inconsistent efficacy and concern about seizure exacerbation (in particular, aggravation of myoclonic seizures) [186]. GBP may significantly ameliorate dystonia severity and improve activities of daily living and quality of life in children [187].

- **Sodium valproate (VPA)** acts through a combination of several mechanisms. Among the mechanisms through which valproate exerts its anticonvulsant properties, an increase in GABA turnover is included by significantly enhanced GABA inhibition in the cerebral cortex, an action which is independent of its effect on spontaneous activity [188]. Thereby, it potentiates GABAergic functions in some specific brain regions, such as substantia nigra, thought to be involved in the control of seizure generation and propagation [189]. In children, and especially in infants with epileptic encephalopathies, treatment with valproate is preferred when proper diagnosis is not achieved [190].

- **Pregabalin:** GBP and pregabalin are structurally related to the inhibitory neurotransmitter GABA, and can modulate voltage-activated Ca^{2+} channels. The pharmacological activity of pregabalin is similar but not identical to that of GBP. Pregabalin reduces excitatory properties by modulating voltage-activated Ca^{2+} and K^{+} channels. The actions of pregabalin may involve both extracellular and intracellular drug target sites and modulation of a variety of neuronal conductances, by direct interactions and through intracellular signaling involving protein kinase A [191]. Pregabalin is remarkable for seizure control in children with intractable epilepsy, and reduced more than 50% of seizure intensity in 40.2% of patients [192], although there are no references to support the use of pregabalin in Ohtahara syndrome.

7.2. Non-GABAergic antiepileptic drugs

7.2.1. Sodium channel blockers

With the increasing knowledge of the involvement of ion channels in the origin of epilepsy, a greater number of publications that establish optimal treatment based on the genetic defect have been appearing. This evidence may allow in the future to establish a "treatment on demand." This is particularly important for genes encoding ion channels and sodium channel blockers, such as:

- First generation: phenytoin (PHT), carbamazepine (CBZ);
- Second generation: oxcarbazepine (OXC), zonisamide (ZNS), lamotrigine (LTG);
- Third generation: eslicarbazepine, lacosemide.

Concerning Dravet's syndrome (caused in 80% of cases by mutations in SCN1A), there is some evidence showing that early aggressive therapy improves outcome, so genetic testing should be considered early. The SCN1A protein appears to be mainly on inhibitory interneurons, and treatment with sodium channel blockers such as lamotrigine and carbamazepine should be avoided, whereas valproic acid, topiramate, clobazam, and stiripentol appear to be beneficial [193, 194]. By contrast, in the epileptic encephalopathies associated with mutations in SCN2A and SCN8A, their profile of drug responsiveness may be different since the proteins encoded by these genes are localized in excitatory neurons. In fact, for SCN8A encephalopathy, sodium channel blockers may be effective in some cases [195].

Regarding the Ohtahara syndrome caused by mutations in the KCNQ2 channel, recent experience suggests that sodium channel blockers, carbamazepine, and phenytoin (40 and 33%, respectively, were seizure-free), are effective in this disorder. An effective treatment may be important for reducing the neurodevelopmental impairment associated with this disorder [60, 196].

Besides the known use of phenytoin for the treatment of neonatal seizures, other AEDs second generation such as oxcarbazepine and zonisamide have been relatively well studied in pediatric seizure patients, including their use as monotherapy. Both agents have demonstrated good efficacy and tolerability for patients as young as 1 month old. Zonisamide is efficacious in pediatric epilepsy syndromes, including LGS, WS, OS [197], and for seizure control in children with intractable epilepsy [192].

7.2.2. Calcium current inhibitors

- In addition to ethosuximide (ESM), other drugs such as topiramate (TPM) and LTG also act as calcium currents inhibitors. Childhood absence epilepsy (CAE) is one of the most common types of pediatric epilepsy. It is generally treated with ESM, VPA, or LTG. VPA-LTG combination therapy has a good efficacy and fewer side effects than other treatments, and it should thus be considered as a first-line therapy in absence of epilepsy [198]. ESM next to clobazam and sulthiame is the most commonly used treatment in patients with Landau-Kleffner syndrome (LKS), but it has no use in EIEE.

7.2.3. Glutamate blockers

7.2.3.1. NMDA antagonist

- **Felbamate:** Although felbamate has multiple mechanisms of action, it is thought to have its most potent antiepileptic effects through the inhibition of the N-methyl-D-aspartate receptor (NMDAR). Felbamate was approved in 1993 as a novel antiepileptic drug to be used both as monotherapy and as an adjunctive therapy to treat partial seizures with and without generalization in adults and as an adjunctive therapy for LGS. Despite its favorable efficacy, there has been restricted approval of felbamate only for adjunctive therapy in patients with LGS because of the occurrence of felbamate-related hepatotoxicity and idiosyncratic aplastic anemia. Our current understanding of clinical data on the risk: benefit of felbamate therapy supports its use as an important therapeutic option for some patients with refractory epilepsy [199]. Early initiation of felbamate is recommended for children with refractory epilepsy [200]. Felbamate monotherapy was able to achieve relevant antiepileptic effects in a unique patient with neurofibromatosis type 1 (NF1) and tuberous sclerosis complex (TSC) [201].

- **Memantine:** In a patient with a mutation in GRIN2A, encoding a glutamate NMDA receptor subunit, memantine therapy (acting on the glutamatergic system by blocking NMDA receptors) appeared effective [202]. This case exemplifies the potential for personalized genomics and therapeutics to be utilized for early diagnosis and treatment of infantile-onset neurological diseases.

7.2.3.2. AMPA/KAINATE antagonist

- **Topiramate (TPM)** exerts an antiepileptic effect via four mechanisms: (1) blockade of voltage-dependent sodium channels, (2) $GABA_A$ agonist, (3) AMPA/kainate glutamate receptor subtype, and (4) inhibition of carbonic anhydrase isoenyzmes type I and IV. In the United States, topiramate currently is approved for (1) partial-onset and secondarily GTCs, (2) primary GTCs, and (3) LGS. Currently, its use for the EOEE has not been established. Although TPM is well studied in adults and older children, limited data exist for the application to neonates. The use of TPM in neonates has met with two significant challenges: first, to date no intravenous formulation is commercially available, and second, there is significant concern that TPM adversely affects language development [203]. TPM is a good add-on drug in patients with epileptic encephalopathies such as LGS and myoclonic astatic epilepsy. Regarding treatment options for ISS, TPM can be used when first-line drugs have proven ineffective. Cessation of all spasms occurred in 32 [204] to 48% infants treated with TPM [205]. In our experience (unpublished data), initial polytherapy with low dose of ACTH and TPM was effective to suppress ISS in most patients, allowing to leave TPM—after removal of ACTH—as AEDs of choice to prevent recurrence of the ISS. This combined treatment has been endorsed by other authors [206, 207].

- **Perampanel (PER):** PER is a newer antiepileptic drug, first-in-class orally active, selective noncompetitive AMPA receptor antagonist. In 2012, the European Union approved usage for adjunctive therapy in partial-onset seizures (for patients age >12 years), with US approval following in 2013 [208]. PER seems to be effective also in children and adolescents with pharmaco-refractory epilepsies. Tolerability was acceptable [209]. But randomized controlled trials in children are necessary to support its use.

7.2.4. Neuronal potassium channel openers

- **Retigabine (RTG)/ezogabine:** The new-generation drugs retigabine (RTG (international nonproprietary name)) and ezogabine (EZG (US adopted name)) are the first neuronal potassium (K_V7_2-7_5) channel openers (act uniquely by enhancing the M-type potassium current), and they are used as an adjunctive treatment for partial epilepsies in adult patients. Mutations in KCNQ2 and KCNQ3, encoding the voltage-gated potassium channels KV 7.2 and KV 7.3, are known to cause BFNS1 and severe epileptic encephalopathy with pharmacoresistant seizures. Application of RTG partially reversed these effects for the majority of the analyzed mutations. Thus, RTG or similar drugs have been proposed for use as a personalized therapy for this severe disease [210]. But unfortunately toxicity may limit its use, and there are few data available on its effectiveness in KCNQ2 encephalopathy.

7.2.5. Carbonic anhydrase inhibitors

In humans, 16 different isozymes of the zinc enzyme carbonic anhydrases (CA) have been described and are considered as drug targets, some of them being involved in various pathological disorders such as glaucoma, epilepsy, and cancer.

Triggering mechanisms of seizures includes an increase of intracellular potassium concentration and a pH shift within the brain. pH buffering of extra- and intracellular spaces is mainly carried out by the CO_2/HCO_3^- buffer, the equilibration of the two species being assured by the zinc enzyme CA [211]. Neuronal excitability is related to GABAergic depolarization via $GABA_A$ receptor and contributed by HCO_3^- efflux, playing a role in initiating ictal-like epileptiform events in several cortical structures. HCO_3^--dependent depolarization can be suppressed by membrane-permeable inhibitors of CA such as acetazolamide, methazolamide, zonisamide, topiramate, and sulthiame, which can reduce seizures through perturbation of the CO_2 equilibrium and/or the inhibition of ion channels [212], leading to diminished depolarization of principal cells and, perhaps, interneurons [213].

- **Acetazolamide** has been approved for the treatment of epilepsy since 1953, and should be considered when there is a poor response to conventional antiepileptic drugs or refractory epilepsy. They have been used in various diseases including LKS [214], dominant paroxysmal ataxia, juvenile myoclonic epilepsy, newborn with Arnold-Chiari malformation with central apneas, or in epileptic apnea in MMPSI resulting in complete disappearance of epileptic seizures [215].

- **Sulthiame** is an inhibitor of CA and a widely used add-on antiepileptic drug for the treatment of intractable epilepsy, WS, status epilepticus during sleep (ESES), continuous spikes and waves during slow sleep (CSWS) syndrome, and LKS, which was refractory to other AEDs. Sulthiame may lead to a cessation of seizures when used as an add-on therapy to pyridoxine in patients with WS. No evidence exists for the use of sulthiame as an add-on therapy in patients with epilepsy outside WS. Large, multicenter randomized controlled trials are necessary to inform clinical practice if sulthiame is to be used as an add-on therapy for epilepsy [216]. Sulthiame was associated with deterioration in cognitive function in children with benign epilepsy of childhood with central temporal spikes [217].

7.3. Others

7.3.1. Drugs with unknown mechanisms of action

- **Levetiracetam (LEV):** Although the mechanism of action of LEV is still not well defined, new hypotheses propose that LEV and brivaracetam act by accelerating the induction of supply rate depression in synaptic vesicle trafficking, mainly synaptic vesicle glycoprotein 2a (SV2a) during incipient epileptic activity [218]. SV2 (encoded by the SV2A gene -OMIM 185860-) might mediate the uptake of NTs into vesicles. Loss of SV2A leads to a reduction in action potential-dependent gamma-aminobutyric acid (GABA)ergic neurotransmission [219]. LEV is utilized for the treatment of seizures, including neonatal seizures. There is strong evidence that LEV is effective in the treatment of focal seizures, whereas for generalized seizures, there is weak evidence to support the use of levetiracetam, valproate, lamotrigine, topiramate, and clobazam uses [167]. Treatment with intravenous levetiracetam is the new option for patients with refractory status epilepticus, even in patients younger than 2 years old (off-label use) [220]. Status epilepticus is characterized by downregulation of the inhibitory gamma-aminobutyric acid system, and LEV acting via different mechanisms could slow the epileptogenesis. Lately, LEV has been considered as the first-choice treatment for patients with early-onset epileptic encephalopathy due to an STXBP1 mutation and refractory to other antiepileptic drugs [221, 222].

- **Rufinamide** is a triazole derivative that is structurally unrelated to any currently marketed AEDs. It was approved by the FDA in December 2008 for adjunctive treatment of seizures associated with LGS for children 4 years or older and for adults. The precise mechanism by which rufinamide exerts its antiepileptic effect is unknown. In vitro studies suggest that the principal mechanism of action of rufinamide is modulation of the activity of sodium channels and, in particular, prolongation of the inactive state of the channel. Placebo-controlled studies for rufinamide that have efficacy data include studies involving (1) patients with LGS in children aged 1 year or older, (2) pediatric partial-onset seizures as adjunctive therapy, (3) adult partial-onset seizures (for both monotherapy and adjunctive therapy), and (4) patients with refractory GTCs [223]. Few studies in children with epileptic encephalopathies (EE) aged <4 years show that RUF is efficacious (60% were responders) and well tolerated. Therefore, for controlling seizures in this very severe form of epilepsy, the off-label use of RUF is justified [224].

7.3.2. Steroid hormones and neurosteroids

Steroid hormones and neurosteroids play an important role in children and adults with epilepsy, and act on both synaptic and extrasynaptic $GABA_A$ receptors. Corticosteroids, progesterone, estrogens, and neurosteroids have been shown to affect seizure activity in animal models and in clinical studies (for a review, see [225]).

- **Sex-steroid hormones** influence brain excitability and could explain sex differences in seizure susceptibility. Androgens are mainly anticonvulsant (mainly enhance GABA-activated currents), but the effects are more varied. For the female gender, progesterone and its metabolites are anticonvulsant, while estrogens are mainly proconvulsant (e.g., catamenial epilepsy). Estrogens reduce chloride conductance and potentiate glutamate receptor-mediated excitotoxicity responses (by potentiating NMDA receptor activity), but also affect GABAergic mechanisms and alter brain morphology by enhancing the density dendrite spine. Progesterone is a natural endogenous anticonvulsant hormone with substantial impact on seizure susceptibility that acts mainly to enhance postsynaptic GABAergic activity by increasing chloride conductance at $GABA_A$ receptors and attenuates the glutamate excitatory response. It also alters messenger RNA for glutamic acid decarboxylase and $GABA_A$ receptor subunits (for a review, see [226]).
- **Adrenocorticotrophic hormone and oral corticosteroids:** Pituitary-adrenal hormones have long been known to affect epileptogenesis. Even though the mechanism behind the efficacy of ACTH is mediated by biochemical processes that remain unknown, a reduction in glutamine/glutamate levels in the cerebral cortex after ACTH therapy in patients with WS has been shown [227]. Systemic administration of ACTH causes an increase in midbrain and striatal GABA receptor binding [228]. ACTH, oral corticosteroids, and VGB are now first-line treatments for IS in the United States and Europe. The current literature suggests that short-term, low-dose ACTH (versus high dose) should be considered first-line treatment of IS [229], and is more effective than oral corticosteroids and VGB for the cessation of spasms. ACTH is preferred for short-term control of epileptic spasms not due to tuberous sclerosis (level B recommendation). Oral steroids are probably effective in short-term control of spasms (level C recommendation), and a shorter interval from the onset of spasms to treatment initiation may improve long-term neurodevelopmental outcome (level C recommendation) [167]. Nevertheless, some clinicians use corticosteroids, VGB, and TPM as first-line treatments for this group. As we have already mentioned above, initial combined

treatment with low-dose ACTH and TPM was effective in treating ISS in most patients. After removing ACTH from the treatment regimen, TPM can be left as the AED of choice to prevent recurrence of the ISS. For refractory infantile spasms, other antiepileptic drugs have been used (i.e., valproate, zonisamide, sulthiame, levetiracetam, lamotrigine, pyridoxine, and ganaxolone) as well as adjunctive flunarizine and novel drugs not yet in clinical use (i.e., pulse rapamycin and melanocortin receptor agonists) [230].

- **Neurosteroids: Ganaxolone (GNX)** is the 3-beta-methylated synthetic analog of allopregnanolone; it belongs to a class of compounds referred to as neurosteroids. GNX is an allosteric modulator of GABA(A) receptors, acting through binding sites, which are distinct from the benzodiazepine-binding site [231]. In children with refractory ISS, or with continuing seizures after a prior history of ISS, ganaxolone has been used as a second-line drug [232].

7.3.3. Other drugs

- **Quinidine** reverses the in vitro functional gain seen with KCNT1 mutations implicated in EIEE 14, and a clinical response to quinidine has been observed [233, 234].
- **Rapamycin:** The recent discovery of the importance of mutations in DEPDC5 (OMIM 614191, "Dep domain-containing protein 5") for familial focal epilepsy with variable foci (OMIM 604364), associated with both lesional (focal cortical dysplasia, band heterotopia, hemimegalencephaly, etc.) and non-lesional epilepsies, whose expression occurred throughout neurons and GABAergic interneurons in brain development, has provided a new source for therapeutic targets. Since DEPDC5 is now known to be a regulator of the mTOR (mammalian target of rapamycin) pathway, this raises the possibility of treatment with rapamycin analogs [235]. Modulation of the mammalian target of rapamycin pathway may hold promise for malformation-associated epilepsy. All of these observations will need careful double-blind trials to establish efficacy [236].
- **Potassium bromide**, an old antiepileptic drug, should have a place as a drug of tertiary choice in the treatment of children with refractory epilepsy. Its main use is in the treatment of MMPS [237] and Dravet's syndrome [238].

8. Conclusion

The distinction between early infantile epileptic encephalopathy (EIEE) —mostly known as Ohtahara syndrome—and early myoclonic encephalopathy (EME), unfortunately, is not always easy due to clinical and etiological overlap. Thus, different authors suggest that both entities are actually the same entity.

The main differences lie in the type of crisis, which may correspond with the underlying activity of the GABAergic system. Acute noxa in the newborn with a still immature cortical brain produces a strong release of GABA. Due to the more depolarized Cl^- reversal potential in the neonatal neurons, the binding of GABA to ligand-gated $GABA_A$ receptor-associated Cl

$^{-}$ channels triggers Cl^{-} efflux and a depolarizing excitation leading to severe and early myoclonic seizures. However, when impairments in the proper migration of GABAergic interneurons occur, a longer period without epileptogenic activity would be expected. Tonic seizures would appear later associated with the severity of the brainstem dysfunction. According to this view, this second type would not be so much an "age-dependent encephalopathy" but rather a "damage-dependent encephalopathy". Therefore, it is possible that these syndromes represent different stages of a progressive neuronal-dysfunction epileptic "continuum of pathology" with a suppression-burst pattern.

A greater knowledge of the genes involved in the origins of epilepsy may lead to a future with improved treatments for patients with early encephalopathies.

Nomenclature/abbreviations

ACTH	adrenocorticotrophic hormone
ADNFLE	autosomal dominant nocturnal frontal lobe epilepsy
AEDs	antiepileptic drugs
AMPA	alpha-amino-3-hydroxy-5-methyl-4-isoxazole propionic acid
ARX	aristaless-related homeobox gene
Array-CGH	array-comparative genomic hybridization
ASDs	autism spectrum disorders
BFNS1	benign familial neonatal seizures-1
BFIS3	benign familial infantile seizures-3
BLBP	brain lipid-binding protein
BS	burst suppression
CA	carbonic anhydrases
CAE	childhood absence epilepsy
CBZ	carbamazepine
CLB	clobazam
CNS	central nervous system
CNVs	copy number variations
CSWS	continuous spikes and waves during sleep
DS	Dravet's syndrome
EAA	excitatory amino acids
EEG	electroencephalogram
EEs	epileptic encephalopathies
EIEE	early infantile epileptic encephalopathy

http://dx.doi.org/10.5772/64458

EEIE	early *epileptic* infantile *encephalopathy*
EIMFS	epilepsy of infancy with migrating focal seizures
EME	early myoclonic encephalopathy
EOEEs	early-onset epileptic encephalopathies
ESES	status epilepticus during sleep
ESM	ethosuximide
EZG	ezogabine
GABA	gamma-aminobutyric acid
$GABA_ARs$	GABA subtype A receptor channel chloride currents
GABA-T	GABA aminotransferase
GBP	gabapentin
GNX	ganaxolone
GPI	glycosylphosphatidylinositol
GTCs	generalized tonic-clonic seizures
HIE	hypoxic-ischemic encephalopathy
iGluRs	ionotropic glutamate receptors
ID	intellectual disability
ILAE	International League Against Epilepsy
ISS	infantile spasms
LCRs	low-copy repeats
LGS	Lennox-Gastaut syndrome
LKS	Landau-Kleffner syndrome
LTG	lamotrigine
MEI	myoclonic epilepsy in infancy
mGlu	metabotropic glutamate
MMPSI	malignant migrating partial seizures in infancy
MRI	magnetic resonance imaging
NAHR	non-allelic homologous recombination
NBs	newborns
NMDA	N-methyl-D-aspartic acid
NS	nervous system
NSID	nonsyndromic intellectual disability
NT	neurotransmitters
OLs	oligodendrocytes

OMIM	online Mendelian inheritance in man
OS	Ohtahara syndrome
OXC	oxcarbazepine
PER	perampanel
PB	phenobarbital
PCW	postconceptional weeks
PHT	phenytoin
RTG	retigabine
SBP	suppression-burst patterns
SDs	segmental duplication
SLC25A22	solute carrier family 25, member 22 gene
SMEN	severe myoclonic epilepsy in infancy
STN	subthalamic nucleus
SPZ	subplate zone
STP	stiripentol
S- XLMR	syndromic X-linked mental retardation
TARPs	transmembrane AMPA regulatory proteins
TGB	tiagabine
TPM	topiramate
VPA	sodium valproate
VGB	vigabatrin
WM	white matter
WS	West syndrome
XLMR	X-linked mental retardation
ZNS	zonisamide

Author details

María Carmen Carrascosa-Romero[1,3] and Carlos De Cabo De La Vega[2,3*]

*Address all correspondence to: carlosd@sescam.jccm.es

1 Department of Neuropediatrics, Albacete General Hospital, Albacete, Spain

2 Neuropsychopharmacology Unit, Albacete General Hospital, Albacete, Spain

3 Complejo Hospitalario Universitario De Albacete, c/Hermanos Falcó, Albacete, Spain

References

[1] Lanska MJ, Lanska DJ. Neonatal seizures in the United States: results of the National Hospital Discharge Survey, 1980–1991. Neuroepidemiology. 1996; 15(3): 117–25

[2] Carrascosa MC, Martínez-Gutiérrez A, Onsurbe I, Vázquez MS, Catalán B, Tébar R. Neonatal convulsions in health care. I. Incidence, etiology and clinical aspects. Rev Neurol. 1996; 24(134): 1258–62

[3] Sankar MJ, Agarwal R, Aggarwal R, Deorari AK, Paul VK. Seizures in the newborn. Indian J Pediatr. 2008; 75(2): 149–55

[4] Wasterlain CG, Niquet J, Thompson KW, Baldwin R, Liu H, Sankar R. Seizure-induced neuronal death in the immature brain. Prog Brain Res. 2002; 135: 335–53

[5] Kang SK, Kadam SD. Neonatal seizures: impact on neurodevelopmental outcomes. Front Pediatr. 2015;3:101. doi: 10.3389/fped.2015.00101. eCollection 2015.

[6] Ben-Ari Y. Basic developmental rules and their implications for epilepsy in the immature brain. Epileptic Disord. 2006; 8(2):91–102

[7] Holliday MA. Body composition and energy needs during growth. In: Falkner F., Tanner J. M. (eds.), Human Growth: A Comprehensive Treatise, Vol. 2, 2nd edn. Plenum, New York, NY, 1986. pp. 101–117

[8] Lombroso CT. Neonatal seizures: a clinician's overview. Brain Dev. 1996; 18(1): 1–28

[9] Manent JB, Represa A. Neurotransmitters and brain maturation: early paracrine actions of GABA and glutamate modulate neuronal migration. Neuroscientist. 2007; 13(3): 268–79

[10] Engel JJr. International League Against Epilepsy (ILAE). A proposed diagnostic scheme for people with epileptic seizures and with epilepsy: report of the ILAE Task Force on Classification and Terminology. Epilepsia. 2001; 42: 796–803

[11] Auvin S, Cilio MR, Vezzani A. Current understanding and neurobiology of epileptic encephalopathies. Neurobiol Dis. 2016 Mar 16. pii: S0969-9961(16)30051-1.

[12] Parisi P, Verrotti A, Paolino MC, Castaldo R, Ianniello F, Ferretti A, et al. "Electro-clinical syndromes" with onset in paediatric age: the highlights of the clinical-EEG, genetic andtherapeutic advances. Ital J Pediatr. 2011 Dec 19; 37: 58. doi: 10.1186/1824-7288-37-58.

[13] Berg AT, Berkovic SF. Brodie MJ. Buchhalter J. Cross JH. van Emde Boas W, et al. Revised terminology and concepts for organization of seizures and epilepsies: report of the ILAE Commission on Classification and Terminology, 2005–2009. Epilepsia. 2010; 51(4): 676–85

[14] ILAE. Epilepsy-syndromes in https://www.epilepsydiagnosis.org/syndrome/epilepsy-syndrome-groupoverview.html [10.05.2016].

[15] Fusco L, Pachatz C, Di Capua M, Vigevano F. Video/EEG aspects of early-infantile epileptic encephalopathy with suppression-bursts (Ohtahara syndrome). Brain Dev. 2001; 23(7): 708–14

[16] Aicardi J, Ohtahara S. Severe neonatal epilepsies with suppression-burst pattern. In: Roger J., Bureau M., Dravet C.H., Genton P., Tassinari C.A., Wolf P. (eds.), Epileptic Syndromes in Infancy, Childhood and Adolescence, 3rd edn. John Libbey, London, UK, 2002. pp. 33–44

[17] Murakami N, Ohtsuka Y, Ohtahara S. Early infantile epileptic syndromes with suppression-bursts: early myoclonic encephalopathy vs. Ohtahara syndrome. Jpn J Psychiatry Neurol. 1993;47(2): 197–200

[18] Aicardi J, Goutieres F. Encephalopathie myoclonique neonatale. Rev Electroencephalogr Neurophysiol Clin. 1978; 8: 99–101

[19] Aicardi J. Early myoclonic encephalopathy (neonatal myoclonic encephalopathy). In: Roger J., Bureau M., Dravet C., Dreifuss F., Perret A., Wolf P. (Eds.), Epileptic Syndromes in Infancy, Childhood and Adolescence. John Libbey & Co. Ltd., London, 1992. pp. 13–23.

[20] Dalla Bernardina B, Dulac O, Fejerman N, Dravet C, Capovilla G, Bondavalli S, Colamaria V, Roger J. Early myoclonic epileptic encephalopathy (EMEE). Eur J Pediatr. 1983; 140: 248–52

[21] Djukic A, Lado FA, Shinnar S, Moshé SL. Are early myoclonic encephalopathy (EME) and the Ohtahara syndrome (EIEE) independent of each other? Epilepsy Res. 2006;70: S68–76

[22] Ohtahara S, Ishida T, Oka E. On the specific age dependent epileptic syndromes: The early-infantile epilepstic encephalopathy with suppression-burst. No To Hattatsu (Tokyo) 1976; 8: 270–80

[23] Ohtahara S, Yamatogi Y. Epileptic encephalopathies in early infancy with suppression-burst. J Clin Neurophysiol. 2003; 20: 398–407

[24] Ohtahara S, Yamatogi Y. Ohtahara syndrome: with special reference to its developmental aspects for differentiating from early myoclonic encephalopathy. Epilepsy Res. 2006; 70 (Suppl 1): S58–67

[25] Martin HJ, Deroubaix-Tella P, Thelliez P. Neonatal epileptic encephalopathy with suppression bursts (author's transl). Rev Electroencephalogr Neurophysiol Clin. 1981; 11(3–4): 397–403

[26] Donat JF. The age-dependent epileptic encephalopathies. J Child Neurol. 1992; 7(1): 7–21

[27] Yelin K, Alfonso I, Papazian O. Syndrome of Ohtahara. Rev Neurol. 1999; 29(4): 340–2

[28] Ohtahara S. Seizure disorders in infancy and childhood. Brain Dev 1984; 6: 509–19

[29] Rufo-Campos M. Inter-relationships of the epileptic encephalopathies of infancy. Rev Neurol. 2000; 30(Suppl 1):S74–80.

[30] Lombroso CT. Early myoclonic encephalopathy, early infantile epileptic encephalopathy, and benign and severe infantile myoclonic epilepsies: a critical review and personal contributions. J Clin Neurophysiol. 1990; 7(3): 380–408

[31] Ohtahara S, Ohtsuka Y, Yamatogi Y, Oka E. The early infantile epileptic encephalopathy with suppression-burst: developmental aspects. Brain Dev. 1987; 9: 371–6

[32] Wang PJ, Lee WT, Hwu WL, Young C, Yau KI, Shen YZ. The controversy regarding diagnostic criteria for early myoclonic encephalopathy. Brain Dev.1998; 20: 530–5

[33] Vigevano F, Bartuli A. Infantile epileptic syndromes and metabolic etiologies. J Child Neurol. 2002; 17(Suppl. 3): 3S9–13

[34] Prasad AN, Hoffman GF. Early onset epilepsy and inherited metabolic disorder: diagnosis and management. Can J Neurol Sci. 2010; 37: 350–8

[35] Rahman S, Footitt ET, Varadkar S, Clayton PT. Inborn errors of metabolism causing epilepsy. Dev Med Child Neurol. 2013; 55: 23–6

[36] Martínez-Bermejo A, Roche C, López-Martín V, Arcas J, Tendero A. Neonatal EEG trace of burst suppression. Etiological and evolutionary factors. Rev Neurol. 2001;33(6): 514–8

[37] Pardal-Fernández JM, Carrascosa-Romero MC, de Cabo-de la Vega C, Iniesta-López I, Gil-Pons E, Martínez-Gutiérrez A. Atypical glycine encephalopathy in an extremely low birth weight infant: description of a new mutation and clinical and electroencephalographic analysis. Epileptic Disord. 2009;11(1): 48–53

[38] Knezevic-Pogancev M. Ohtahara syndrome—early infantile epileptic encephalopathy. Med Pregl. 2008; 61: 581–5

[39] Hildebrand MS, Dahl HH, Damiano JA, Smith RJ, Scheffer IE, Berkovic SF. Recent advances in the molecular genetics of epilepsy. J Med Genet. 2013;50: 271–9

[40] Nieh SE, Sherr EH. Epileptic encephalopathies: new genes and new pathways. Neurotherapeutics. 2014; 11(4):796–806

[41] Pong AW, Pal DK, Chung WK. Developments in molecular genetic diagnostics: an update for the pediatric epilepsy specialist. Pediatr Neurol. 2011; 44: 317–27

[42] Mastrangelo M, Leuzzi V. Genes of early-onset epileptic encephalopathies: from genotype to phenotype. Pediatr Neurol. 2012; 46: 24–31

[43] Mastrangelo M. Novel genes of early-onset epileptic encephalopathies: from genotype to phenotypes. Pediatr Neurol. 2015; 53(2):119–29

[44] Online Catalog of Human Genes and Genetic Disorders "Online Mendelian Inheritance in Man" (OMIM) in http://www.omim.org [10.05.2016]

[45] Trump N, McTague A, Brittain H, Papandreou A, Meyer E, Ngoh A, et al. Improving diagnosis and broadening the phenotypes in early-onset seizure and severe developmental delay disorders through gene panel analysis. J Med Genet. 2016; Mar 18. pii: jmedgenet-2015-103263.

[46] Kitamura K, Yanazawa M, Sugiyama N, Miura H, Iizuka-Kogo A, Kusaka M, et al. Mutation of ARX causes abnormal development of forebrain and testes in mice and X-linked lissencephaly with abnormal genitalia in humans. Nat Genet. 2002; 32(3): 359–69

[47] Poirier K, Van Esch H, Friocourt G, Saillour Y, Bahi N, Backer S, et al. Neuroanatomical distribution of ARX in brain and its localisation in GABAergic neurons. Brain Res Mol Brain Res. 2004; 122(1): 35–46

[48] Colombo E, Collombat P, Colasante G, Bianchi M, Long J, Mansouri A, et al. Inactivation of Arx, the murine ortholog of the X-linked lissencephaly with ambiguous genitalia gene, leads to severe disorganization of the ventral telencephalon with impaired neuronal migration and differentiation. J Neurosci. 2007; 27(17): 4786–98

[49] Friocourt G, Parnavelas JG. Mutations in ARX result in several defects involving GABAergic neurons. Front Cell Neurosci. 2010; 4: 1–11

[50] Colasante G, Collombat P, Raimondi V, Bonanomi D, Ferrai C, Maira M, et al. Arx is a direct target of Dlx2 and thereby contributes to the tangential migration of GABAergic interneurons. J Neurosci. 2008; 28(42): 10674–86

[51] Beguin S, Crépel V, Aniksztejn L, Becq H, Pelosi B, Pallesi-Pocachard E, et al. An epilepsy-related ARX polyalanine expansion modifies glutamatergic neurons excitability and morphology without affecting GABAergic neurons development. Cereb Cortex. 2013; 23(6): 1484–94

[52] Gécz J, Cloosterman D, Partington M. ARX: a gene for all seasons. Curr Opin Genet Dev. 2006; 16(3): 308–16

[53] Shoubridge C, Fullston T, Gécz J. ARX spectrum disorders: making inroads into the molecular pathology. Hum Mutat. 2010; 31(8): 889–900

[54] Suri M. The phenotypic spectrum of ARX mutations. Dev Med Child Neurol. 2005; 47(2): 133–7

[55] Quillé ML, Carat S, Quéméner-Redon S, Hirchaud E, Baron D, Benech C, et al. High throughput analysis of promoter occupancy reveals new targets for

Arx, gene mutated in mental retardation and interneuronopathies. PLoS One. 2011; 6(9): e25181

[56] Sherr EH. The ARX story (epilepsy, mental retardation, autism, and cerebral malformations): one gene leads to many phenotypes. Curr Opin Pediatr. 2003; 15(6): 567–71

[57] D'Adamo MC, Catacuzzeno L, Di Giovanni G, Franciolini F, Pessia M. K(+) channelepsy: progress in the neurobiology of potassium channels and epilepsy. Front Cell Neurosci. 2013; 7: 134. doi: 10.3389/fncel.2013.00134

[58] Villa C, Combi R. Potassium channels and human epileptic phenotypes: an updated overview. Front Cell Neurosci. 2016; 10: 81. doi: 10.3389/fncel.2016.00081. eCollection 2016.

[59] Miceli F, Soldovieri MV, Ambrosino P, Barrese V, Migliore M, Cilio MR, Taglialatela M. Genotype-phenotype correlations in neonatal epilepsies caused by mutations in the voltage sensor of Kv7.2 potassium channel subunits. Proc Natl Acad Sci U S A. 2013; 110: 4386–91

[60] Kato M, Yamagata T, Kubota M, Arai H, Yamashita S, Nakagawa T, et al. Clinical spectrum of early onset epileptic encephalopathies caused by KCNQ2 mutation. Epilepsia. 2013; 54(7): 1282–7

[61] Weckhuysen S, Mandelstam S, Suls A, Audenaert D, Deconinck T, Claes LR, et al. KCNQ2 encephalopathy: emerging phenotype of a neonatal epileptic encephalopathy. Ann Neurol. 2012; 71(1): 15–25

[62] Martin HC, Kim GE, Pagnamenta AT, Murakami Y, Carvill GL, Meyer E, et al. Clinical whole-genome sequencing in severe early-onset epilepsy reveals new genes and improves molecular diagnosis. Hum Mol Genet. 2014; 23: 3200–11

[63] Malo D, Schurr E, Dorfman J, Canfield V, Levenson R, Gros P. Three brain sodium channel alpha-subunit genes are clustered on the proximal segment of mouse chromosome 2. Genomics. 1991; 10: 666–72.

[64] Shi X, Yasumoto S, Kurahashi H, Nakagawa E, Fukasawa T, Uchiya S, Hirose S. Clinical spectrum of SCN2A mutations. Brain Dev. 2012; 34: 541–5

[65] Ogiwara I, Ito K, Sawaishi Y, Osaka H, Mazaki E, Inoue I, et al. De novo mutations of voltage-gated sodium channel alphaII gene SCN2A in intractable epilepsies. Neurology. 2009; 73(13): 1046–53

[66] Swanson DA, Steel JM, Valle D. Identification and characterization of the human ortholog of rat STXBP1, a protein implicated in vesicle trafficking and neurotransmitter release. Genomics. 1998; 48(3): 373–6

[67] Otsuka M, Oguni H, Liang JS, Ikeda H, Imai K, Hirasawa K, et al. STXBP1 mutations cause not only Ohtahara syndrome but also West syndrome: result of Japanese cohort study. Epilepsia. 2010; 51: 2449–52

[68] Deprez L, Weckhuysen S, Holmgren P, Suls A, Van Dyck T, Goossens D, et al. Clinical spectrum of early onset epileptic encephalopathies associated with STXBP1 mutations. Neurology. 2010; 75: 1159–64

[69] Saitsu H, Kato M, Mizuguchi T, Hamada K, Osaka H, Tohyama J, et al. De novo mutations in the gene encoding STXBP1 (MUNC18-1) cause early infantile epileptic encephalopathy. Nat Genet. 2008; 40(6): 782–8

[70] Liu LL, Hou XL, Zhou CL, Tang ZZ, Bao XH, Jiang Y. STXBP1 gene mutation in newborns with refractory seizures]. Zhongguo Dang Dai Er Ke Za Zhi. 2014; 16(7): 701–4

[71] Hamdan FF, Piton A, Gauthier J, Lortie A, Dubeau F, Dobrzeniecka S, et al. De novo STXBP1 mutations in mental retardation and nonsyndromic epilepsy. Ann Neurol. 2009; 65(6): 748–53

[72] Hamdan FF, Gauthier J, Dobrzeniecka S, Lortie A, Mottron L, Vanasse M, et al. Intellectual disability without epilepsy associated with STXBP1 disruption. Eur J Hum Genet. 2011; 19(5): 607–9

[73] Nakamura K, Kodera H, Akita T, Shiina M, Kato M, Hoshino H, et al. De novo mutations in GNAO1, encoding a Gαo subunit of heterotrimeric G proteins, cause epileptic encephalopathy. Am J Hum Genet. 2013; 93(3): 496–505

[74] Law CY, Chang ST, Cho SY, Yau EK, Ng GS, Fong NC, et al. Clinical whole-exome sequencing reveals a novel missense pathogenic variant of GNAO1 in a patient with infantile-onset epilepsy. Clin Chim Acta. 2015; 451(Pt B): 292–6

[75] Saitsu H, Fukai R, Ben-Zeev B, Sakai Y, Mimaki M, Okamoto N, et al. Phenotypic spectrum of GNAO1 variants: epileptic encephalopathy to involuntary movements with severe developmental delay. Eur J Hum Genet. 2016; 24(1): 129–34

[76] Molinari F, Kaminska A, Fiermonte G, Boddaert N, Raas-Rothschild A, Plouin P, et al. Mutations in the mitochondrial glutamate carrier SLC25A22 in neonatal epileptic encephalopathy with suppression bursts. Clin Genet. 2009; 76: 188–94

[77] Poduri A, Heinzen EL, Chitsazzadeh V, Lasorsa FM, Elhosary PC, LaCoursiere CM, et al. SLC25A22 is a novel gene for migrating partial seizures in infancy. Ann Neurol. 2013; 74(6): 873–82

[78] Johnston JJ, Gropman AL, Sapp JC, Teer JK, Martin JM, Liu CF, et al. The phenotype of a germline mutation in PIGA: the gene somatically mutated in paroxysmal nocturnal hemoglobinuria. Am J Hum Genet. 2012; 90(2): 295–300

[79] Liu Y, Poon V, Sanchez-Watts G, Watts AG, Takemori H, Aguilera G. Salt-inducible kinase is involved in the regulation of corticotropin-releasing hormone transcription in hypothalamic neurons in rats. Endocrinology. 2012;153: 223–33

[80] Hansen J, Snow C, Tuttle E, Ghoneim DH, Yang CS, Spencer A, et al. De novo mutations in SIK1 cause a spectrum of developmental epilepsies. Am J Hum Genet. 2015; 96(4): 682–90

[81] Backx L, Ceulemans B, Vermeesch JR, Devriendt K, Van Esch H. Early myoclonic encephalopathy caused by a disruption of the neuregulin-1 receptor ErbB4. Eur J Hum Genet. 2009; 17(3): 378–82

[82] Yau HJ, Wang HF, Lai C, Liu FC. Neural development of the neuregulin receptor ErbB4 in the cerebral cortex and the hippocampus: preferential expression by interneurons tangentially migrating from the ganglionic eminences. Cereb Cortex. 2003; 13: 252–64

[83] Flames N, Long JE, Garratt AN, Fischer TM, Gassmann M, Birchmeier C, et al. Short- and long-range attraction of cortical GABAergic interneurons by neuregulin-1. Neuron. 2004; 44(2): 251–61

[84] Poluch S, Juliano SL. Populations of radial glial cells respond differently to reelin and neuroregulin 1 in a ferret model of cortical dysplasia. PLoS One. 2010; 5(10): e13709

[85] Sardi SP, Murtie J, Koirala S, Patten BA, Corfas G. Presenilin-dependent ErbB4 nuclear signaling regulates the timing of astrogenesis in the developing brain. Cell 2006; 127 (1): 185–97

[86] Britsch S. The neuregulin-I/ErbB signaling system in development and disease. Adv Anat Embryol Cell Biol. 2007; 190: 1–65

[87] Mulley JC, Mefford HC. Epilepsy and the new cytogenetics. Epilepsia 2011; 52: 423–32

[88] Mefford HC, Yendle SC, Hsu C, Cook J, Geraghty E, McMahon JM, et al. Rare copy number variants are an important cause of epileptic encephalopathies. Ann Neurol 2011; 70: 974–85

[89] Ma Y, Chen C, Wang Y, Wu L, He F, Chen C, et al. Analysis copy number variation of Chinese children in early onset epileptic encephalopathies with unknown cause. Clin Genet. 2016 Mar 1. doi: 10.1111/cge.12768. [Epub ahead of print]

[90] Manent JB, Represa A. Neurotransmitters and brain maturation: early paracrine actions of GABA and glutamate modulate neuronal migration. Neuroscientist. 2007; 13(3): 268–79.

[91] Nadarajah B, Parnavelas JG. Modes of neuronal migration in the developing cerebral cortex. Nat Rev Neurosci. 2002; 3(6): 423–32

[92] Cooper JA. Mechanisms of cell migration in the nervous system. JCB. 2013; 202(5): 725–34

[93] Wu C, Sun D. GABA receptors in brain development, function, and injury. Metab Brain Dis. 2015; 30(2): 367–79

[94] Luskin MB, Coskun V. The progenitor cells of the embryonic telencephalon and the neonatal anterior subventricular zone differentially regulate their cell cycle. Chem Senses. 2002; 27(6): 577–80

[95] Judaš M, Sedmak G, Pletikos M, Jovanov-Milošević N. Populations of subplate and interstitial neurons in fetal and adult human telencephalon. J Anat. 2010; 217(4): 381–99

[96] Kostovic I, Judas M. Prolonged coexistence of transient and permanent circuitry elements in the developing cerebral cortex of fetuses and preterm infants. Dev Med Child Neurol. 2006; 48(5): 388–93

[97] Butt AM, Fern RF, Matute C. Neurotransmitter signaling in white matter. Glia. 2014; 62(11): 1762–79

[98] Káradóttir R, Attwell D. Neurotransmitter receptors in the life and death of oligodendrocytes. Neuroscience. 2007; 145(4):1426–38

[99] Williamson AV, Mellor JR, Grant AL, Randall AD. Properties of GABA(A) receptors in cultured rat oligodendrocyte progenitor cells. Neuropharmacology. 1998;37: 859–73

[100] Lin SC, Bergles DE. Synaptic signaling between GABAergic interneurons and oligodendrocyte precursor cells in the hippocampus. Nat Neurosci. 2004;7:24–32

[101] Robinson S, Li Q, Dechant A, Cohen ML. Neonatal loss of γ-aminobutyric acid pathway expression after human perinatal brain injury. J Neurosurg. 2006; 104(6 Suppl):396–408

[102] Abraham J, Fox PD, Condello C, Bartolini A, Koh S. Minocycline attenuates microglia activation and blocks the long-term epileptogenic effects of early-life seizures. Neurobiol Dis. 2012; 46(2): 425–30

[103] Druga R. Neocortical inhibitory system. Folia Biol (Praha). 2009; 55(6): 201–17

[104] Rossignol E. Genetics and function of neocortical GABAergic interneurons in neurodevelopmental disorders. Neural Plast. 2011; 2011:649325. doi: 10.1155/2011/649325

[105] Petanjek Z, Dujmović A, Kostović I, Esclapez M. Distinct origin of GABA-ergic neurons in forebrain of man, nonhuman primates and lower mammals. Coll Antropol. 2008; 32 (Suppl 1): 9–17

[106] Nguyen L, Rigo JM, Rocher V, Belachew S, Malgrange B, Rogister B, et al. Neurotransmitters as early signals for central nervous system development. Cell Tissue Res. 2001; 305(2): 187–202

[107] Heng JI, Moonen G, Nguyen L. Neurotransmitters regulate cell migration in the telencephalon. Eur J Neurosci. 2007; 26(3): 537–46

[108] Inada H, Watanabe M, Uchida T, Ishibashi H, Wake H, Nemoto T. GABA regulates the multidirectional tangential migration of GABAergic interneurons in living neonatal mice. PLoS One. 2011; 6(12): e27048

[109] Laurén HB, Ruohonen S, Kukko-Lukjanov TK, Virta JE, Grönman M, Lopez-Picon FR, et al. Status epilepticus alters neurogenesis and decreases the number of GABAergic neurons in the septal dentate gyrus of 9-day-old rats at the early phase of epileptogenesis. Brain Res. 2013; 1516: 33–44

[110] Lévesque M, Herrington R, Hamidi S, Avoli M. Interneurons spark seizure-like activity in the entorhinal cortex. Neurobiol Dis. 2016; 87: 91–101

[111] Zhou Y, Danbolt NC. GABA and glutamate transporters in Brain. Front Endocrinol (Lausanne). 2013; 4: 165. doi: 10.3389/fendo.2013.00165. eCollection 2013.

[112] Traynelis SF, Wollmuth LP, McBain CJ, Menniti FS, Vance KM, Ogden KK, et al. Glutamate receptor ion channels: structure, regulation, and function. Pharmacol Rev. 2010; 62: 405–96

[113] Wolszon LR, Pereda AE, Faber DS. A fast synaptic potential mediated by NMDA and non-NMDA receptors. J Neurophysiol. 1997; 78(5): 2693–706

[114] Nicoletti F, Bockaert J, Collingridge GL, Conn PJ, Ferraguti F, Schoepp DD, et al. Metabotropic glutamate receptors: from the workbench to the bedside. Neuropharmacology. 2011; 60: 1017–41

[115] Hunt DL, Castillo PE. Synaptic plasticity of NMDA receptors: mechanisms and functional implications. Curr Opin Neurobiol. 2012; 22: 496–508

[116] Malenka RC, Nicoll RA. NMDA-receptor-dependent synaptic plasticity: multiple forms and mechanisms. Trends Neurosci. 1993; 16: 521–7

[117] Johnston MV. Excitotoxicity in neonatal hypoxia. Ment Retard Dev Disabil Res Rev. 2001; 7: 229–34

[118] Johnston MV, Trescher WH, Ishida A, Nakajima W. Neurobiology of hypoxic–ischemic injury in the developing brain. Pediatr Res. 2001; 49: 735–41

[119] Desfeux A, El Ghazi F, Jégou S, Legros H, Marret S, Laudenbach V. Dual effect of glutamate on GABAergic interneuron survival during cerebral cortex development in miceneonates. Cereb Cortex. 2010; 20(5): 1092–108

[120] Vyklicky V, Korinek M, Smejkalova T, Balik A, Krausova B, Kaniakova M, et al. Structure, function, and pharmacology of NMDA receptor channels. Physiol Res. 2014; 63 (Suppl 1): S191–203

[121] Köles L, Kató E, Hanuska A, Zádori ZS, Al-Khrasani M, Zelles T, et al. Modulation of excitatory neurotransmission by neuronal/glial signalling molecules: interplay between purinergic and glutamatergic systems. Purinergic Signal. 2016;12(1):1–24

[122] Carrascosa-Romero MC, De Cabo-De La Vega C. Neuroprotection in Perinatal Hypoxic-Ischemic Encephalopathy. Pharmacologic Combination Therapy. In: Emira S. (ed.) "Cerebral Palsy – Challenges for the Future". InTech– Open Access Publisher. ISBN: 978-953-51-1234-1, pp. 123–192, 2014.

[123] Rakhade SN, Zhou C, Aujla PK, Fishman R, Sucher NJ, Jensen FE. Early alterations of AMPA receptors mediate synaptic potentiation induced by neonatal seizures. J Neurosci. 2008; 28(32): 7979–90

[124] Henley JM, Wilkinson KA. AMPA receptor trafficking and the mechanisms underlying synaptic plasticity and cognitive aging. Dialogues Clin Neurosci 2013; 15: 11–27

[125] Jensen FE. The role of glutamate receptor maturation in perinatal seizures and brain injury. Int J Dev Neurosci. 2002; 20(3–5): 339–47

[126] Wang DD, Kriegstein AR. Defining the role of GABA in cortical development. J Physiol. 2009; 587(Pt 9): 1873–9

[127] Castillo PE, Chiu CQ, Carroll RC. Long-term plasticity at inhibitory synapses. Curr Opin Neurobiol. 2011; 21(2): 328–38.

[128] Roth FC, Draguhn A. GABA metabolism and transport: effects on synaptic efficacy. Neural Plast. 2012; 2012: 805830. doi: 10.1155/2012/805830

[129] Allain AE, Le Corronc H, Delpy A, Cazenave W, Meyrand P, Legendre P, et al. Maturation of the GABAergic transmission in normal and pathologic motoneurons. Neural Plast. 2011; 2011: 905624. doi: 10.1155/2011/905624

[130] Jin XT, Galvan A, Wichmann T, Smith Y. Localization and function of GABA transporters GAT-1 and GAT-3 in the basal ganglia. Front Syst Neurosci. 2011; 5: 63. doi: 10.3389/fnsys.2011.00063. eCollection 2011

[131] Sarup A, Larsson OM, Schousboe A. GABA transporters and GABA-transaminase as drug targets. Curr Drug Targets CNS Neurol Disorder. 2003; 2(4): 269–77

[132] Couve A, Moss SJ, Pangalos MN. GABAB receptors: a new paradigm in G protein signaling. Mol Cell Neurosci. 2000; 16(4): 296–312

[133] Briggs SW, Galanopoulou AS. Altered GABA signaling in early life epilepsies. Neural Plast. 2011; 2011: 527605. doi: 10.1155/2011/527605

[134] Plotkin MD, Snyder EY, Hebert SC, Delpire E. Expression of the Na-K-2Cl cotransporter is developmentally regulated in postnatal rat brains: a possible mechanism underlying GABA's excitatory role in immature brain. J Neurobiol. 1997; 33: 781–95

[135] De Cabo-de la Vega C, Villanueva-Hernandez P, Prieto-Martin A. The neurochemistry of epilepsy, inhibitory neurotransmission and experimental models: new perspectives. Rev Neurol. 2006; 42(3): 159–68

http://dx.doi.org/10.5772/64458

[136] Sperber EF, Velísková J, Germano IM, Friedman LK, Moshé SL. Age-dependent vulnerability to seizures. Adv Neurol. 1999; 79:161–9

[137] Ben-Ari Y. Seizures beget seizures: the quest for GABA as a key player. Crit Rev Neurobiol. 2006; 18(1–2): 135–44

[138] Staley K. Enhancement of the excitatory actions of GABA by barbiturates and benzodiazepines. Neurosci Lett. 1992; 146(1): 105–7

[139] Moshé SL, Sperber EF, Brown LL, Tempel A. Age-dependent changes in substantia nigra GABA-mediated seizure suppression. Epilepsy Res Suppl. 1992;8: 97–106

[140] Chudomel O, Herman H, Nair K, Moshé SL, Galanopoulou AS. Age- and gender-related differences in GABAA receptor-mediated postsynaptic currents in GABAergic neurons of the substantia nigra reticulata in the rat. Neuroscience. 2009; 163(1):155–67

[141] Lukatch HS, Kiddoo CE, Maciver MB. Anesthetic-induced burst suppression EEG activity requires glutamate-mediated excitatory synaptic transmission. Cereb Cortex. 2005; 15(9): 1322–31

[142] Grenier F, Timofeev I, Steriade M. Neocortical very fast oscillations (ripples, 80–200 Hz) during seizures: intracellular correlates. J Neurophysiol. 2003; 89(2): 841–52

[143] Papandreou A, McTague A, Trump N, Ambegaonkar G, Ngoh A, Meyer E, et al. GABRB3 mutations: a new and emerging cause of early infantile epileptic encephalopathy. Dev Med Child Neurol. 2015; doi: 10.1111/dmcn.12976 [Epub ahead of print]

[144] Macdonald RL, Kang JQ, Gallagher MJ. Mutations in GABAA receptor subunits associated with genetic epilepsies. J Physiol. 2010; 588(Pt 11): 1861–9

[145] Hirose S. Mutant GABA(A) receptor subunits in genetic (idiopathic) epilepsy. Prog Brain Res. 2014; 213: 55–85

[146] Olivetti PR, Noebels JL. Interneuron, interrupted: molecular pathogenesis of ARX mutations and X-linked infantile spasms. Curr Opin Neurobiol. 2012; 22(5):859–65

[147] Williams CA, Battaglia A. Molecular biology of epilepsy genes. Exp Neurol. 2013; 244: 51–8

[148] Kato M, Dobyns WB. X-linked lissencephaly with abnormal genitalia as a tangential migration disorder causing intractable epilepsy: proposal for a new term, "interneuronopathy". J Child Neurol. 2005; 20(4): 392–7

[149] Kato M. Topics of brain malformation and epilepsy – age-dependent epileptic encephalopathies and interneuronopathies. No To Hattatsu. 2010; 42(5): 333–8

[150] Ruggieri M, Pavone P, Scapagnini G, Romeo L, Lombardo I, Li Volti G, et al. The aristaless (Arx) gene: one gene for many "interneuronopathies". Front Biosci (Elite Ed). 2010; 2: 701–10

[151] Molinari F. Mitochondria and neonatal epileptic encephalopathies with suppression burst. J Bioenerg Biomembr. 2010; 42 (6): 467–71

[152] Perrault I, Hamdan FF, Rio M, Capo-Chichi JM, Boddaert N, Décarie JC, et al. Mutations in DOCK7 in individuals with epileptic encephalopathy and cortical blindness. Am J Hum Genet. 2014; 94(6): 891–7

[153] van den Pol AN, Gao XB, Patrylo PR, Ghosh PK, Obrietan K. Glutamate inhibits GABA excitatory activity in developing neurons. J Neurosci. 1998; 18(24):10749–61

[154] Obrietan K, van den Pol AN. GABAB receptor-mediated inhibition of GABAA receptor calcium elevations in developing hypothalamic neurons. J Neurophysiol. 1998; 79(3): 1360–70

[155] Xu G, Broadbelt KG, Haynes RL, Folkerth RD, Borenstein NS, Belliveau RA, Trachtenberg FL, Volpe JJ, Kinney HC. Late development of the GABAergic system in the human cerebral cortex and white matter. J Neuropathol Exp Neurol. 2011; 70 (10): 841–58

[156] Kilb W. Development of the GABAergic system from birth to adolescence. Neuroscientist. 2012; 18(6): 613–30

[157] Corbin JG, Butt SJ. Developmental mechanisms for the generation of telencephalic interneurons. Dev Neurobiol. 2011; 71(8): 710–32

[158] Briggs SW, Galanopoulou AS. Altered GABA signaling in early life epilepsies. Neural Plast. 2011; 2011: 527605. doi: 10.1155/2011/527605.

[159] DeFelipe J. Chandelier cells and epilepsy. Brain. 1999; 122(Pt 10): 1807–22

[160] Baraban SC, Southwell DG, Estrada RC, Jones DL, Sebe JY, Alfaro-Cervello C. Reduction of seizures by transplantation of cortical GABAergic interneuron precursors into Kv1.1 mutant mice. Proc Natl Acad Sci U S A. 2009; 106(36): 15472–7

[161] Sebe JY, Baraban SC. The promise of an interneuron-based cell therapy for epilepsy. Dev Neurobiol. 2011; 71(1):107–17.

[162] Levy RH, Mattson RH, Meldrum BS, Perucca E, eds. Antiepileptic Drug. Lippincott Williams & Wilkins, Philadelphia, 2002

[163] Hwang H, Kim KJ. New antiepileptic drugs in pediatric epilepsy. Brain Dev. 2008; 30: 549–55

[164] Chung AM, Eiland LS. Use of second-generation antiepileptic drugs in the pediatric population. Paediatr Drugs. 2008; 10(4): 217–54

[165] Parisi P, Spalice A, Nicita F, Papetti L, Ursitti F, Verrotti A, et al. "Epileptic encephalopathy" of infancy and childhood: electro-clinical pictures and recent understandings. Curr Neuropharmacol. 2010; 8(4): 409–21

[166] Connock M, Frew E, Evans BW, Bryan S, Cummins C, Fry-Smith A, et al. The clinical effectiveness and cost-effectiveness of newer drugs for children with epilepsy. A systematic review. Health Technol Assess. 2006; 10(7): iii, ix–118

[167] Wilmshurst JM, Gaillard WD, Vinayan KP, Tsuchida TN, Plouin P, Van Bogaert P, et al. Summary of recommendations for the management of infantile seizures: Task Force Report for the ILAE Commission of Pediatrics. Epilepsia. 2015; 56(8): 1185–97

[168] Berkovic SF. Genetics of epilepsy in clinical practice. Epilepsy Curr. 2015; 15(4): 192–6

[169] Khanna A, Walcott BP, Kahle KT. Limitations of current GABA agonists in neonatal seizures: toward GABA modulation via the targeting of neuronal Cl(-) transport. Front Neurol. 2013; 25(4): 78.

[170] Slaughter LA, Anup D, Patel AD, Slaughter JL. Pharmacological treatment of neonatal seizures: a systematic review. J Child Neurol. 2013; 28(3) 351–64

[171] Painter MJ, Scher MS, Stein AD, Armatti S, Wang Z, Gardiner JC, et al. Phenobarbital compared with phenytoin for the treatment of neonatal seizures. N Engl J Med. 1999; 341:485–9

[172] Dzhala VI, Brumback AC, Staley KJ. Bumetanide enhances phenobarbital efficacy in a neonatal seizure model. Ann Neurol. 2008; 63: 222–35

[173] Kahle KT, Staley KJ. The bumetanide-sensitive Na-K-2Cl cotransporter NKCC1 as a potential target of a novel mechanism based treatment strategy for neonatal seizures. Neurosurg Focus. 2008; 25(3): E22. doi: 10.3171/FOC/2008/25/9/E22

[174] Kahle KT, Barnett SM, Sassower KC, Staley KJ. Decreased seizure activity in a human neonate treated with bumetanide, an inhibitor of the NaC-KC-2Cl- cotransporter NKCC1. J Child Neurol. 2009; 24:572–6

[175] Inoue Y, Ohtsuka Y, STP-1 Study Group. Long-term safety and efficacy of stiripentol for the treatment of Dravet syndrome: a multicenter, open-label study in Japan. Epilepsy Res. 2015; 113: 90–7

[176] Thanh TN, Chiron C, Dellatolas G, Rey E, Pons G, Vincent J, et al. Long-term efficacy and tolerance of stiripentaol in severe myoclonic epilepsy of infancy (Dravet's syndrome). Arch Pediatr. 2002; 9(11):1120–7

[177] Ochoa JG, Riche W. Antiepileptic Drugs. In: http://emedicine.medscape.com/article/1187334-overview#showall. Medscape Reference © 2011 WebMD, LLC. Updated: Mar 08, 2016.

[178] FDA medwatch. in www.fda.gov/cder/drug/infopage/tiagabine/tiagabine/default.htm [10.05.2016]

[179] Sabers A, Gram L. Pharmacology of vigabatrin. Pharmacol Toxicol. 1992; 70: 237–43

[180] Gey L, Gernert M, Löscher W. Continuous bilateral infusion of vigabatrin into the subthalamic nucleus: effects on seizure threshold and GABA metabolism in two rat models. Neurobiol Dis. 2016; 91: 194–208

[181] Korff CM, Vulliemoz S, Picard F, Fluss J. Ohtahara syndrome or early-onset West syndrome? A case with overlapping features and favorable response tovigabatrin. Eur J Paediatr Neurol. 2012; 16(6): 753–7

[182] Romaniello R, Zucca C, Tenderini E, Arrigoni F, Ragona F, Zorzi G, et al. A novel mutation in STXBP1 gene in a child with epileptic encephalopathy and an atypical electroclinical pattern. J Child Neurol. 2014; 29(2): 249–53

[183] Sidhu RS, Del Bigio MR, Tuor UI, Seshia SS. Low-dose vigabatrin (gamma-vinyl GABA)-induced damage in the immature rat brain. Exp Neurol. 1997; 144(2): 400–5

[184] Taylor CP, Gee NS, Su TZ, Kocsis JD, Welty DF, Brown JP, et al. A summary of mechanistic hypotheses of gabapentin pharmacology. Epilepsy Res. 1998; 29(3): 233–49

[185] Haney AL, Garner SS, Cox TH. Gabapentin therapy for pain and irritability in a neurologically impaired infant. Pharmacotherapy. 2009; 29(8): 997–1001

[186] Asconape J, Diedrich A, DellaBadia J. Myoclonus associated with the use of gabapentin. Epilepsia. 2000; 41(4): 479–81

[187] Liow NY, Gimeno H, Lumsden DE, Marianczak J, Kaminska M, Tomlin S, et al. Gabapentin can significantly improve dystonia severity and quality of life in children. Eur J Paediatr Neurol. 2016; 20(1): 100–7

[188] Baldino F Jr, Geller HM. Sodium valproate enhancement of gamma-aminobutyric acid (GABA) inhibition: electrophysiological evidence for anticonvulsant activity. J Pharmacol Exp Ther. 1981; 217(2): 445–50

[189] Löscher W. Effects of the antiepileptic drug valproate on metabolism and function of inhibitory and excitatory amino acids in the brain. Neurochem Res. 1993; 18(4): 485–502

[190] Dulac O. Epileptic encephalopathy. Epilepsia. 2001; 42 (Suppl 3): 23–6

[191] McClelland D, Evans RM, Barkworth L, Martin DJ, Scott RH. A study comparing the actions of gabapentin and pregabalin on the electrophysiological properties of cultured DRG neurones from neonatal rats. BMC Pharmacol. 2004; 4(4): 14

[192] Taghdiri MM, Bakhshandeh Bali MK, Karimzadeh P, Ashrafi MR, Tonekaboni SH, Ghofrani M. Comparative efficacy of zonisamide and pregabalin as an adjunctive therapy in children with refractory epilepsy. Iran J Child Neurol. 2015; 9(1): 49–55

[193] Chiron C, Dulac O. The pharmacologic treatment of Dravet syndrome. Epilepsia 2011; 52(Suppl 2): 72–5

[194] Brunklaus A, Ellis R, Reavey E, Forbes GH, Zuberi SM. Prognostic, clinical and demographic features in SCN1A mutation-positive Dravet syndrome. Brain 2012; 135: 2329–36

[195] Larsen J, Carvill GL, Gardella E, Kluger G, Schmiedel G, Barisic N, et al. EuroEPI-NOMICS RES Consortium CRP. The phenotypic spectrum of SCN8A encephalopathy. Neurology 2015; 84: 480–9

[196] Pisano T, Numis AL, Heavin SB, Weckhuysen S, Angriman M, Suls A, et al. Early and effective treatment of KCNQ2 encephalopathy. Epilepsia. 2015 May; 56(5): 685–91

[197] Ohtahara S. Zonisamide in the management of epilepsy. Japanese experience. Epilepsy Res 2006; 68(Suppl 2): S25–33

[198] Kim HR, Kim GH, Eun SH, Eun BL, Byeon JH. Therapeutic outcomes and prognostic factors in childhood absence epilepsy. J Clin Neurol. 2016; 12(2): 160–5

[199] Pellock JM, Faught E, Leppik IE, Shinnar S, Zupanc ML. Felbamate: consensus of current clinical experience. Epilepsy Res. 2006; 71(2–3): 89–101

[200] Heyman E, Levin N, Lahat E, Epstein O, Gandelman-Marton R. Efficacy and safety of felbamate in children with refractory epilepsy. Eur J Paediatr Neurol. 2014; 18(6): 658–62

[201] Mishal NM, Arkilo D, Tang J, Crawford JR, Wang SG. A potential role for felbamate in TSC- and NF1-related epilepsy: a case report and review of the literature. Case Rep Neurol Med. 2015; 2015: 960746. doi: 10.1155/2015/960746

[202] Pierson TM, Yuan H, Marsh ED, Fuentes-Fajardo K, Adams DR, Markello T. GRIN2A mutation and early-onset epileptic encephalopathy: personalized therapy with memantine. Ann Clin Transl Neurol 2014; 1: 190–8

[203] Ortinski P, Meador KJ. Cognitive side effects of antiepileptic drugs. Epilepsy Behav EB. 2004; 5(Suppl 1): S60–65

[204] Lee GM, Lee KS, Lee EH, Chung S. Short term outcomes of topiramate monotherapy as a first-line treatment in newly diagnosed West syndrome. Korean J Pediatr. 2011; 54(9): 380–4

[205] Fallah R, Salor F, Akhavan Karbasi S, Motaghipisheh H. Randomised clinical efficacy trial of topiramate and nitrazepam in treatment of infantile spasms. Iran J Child Neurol. 2014; 8(1): 12–9

[206] Jia F, Jiang H, Du L, Li N, Sun J, Niu C. An effective initial polytherapy for children with West syndrome. Neural Regen Res. 2013; 8(17): 1623–30

[207] Zhu X, Chen O, Zhang D, Jin R, Li F, Wang Y, Sun R. A prospective study on the treatment of infantile spasms with first line topiramate followed by low-dose ACTH. Epilepsy Res. 2011; 93 (2–3): 149–54

[208] Steinhoff BJ, Ben-Menachem E, Ryvlin P, Shorvon S, Kramer L, Satlin A, et al. Efficacy and safety of adjunctive perampanel for the treatment of refractory partial seizures: a pooled analysis of three phase III studies. Epilepsia. 2013; 54(8):1481–9

[209] Biró A, Stephani U, Tarallo T, Bast T, Schlachter K, Fleger M,et al. Effectiveness and tolerability of perampanel in children and adolescents with refractory epilepsies: first experiences. Neuropediatrics. 2015; 46(2): 110–6

[210] Orhan G, Bock M, Schepers D, Ilina EI, Reichel SN, Löffler H, et al. Dominant-negative effects of KCNQ2 mutations are associated with epileptic encephalopathy. Ann Neurol. 2014; 75(3): 382–94

[211] Thiry A, Dogné JM, Supuran CT, Masereel B. Carbonic anhydrase inhibitors as anticonvulsant agents. Curr Top Med Chem. 2007; 7(9): 855–64

[212] Aggarwal M, Kondeti B, McKenna R. Anticonvulsant/antiepilectic carbonic anhydrase inhibitors: a patent review. Expert Opin Ther Pat. 2013; 23(6): 717–24

[213] Hamidi S, Avoli M. Carbonic anhydrase inhibition by acetazolamide reduces in vitro epileptiform synchronization. Neuropharmacology. 2015;95: 377–87

[214] Pisani F, Seri S, Pelliccia A. Landau-Kleffner syndrome and atypical benign partial epilepsy of childhood: the effectiveness of acetazolamide. Neuropediatrics. 1999; 30(3):164

[215] Irahara K, Saito Y, Sugai K, Nakagawa E, Saito T, Komaki H, et al. Effects of acetazolamide on epileptic apnea in migrating partial seizures in infancy. Epilepsy Res. 2011; 96(1–2): 185–9

[216] Milburn-McNulty P, Powell G, Sills GJ, Marson AG. Sulthiame add-on therapy for epilepsy. Cochrane Database Syst Rev. 2015; 10: CD009472

[217] Wirrell E, Sherman EM, Vanmastrigt R, Hamiwka L. Deterioration in cognitive function in children with benign epilepsy of childhood with central temporal spikes treated with sulthiame. J Child Neurol. 2008; 23(1): 14–21

[218] García-Pérez E, Mahfooz K, Covita J, Zandueta A, Wesseling JF. Levetiracetam accelerates the onset of supply rate depression in synaptic vesicle trafficking. Epilepsia. 2015; 56(4): 535–45

[219] Crowder KM, Gunther JM, Jones TA, Hale BD, Zhang HZ, Peterson MR, et al. Abnormal neurotransmission in mice lacking synaptic vesicle protein 2A (SV2A). Proc Natl Acad Sci U S A. 1999; 96(26): 15268–73

[220] Kim JS, Lee JH, Ryu HW, Lim BC, Hwang H, Chae JH, et al. Effectiveness of intravenous levetiracetam as an adjunctive treatment in pediatric refractory status epilepticus. Pediatr Emerg Care. 2014; 30(8): 525–8

[221] Vatta M, Tennison MB, Aylsworth AS, Turcott CM, Guerra MP, Eng CM, et al. A novel STXBP1 mutation causes focal seizures with neonatal onset. J Child Neurol. 2012; 27(6): 811–4

[222] Dilena R, Striano P, Traverso M, Viri M, Cristofori G, Tadini L, et al. Dramatic effect of levetiracetam in early-onset epileptic encephalopathy due to STXBP1 mutation. Brain Dev. 2016; 38(1): 128–31

[223] Wheless JW, Vazquez B. Rufinamide: a novel broad spectrum antiepileptic drug. Epilepsy Curr. 2010; 10(1): 1–6

[224] la Marca G, Rosati A, Falchi M, Malvagia S, Della Bona ML, Pellacani S, et al. A pharmacokinetic study and correlation with clinical response of rufinamide in infants with epileptic encephalopathies. Pharmacology. 2013; 91(5–6): 275–80

[225] Reddy DS. Role of hormones and neurosteroids in epileptogenesis. Front Cell Neurosci. 2013; 7: 115. doi: 10.3389/fncel.2013.00115. eCollection 2013.

[226] Taubøll E, Sveberg L, Svalheim S. Interactions between hormones and epilepsy. Seizure. 2015; 28: 3–11

[227] Munakata M, Togashi N, Sakamoto O, Haginoya K, Kobayashi Y, Onuma A, et al. Reduction in glutamine/glutamate levels in the cerebral cortex after adrenocorticotropic hormone therapy in patients with west syndrome. Tohoku J Exp Med. 2014; 232(4): 277–83

[228] Kendall DA, McEwen BS, Enna SJ. The influence of ACTH and corticosterone on [3H]GABA receptor binding in rat brain. Brain Res. 1982; 236(2):365–74

[229] Shumiloff NA, Lam WM, Manasco KB. Adrenocorticotropic hormone for the treatment of West Syndrome in children. Ann Pharmacother. 2013; 47(5): 744–54

[230] Riikonen R. Recent advances in the pharmacotherapy of infantile spasms. CNS Drugs. 2014; 28(4): 279–90

[231] Nohria V, Giller E. Ganaxolone. Neurotherapeutics. 2007; 4(1): 102–5

[232] Kerrigan JF, Shields WD, Nelson TY, Bluestone DL, Dodson WE, Bourgeois BF, et al. Ganaxolone for treating intractable infantile spasms: a multicenter, open-label, add-on trial. Epilepsy Res. 2000;42 (2–3): 133–9

[233] Milligan CJ, Li M, Gazina EV, Heron SE, Nair U, Trager C, Reid CA, et al. KCNT1 gain of function in 2 epilepsy phenotypes is reversed by quinidine. Ann Neurol. 2014; 75: 581–90.

[234] Bearden D, Strong A, Ehnot J, DiGiovine M, Dlugos D, Goldberg EM. Targeted treatment of migrating partial seizures of infancy with quinidine. Ann Neurol. 2014; 76: 457–61

[235] Scheffer IE, Heron SE, Regan BM, Mandelstam S, Crompton DE, Hodgson BL, Mutations in mammalian target of rapamycin regulator DEPDC5 cause focal epilepsy with brain malformations. Ann Neurol. 2014; 75(5): 782–7

[236] D'Gama AM, Geng Y, Couto JA, Martin B, Boyle EA, LaCoursiere CM Mammalian target of rapamycin pathway mutations cause hemimegalencephaly and focal cortical dysplasia. Ann Neurol. 2015; 77(4): 720–5

[237] Ünver O, Incecik F, Dündar H, Kömür M, Ünver A, Okuyaz Ç. Potassium bromide for treatment of malignant migrating partial seizures in infancy. Pediatr Neurol. 2013; 49(5): 355–7

[238] Tanabe T, Awaya Y, Matsuishi T, Iyoda K, Nagai T, Kurihara M, et al. Management of and prophylaxis against status epilepticus in children with severe myoclonic epilepsy in infancy (SMEI; Dravet syndrome) – a nationwide questionnaire survey in Japan. Brain Dev. 2008; 30(10): 629–35.

Chapter 4

Epilepsy as a Pyridoxine-Dependent Condition: Quantitative Urinary Biomarkers of Epilepsy. Family Disorders of Pyridoxine Metabolism

Svetlana A. Dolina

Additional information is available at the end of the chapter

http://dx.doi.org/10.5772/64691

Abstract

The affected pyridoxine metabolism is discussed as an inborn genetic sign of epilepsy. In children with different forms of epilepsy and matched healthy controls, the urinary parameters of pyridoxal phosphate–dependent tryptophan degradation were measured by high-performance liquid chromatography (HPLC) method with simultaneous ultraviolet and fluorimetric detection. Concentrations of compounds, which are formed in the course of tryptophan degradation, and correlations between them turned out to be quantitative biomarkers useful for evaluation of patient's condition and monitoring individualized antiepileptic treatment. Accumulation of tryptophan, kynurenine, and neurotoxic 3-hydroxykynurenine, along with reduced kynureninase activity, is characteristic of epileptic patients. Growing progressively worse, epilepsy is accompanied by aggravation of pyridoxal phosphate–dependent disturbances of tryptophan metabolism and further inhibition of kynureninase.

In asymptomatic first-degree relatives of epileptic probands, disorders of pyridoxine metabolism are of the same (or even higher) extent as in probands. Long-term pyridoxine treatment (7–10 mg/kg daily) is suggested as safe and effective protective replacement therapy. The protocols of this study have been approved by the ethics committee of Kaplan Hospital (Israel).

Keywords: epilepsy, epileptic families, tryptophan metabolism, vitamin B6 (pyridoxine)-dependent enzymes

1. Quantitative urinary biomarkers for evaluation of patient's state and monitoring antiepileptic treatment

1.1. Introduction

Sixty years ago Hunt et al. [1] described pyridoxine-dependent epilepsy (PDE), which until now is considered as a rare (1:100.000) autosomal recessive genetic disorder, occurring in the uterus, or later in infancy, or early childhood. Most often seizures are observed within the first month of life, even within hours of birth. In atypical (late-onset) PDE seizures start later (up to 2 years). After the first year of life autistic features are often revealed. The resistance to conventional antiepileptic drugs (AEDs) and response to vitamin B6 administration (5–10 mg/kg/day) are accepted as the main characteristic features of PDE [2–5].

Vitamin B6 consists of six different vitamers: pyridoxine (PN), pyridoxal (PL), pyridoxamine (PM), and their phosphate-esterified forms. Pyridoxal phosphate (PLP) is the active B6 vitamer, which is produced from its precursor vitamers (PN, PM, and PL) by phosphorylation and oxidation (PN phosphate, PLP, and PM phosphate) through the actions of pyridoxal kinase and pyridox(am)ine oxidase (PNPO), respectively (**Figure 1**) [6]. Vitamin B6 is broken down to pyridoxic acid (4PA), which is excreted in the urine.

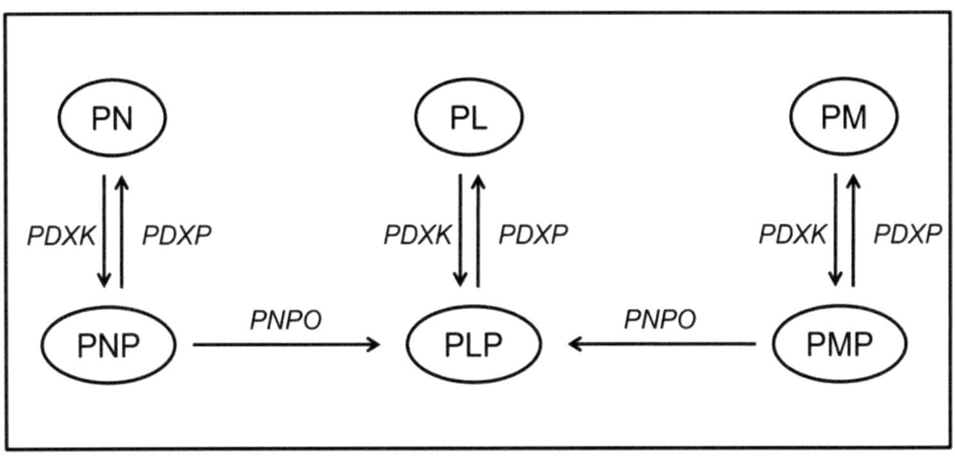

Figure 1. Human vitamin B6 metabolism. PDXK, pyridoxal kinase; PDXR, vitamin B6-specific phosphatase; PNPO, pyridox(am)ine phosphate oxidase.

PLP is a cofactor for numerous enzymatic reactions in the central nervous system (CNS). An inborn abnormality of PLP-dependent GABA synthesis induced by glutamate decarboxylase (GAD) deficiency earlier was postulated as a cause of epilepsy, and lifelong pyridoxine administration was recommended. Later on in the search for the PDE-responsible gene, the primary involvement of the GAD 1 gene on chromosome 2q31 and the GAD 2 on 10p23 was discussed and excluded [7, 8].

http://dx.doi.org/10.5772/64691

At present, PDE is considered as a result of mutations in the ALDH7A1 gene, encoding antiquitin. Antiquitin deficiency in the lysine degradation pathway leads to the accumulation of piperidein-6-carboxylic acid, which inactivates PLP [9, 10]. Recently, several cases of other inborn errors of vitamin B6 metabolism, that is, pyridox(am)ine 5-phospate oxidase deficiency and type 2 hyperprolinemia, have also been described. So, the accumulated data have shown that autosomal recessive pyridoxine-dependent seizures are genetically heterogeneous [11–13].

Nevertheless, neither data accumulation, nor recommendations for pyridoxine administration in early cases of intractable epilepsy [3, 14, 15], or pyridoxine applicability as the first-line drug for infantile spasms [16–19] have changed conventional perception of the strictly limited role of pyridoxine in the pathogenesis of *epilepsy as a whole*.

Meanwhile, disturbances in the metabolism of glutamate, GABA, tryptophan (TRP), serotonin, taurine, dopamine, and norepinephrine, which are synthesized and/or metabolized by PLP-dependent enzymes [20–32], have been repeatedly found in epileptic patients. The increased levels of excitatory amino acids—glutamate, aspartate, and glycine [21–27] along with the reduced levels of inhibitory amino acids and amines—GABA, serotonin, and taurine [28–32] were detected in the plasma, cerebrospinal fluid (CSF), and epileptogenic foci of patients with different forms of epilepsy. Moreover, a moderate increase in the activity of glutamic acid dehydrogenase, the glutamate-synthesizing enzyme, which is specifically inhibited by PLP, has been found in epileptic foci [33].

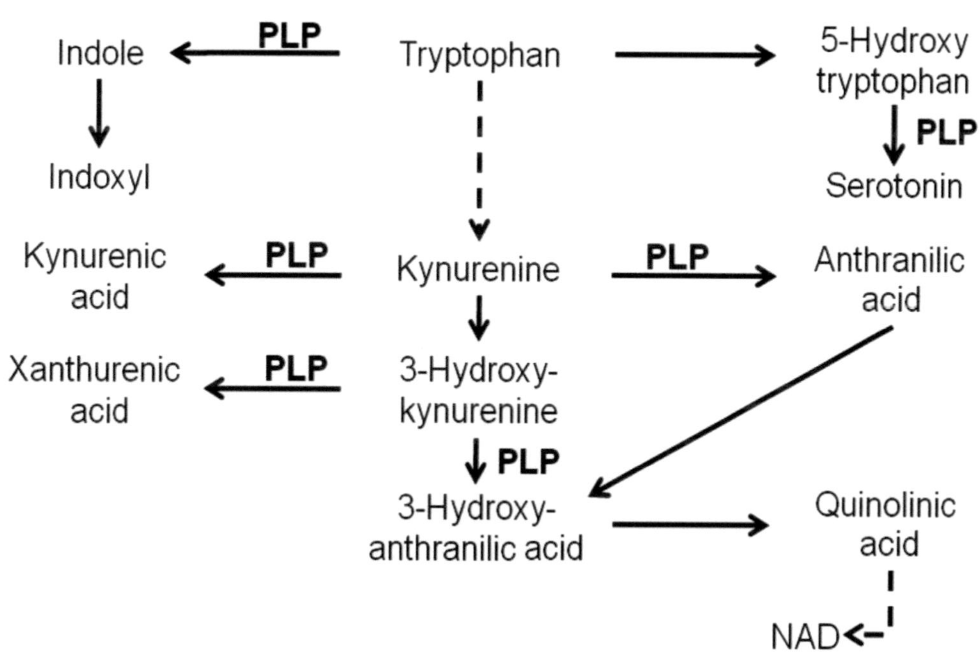

Figure 2. Outline of kynurenic pathway of tryptophan degradation.

These clinical data along with experimental results obtained in genetically epilepsy-prone seizure-naive animals, in comparison with genetically epilepsy resistant [34–37], enable us to hypothesize that an inborn error of pyridoxine metabolism (accentuated by high pyridoxine requirement during early development) is inherent in epilepsy. Being a starting point for neurotransmitter disorders, such an error may be a key determinant of epileptic diathesis. An impairment of GABA (as well as serotonin and taurine)-mediated inhibition along with an enhancement of glutamate (and aspartate)-mediated excitatory transmission evidently facilitates spreading of ictal activity throughout the brain and thereby generation of seizures.

Disturbances of PLP-dependent tryptophan degradation, in particular over-excess of neurotoxic 3-HOKYN, have been repeatedly shown in epileptic patients starting from 50-s [38–41]. Summarizing the data obtained [42–44], we suggested that quantitative correlations between metabolites formed in the course of TRP degradation (**Figure 2**) might be indicative of clinical status in epileptic patients.

Specifically, the ratio of KYN to TRP serves as an index of activity of indoleamine-2, 3-dioxygenase (IDO), the rate-limiting enzyme of TRP degradation, initiating the pathway. (Being heme-containing enzyme, IDO is apparently PLP dependent, inasmuch as heme synthesis is PLP dependent).

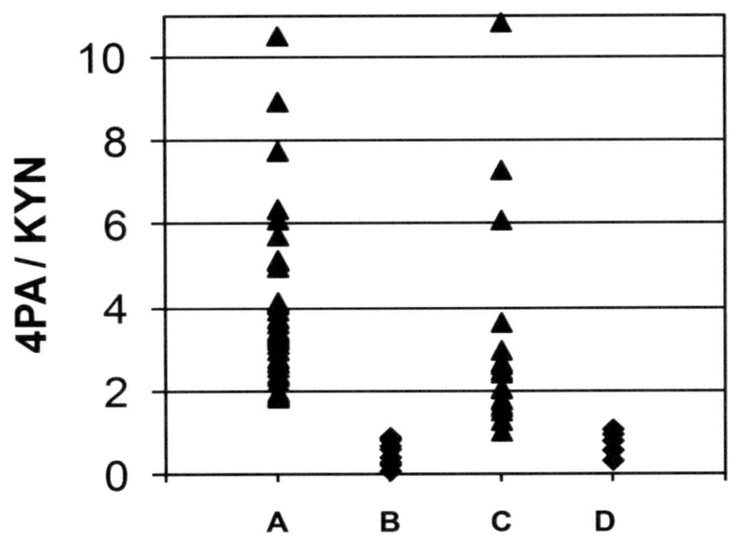

Figure 3. The value of 4PA/KYN ratios in healthy controls (A); patients experienced the first seizure attack (B); AED-treated seizure-free patients (C); partially AED-controlled epileptic patients (D).

The ratio between the levels of 3-HOAA and 3-HOKYN is considered as an index of kynureninase activity, the enzyme of critical sensitivity to PLP supply [45–47]. The ratio between 4-PA and KYN turned out to be an indicator of recently experienced seizure attack (**Figure 3**).

We have used these and other quantitative urinary biomarkers for clarification of patient's state in epilepsy and for tailoring of individual AED treatment.

http://dx.doi.org/10.5772/64691

1.2. Materials and methods

1.2.1. Subjects

Urine samples were analyzed in children of 4–17 years of age with different clinical forms and stages of epilepsy, excluding absence and atonic seizures, healthy in all other respects. Altogether, 109 subjects divided into following groups were comparatively studied:

1. Newly diagnosed epileptic patients, who had experienced their first epileptic attack on the previous day(s) and were never treated with AEDs ($n = 11$);

2. Epileptic patients regardless of the type of epilepsy successfully treated with AED and at present seizure-free for at least 3 months, regardless of the type of epilepsy ($n = 19$);

3. Epileptic patients partially responsive to AED treatment, that is, those having repeated seizure attacks in spite of antiepileptic treatment ($n = 19$);

4. Control group of healthy children matched by sex and age ($n = 37$).

About 270 urine samples were analyzed. Control samples were collected from healthy children in local kindergartens and elementary schools.

1.2.2. Determination of tryptophan and its metabolites in urine by high-performance liquid chromatography with simultaneous ultraviolet and fluorimetric detection

Urinary TRP and its metabolites were determined by high-performance liquid chromatography (HPLC) modified in our laboratory by Rabinkov, Pressman, and Malitsky. In addition to KYN, 3-HOKYN and 3-HOAA detected by Herve et al. [48]; some other TRP metabolites, that is, anthranilic acid (AA), kynurenic acid (KA), indoxyl sulfate (IND), and 4-PA, were also measured [36, 49].

All standards were purchased from Sigma. All solvents were of HPLC grade. The same method of TRP metabolite detection has been used by our collaborators in patients with attention deficit hyperactivity disorder (ADHD), the disease mutually interconnected with epilepsy [50].

1.2.2.1. Sample preparation

Mixed standard solutions (1 mM of each compound) were stored at −80°C for up to 3 months. Urine samples were collected into 20-mL glass scintillation vials and stored in aliquots at −80°C. Samples were acidified by the addition of 100 μL of 2.4 M perchloric acid to 900 μL of urine. After centrifugation (5000 g, 15 min, 4°C), supernatants were filtered (0.22-μL Millipore filter) into HPLC vials and analyzed the same day.

1.2.2.2. Chromatography

Reverse phase HPLC analysis was performed with an Inertsil (C-18, 5 μm) column (250 × 4.6 mm) and Merck Hitachi system equipped with a Quaternary Pump L-7100 and interface D-7000.

Peaks detection and quantification were carried out using a scanning fluorescence detector L-7485 connected to the programmable photodiode array detector L-7450A. Samples were analyzed using the following gradient: 28-min isocratic elution of 100% solvent A, 6-min linear gradient from 100 to 75% of solvent A, 61-min isocratic elution of 75% of solvent A, 2-min linear gradient from 75 to 100% of solvent A, and 8-min isocratic elution of 100% solvent A. Solvent A was 1 M ammonium acetate buffer, pH 5.2. Solvent B was 6% acetonitrile in 1 M ammonium acetate buffer, pH 5.2. The mobile phase was prepared on the day of analysis. Acquisition and processing of chromatograms were performed using HSM software (Merck-Hitachi). Standard compounds showed linearity range from 0.03 to 10 μM. Concentrations were calculated on the basis of peak areas of external standards. TRP, its metabolites, and 4-PA were determined with UV and fluorescence detection at two different excitation and emission wavelengths: 3-HOKYN and KYN were detected by UV absorption at 365 nm and eluted at 14.3, 41.4, and 87.0 min, respectively, while 3-HOAA, 4-PA, AA, TRP, IND, and KA were detected by fluorescence and eluted at 31.6, 58.9, 72.4, 84.5, 92.8, and 99.9 min, respectively.

For 3-HOAA and 4-PA, fluorescence excitation and emission wavelengths were set up as 320/420 nm during the first 60 min of elution; for AA, TRP, IND, and KA the wavelengths were 254/404 nm during the following 45 min of elution.

1.2.3. Statistical analysis

The data were expressed as mean ± SEM. Paired Student's *t*-test was used to assess the difference between groups; $p < 0.05$ was considered as statistically significant difference between values of parameters.

1.3. Urinary biomarkers for detection of the endured first seizure attack

In patients who endured seizures for the first time before admission to the ward, the mean level of TRP, and especially of KYN were sharply increased in comparison with healthy control group, thus providing the elevated mean value of KYN/TRP ratio and decreased value of 3-HOKYN/KYN ratio. The level of KA was twofold elevated, while the IND level was almost twice reduced.

Taken together, these changes in "first seizure attack" children formed a pattern strongly distinguishable from that of healthy controls (**Table 1**). The level of urinary 4-PA was statistically indistinguishable from healthy controls (though in four out of 11 patients it was reduced to 1μM or even lower). The mean value of 4-PA/KYN ratio in children of this group turned out to be almost sevenfold less than in healthy controls (**Table 1** and **Figure 3**) and appeared to be the marker of seizure attack occurred (regardless of its type).

The alterations in the urinary levels of TRP and KYN lead to a rightward shift in the histogram of distribution of the KYN/TRP ratio and a strong leftward shift in the histogram of distribution of the ratio 3-HOKYN/KYN (**Figures 4** and **5**).

http://dx.doi.org/10.5772/64691

Parameters	Epileptic patients								P values between compared groups *p < 0.1; **P ≤ 0.05; ***P ≤ 0.01				
			Non treated		AED treated								
	Group 1: healthy controls (n = 37)		Group 2: after first seizure attack (n = 11)		Group 3: seizure-free (n = 19)		Group 4: partially controlled (n = 19)						
	Mean	SEM	Mean	SEM	Mean	SEM	Mean	SEM	1–2	1–3	2–3	2–4	3–4
TRP, (μM)	23	2	57	20	36	7	58	15	***	**			
KYN, (μM)	1.7	0.2	5.7	1.4	2.4	0.2	3.3	0.3	***	**	***		**
3-HOKYN, (μM)	1.1	0.1	1.8	0.5	1.1	0.2	4.6	0.8	*			**	****
3-OHAA, (μM)	4.5	0.7	3.5	0.6	4.4	1.0	2.4	0.5					*
AA, (μM)	0.20	0.02	0.26	0.09	0.20	0.06	0.30	0.11					
KA, (μM)	3.3	0.4	6.3	1.1	5.3	1.3	8.4	1.3	***	**			*
4PA, (μM)	6.0	0.9	5.0	1.3	6.8	1.2	5.5	1.0					
IND, (μM)	576	53	294	70	289	50	460	77	**	***			*
4PA/KYN	4.1	0.5	0.6	0.1	3.1	0.6	2.5	0.7	***		***	**	
4PA/3HOKYN	8.42	1.45	3.85	0.94	8.6	1.26	4.12	1.53	*		***		**
4PA/(KYN + 3HOKYN)	2,5	0.35	0.76	0.24	1.94	0.28	1.3	0.35	***		***		
KYN/TRP	0.08	0.005	0.226	0.086	0.116	0.029	0.116	0.034	***	*			
3HOKYN/KYN	0.72	0.08	0.35	0.09	0.56	0.12	1.57	0.29	**			***	***
3HOAA/3HOKYN	6.0	1.1	4.4	1.3	5.9	1.5	0.9	0.2				***	***
KA/3HOAA	2.2	0.6	2.9	0.8	1.8	0.3	4.9	1.2					**
KYN/(3HOAA/3HOKYN)	1.06	0.27	4.16	1.74	0.91	0.19	9.73	2.65	***		**	***	****
KA/(3HOAA/3HOKYN)	2.0	0.5	5.3	2.3	1.5	0.3	20.4	4.8	**		*	**	***
TRP/(3HOAA/3HOKYN)	14	3	38	15	13	3	155	53	**		***	**	****
IND/TRP	29.4	2.8	6.7	1.4	13.1	2.3	14.1	5.4	****	***	**		
IND/KYN	433	50	78	23	164	26	210	42	***	***	**	**	

Table 1. Urinary metabolites of tryptophan and correlations between them in epileptic patients in comparison with healthy controls.

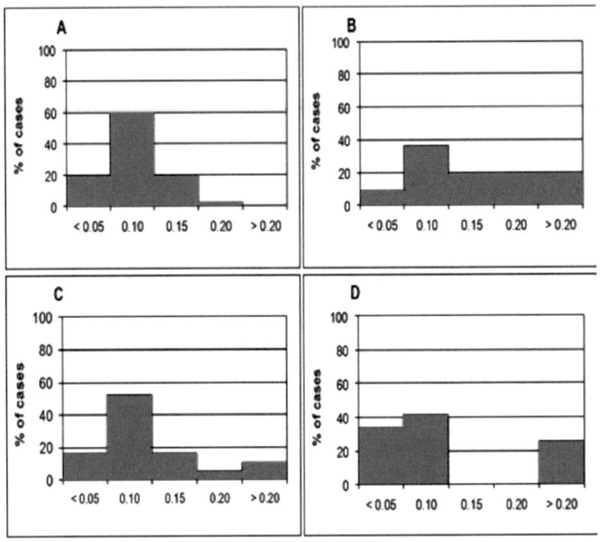

Figure 4. Distribution of KYN/TRP values in epileptic patients, in comparison with healthy controls. Designations: healthy controls (A); patients experienced the first seizure attack (B); AED-treated seizure-free patients (C); partially AED-controlled patients (D).

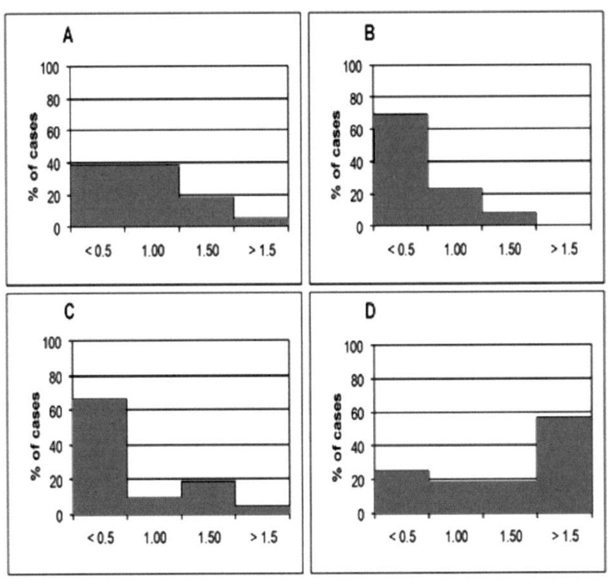

Figure 5. Distribution of 3HOKYN/KYN values in epileptic patients, in comparison with healthy controls. Designations: healthy controls (A); patients experienced the first seizure attack (B); AED-treated seizure-free patients (C); partially AED-controlled patients (D).

At the same time, the histogram of distribution of the 3-HOAA/3-HOKYN ratio tends distinctly to the left (**Figure 6**), reflecting some reduction in kynureninase activity, though the mean value

http://dx.doi.org/10.5772/64691

of this ratio is decreased insignificantly (**Table 1**). The correlations between concentrations of TRP (as well as KYN) and the ratio indicative of kynureninase activity, that is, TRP: (3-HOAA/3-HOKYN) and KYN: (3-HOAA/3-HOKYN), are strongly higher in "first-attack" children than in the control group.

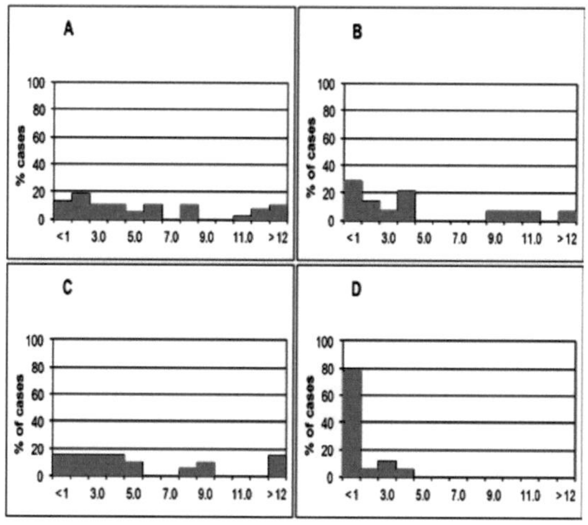

Figure 6. Distribution of 3HOKYN/3HOAA values in epileptic patients, in comparison with healthy controls. Designations: healthy controls (A); patients experienced the first seizure attack (B); AED-treated seizure-free patients (C); partially AED-controlled patients (D).

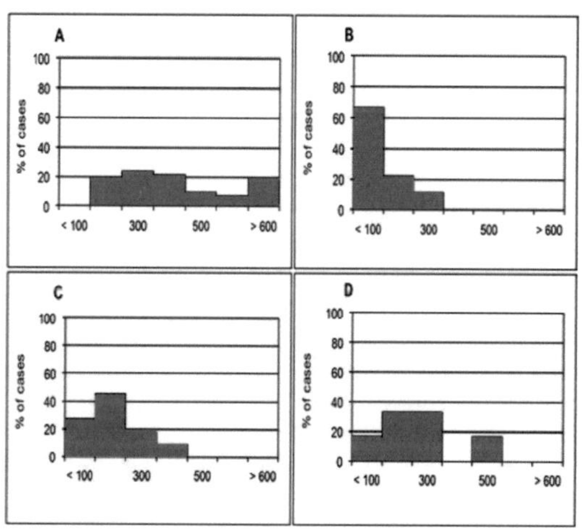

Figure 7. Distribution of IND/KYN values in epileptic patients, in comparison with healthy controls. Designations: healthy controls (A); patients experienced the first seizure attack (B); AED-treated seizure-free patients (C); partially AED-controlled patients (D).

The low value of IND/TRP and especially IND/KYN are also the markers, distinguishing first-attack children from healthy controls. The combination of increased concentrations of TRP and

KYN with decreased concentrations of IND provides drastic diminution in both IND/TRP and IND/KYN ratios in patients who endured the first attack. In approximately 70% of these patients, the IND/KYN ratio is lower than 100, while in healthy children these ratios are always higher than 100; in 60% of the healthy group, these ratios are even higher than 300 (**Table 1** and **Figure** 7).

1.4. Urinary markers in AEDs treated seizure-free patients

In patients well controlled by AEDs (in our study, those who has been seizure-free for at least 3 months) most of the studied parameters are practically similar to those in healthy controls. The mean values of KYN/TRP, 4-PA/KYN, 3- HOKYN/KYN, and 3-HOAA/3-HOKYN ratios coincide with those in the control group (**Table 1**). Though the urinary concentrations of TRP and KYN in seizure-free patients are significantly higher than in the healthy group, the correlations TRP: (3HOAA/3-HOKYN) and KYN: (3HOAA/3-HOKYN) practically coincide with corresponding values in healthy controls.

Histograms of distribution of studied parameters in AED-treated seizure-free children are similar to those in healthy controls (**Figures 4** and **6**), with the exception of histograms of distribution of 3-HOKYN/KYN ratios (**Figure 5**). Similarity between the histogram of distribution of these ratios in seizure-free AED-treated children and the group experienced the first attack signifies that kynureninase activity is not yet restored in AED-treated patients.

The mean concentration of IND in these patients remains as low as in "first-attack" group, but values of IND/TRP and IND/KYN ratios—due to reduction of TRP and KYN levels—are higher than in first-attack group, but far lower than in healthy group. The histogram of the distribution of IND/KYN ratios remains still shifted to the left (**Figure 7**).

1.5. Urinary markers in patients partially responsive to AED treatment

Repeated convulsive attacks, which occur in epileptic patients in spite of AED treatment, result in decreased values of 4-PA/KYN ratio, the marker of recently experienced seizure attacks (**Figure 3**). In three out of five patients, who had seizures shortly before the admission to the hospital, this ratio was less than one, decreasing thereby the mean value of the group (**Table 1**). The fourfold elevated concentration of toxic 3-HOKYN, the twofold elevated ratio of 3-HOKYN/KYN, and the dramatically reduced value of the 3-HOAA/3-HOKYN ratio are the most remarkable signs of the group. The mean value of 3-HOAA/3-HOKYN ratio is reduced to 0.9 and represents only 15% of the corresponding value in seizure-free patients (**Table 1**).

The strongly right-shifted histogram of the distribution of 3-HOKYN/KYN ratios and the strongly left-shifted histogram of the distribution of 3-HOAA/3-HOKYN ratios are apparently the signs of severe disturbances of kynureninase activity in partially AED-controlled patients (**Figures 5** and **6**).

Reduction in the kynureninase activity results also in the accumulation of TRP, KYN, and KA. Accordingly, the correlation of each of these compounds to the 3-HOAA/3-HOKYN ratio, that is, KYN: (3-HOAA/3-HOKYN), KA: (3-HOAA/3-HOKYN), and TRP: (3-HOAA/3-HOKYN), reaches extremely high values in patients partly responsive to AEDs (**Table 1**).

The intensive inpatient AED treatment distinctly changes the examined parameters. First of all, the value of 4-PA/KYN ratio is increased. The value of 3-HOAA/3-HOKYN ratio is also increased, reflecting an increase in kynureninase activity. Accordingly, values of KYN: (3-HOAA/3-HOKYN), KA: (3-HOAA/3-HOKYN), and TRP: (3-HOAA/3-HOKYN) are significantly diminished. In successful cases, favorable changes, once attained, remain stable (**Figure 8**; patients E and K). In unsuccessful cases, the initial increase in the 3-HOAA/3-HOKYN ratio suddenly reverts back, and the related parameters are accordingly changed (**Figure 8**, patient D).

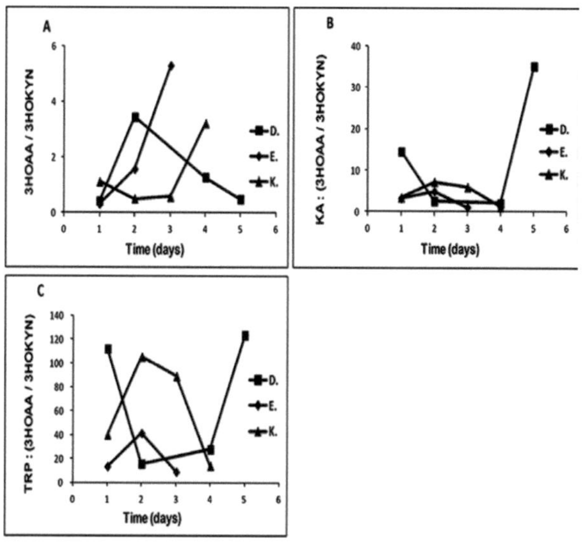

Figure 8. Dynamics of correlations between TRP metabolites under intensive AED treatment in partially AED-controlled patients. Note the difference between successfully (E and K) and unsuccessfully (case D) treated patients.

1.6. Discussion

Disturbances of PLP-dependent TRP degradation revealed in children with different forms of epilepsy confirm the suggestion that **epilepsy as a whole is PLP-dependent disorder**. The data obtained testify that concentrations of compounds formed or metabolized in the course of PLP-dependent TRP degradation, as well as correlations between them, are quantitative urinary biomarkers for the determination of clinical status—from the first seizure attack up to progressively worsening condition. These biomarkers are also indicative for the evaluation of AED treatment effectiveness and its individual monitoring. The parameters reflecting kynureninase activity turned out to be the most sensitive link of this chain.

Once the initial seizure attack has occurred, the drastically increased levels of TRP, KYN, and toxic 3HOKYN, and the drastically reduced level of IND pointed to the disordered PLP-dependent TRP degradation. Low values of IND/TRP and IND/KYN, as well as 4-PA/KYN and 4PA/3-HOKYN ratios, completely change the pattern of TRP metabolites (**Table 1**).

Specifically, the low value of 4-PA/KYN ratio (**Figure 3**) distinguishes an epileptic episode from paroxysmal loss of consciousness of nonepileptic origin. It is important to trace how long this index remains at such a low level after a single seizure episode.

The effective AED treatment normalizes most of the discussed parameters (**Table 1**). The ratio 4-PA/KYN is increased almost up to its control value. We believe that maintaining this ratio within the range between two and four (**Figure 3**) would help to provide adequate seizure control and reduce a risk of pharmacological overtreatment [45, 46]. However, increased levels of TRP, KA, and KYN, reduced concentrations of IND, and diminished IND/TRP and IND/KYN ratios (**Table 1** and **Figure 8**) still clearly distinguish AED-treated seizure-free patients from healthy controls.

The values of IND/KYN and IND/TRP ratios require an additional consideration. Intestinal PLP-dependent tryptophanase of bacterial origin is the key enzyme of alternative IND pathway of TRP degradation, which is inhibited by KYN [20]. A drastic drop in the levels of IND along with increased concentrations of KYN results in diminished IND/KYN and IND/TRP ratios in the studied groups.

Parameters reflecting the activity of kynureninase at the different stages of disease indicate that aggravation of epilepsy is accompanied by expanding inhibition of the enzyme activity [51–53]. The accumulation of toxic 3-HOKYN, along with twofold increase in the 3HOKYN/KYN ratio and sixfold decrease in the 3-HOAA/3-HOKYN ratio, appear to be the most characteristic signs of sharply reduced kynureninase activity in patients partially controlled AEDs (**Table 1**). The decrease in the value of 3HOAA/3HOKYN ratio leads to the accumulation of TRP, KYN, and KA (**Table 1**). The similar pattern is reproduced by kynureninase inhibitors, once even considered as possible anticonvulsants [54].

The intensive inpatient AED treatment of partially controlled patients decreases the 3-HOKYN/KYN ratio and increases the ratio 3-HOAA/3-HOKYN. Stability of attained parameters signifies successful treatment (**Figure 8**). The data obtained indicate that indices of kynureninase activity are the reliable markers for evaluation of clinical status and effectiveness of individual AED therapy.

The effective AED treatment increases alkaline phosphatase (ALP) activity [55–58], the enzyme which dephosphorylates PLP, and thus provides pyridoxal transport through membranes. Intensification of pyridoxine transport normalizes PLP-dependent systems (more details in part 2).

In summary, the suggested quantifiable urinary biomarkers, based on dynamic alterations of TRP metabolites in the course of the disease and antiepileptic treatment, are potentially helpful for

1. Identifying the patients who recently experienced seizure episode regardless of seizure type;

2. Detecting minimal effective doses of AED and gradual improvement of clinical status in the course of AED treatment;

3. Evaluating seizure-free status with greater precision;

4. Identification of inadequate seizure control, and rapid evaluation of the effectiveness of the novel treatment regimen;

5. Tracing the stability of results attained in the course of individualized AED treatment.

Taking into account the overall misdiagnosis rate of epilepsy (26%) and the rate of seizure recurrence after discontinuation of AED treatment ranging from 12 to 66% [59, 60], the use of suggested biomarkers seems to be expedient.

2. Family disorders of pyridoxine metabolism: Urinary TRP metabolites in asymptomatic first-degree relatives of epileptic probands

2.1. Introduction

The results obtained gave us an opportunity to discuss the nature of pyridoxine metabolism derangements in epilepsy. Are they a part of etiology of the disease [61], or consequences of seizures? Namely, are they an inborn error of metabolism, or epiphenomena of seizures, or possibly epiphenomena of seizures superimposed on inherently dysfunctional system of pyridoxine metabolism?

To understand whether dysfunctional vitamin B6 metabolism is an inborn error of metabolism inherent in epileptic families, and thereby a part of etiology of the disease, urinary parameters of vitamin B6–dependent TRP metabolism were HPLC detected in epileptic probands and their first-degree asymptomatic relatives in comparison with healthy controls.

Two non-sanguineous families were studied. Samples of each person were repeatedly analyzed over several (2–8) consecutive days. The mean value of each parameter is presented in **Table 2**.

Family one consisted of AED-treated proband D, an 8-year-old boy with a 3-s/spike-wave epilepsy (the only patient with absence epilepsy included into our study), his asymptomatic 13-year-old sibling brother, their mother affected with bronchial asthma [62], and the healthy stepfather of both children.

Grossly abnormal TRP metabolism in all three closely interconnected relatives, that is, the proband, his sibling (note especially his data), and their mother, clearly distinguished them from healthy controls and their healthy stepfather. Severe hypertryptophanuria and strongly reduced ratio KYN/TRP reflected the low activity of PLP-dependent IDO in all these three relatives. The values of 3-HOAA/3-HOKYN ratios in the proband, his mother, and especially in his asymptomatic sibling brother were 10–25% of the corresponding mean value in healthy controls, coinciding with the mean value of this parameter in epileptic patients ineffectively treated with AED *(see part 1)*. Extremely low values of 3HOAA/3HOKYN ratios along with increased levels of toxic 3-HOKYN testified kynureninase inhibition in all these three interconnected relatives. High levels of urinary 4-PA in siblings apparently meant the elevated PLP plasma level [63]. The combination of hypertryptophanuria (and increased KA levels) with extremely low values of 3-HOAA/3-HOKYN ratios provides drastically increased correlations between these indices. In each of the relatives from this family ratios TRP: (3-HOAA/3-HOKYN) and KA: (3-HOAA/3-HOKYN) were much higher than in control patients. Low concentrations of IND and low values of IND/TRP ratios in all three interconnected relatives (**Table 2**) attest to familial disruption of alternative pathway of TRP degradation as well.

Family two included AED-resistant proband (Sh-T), a 10-year-old boy with frontal lobe epilepsy and secondary generalized convulsions unsuccessfully treated with carbamazepine, phenytoin, and valproic acid, and his asymptomatic sibling brother of 7 years. Diversity of proband's data made us repeat his analyses every 5 consecutive days and to demonstrate the ranges of them.

Parameters		**Family 1**			**Family 2**	
	Healthy controls (n = 37)	**Proband D. (n = 8)**	**Proband's mother M. (n = 8)**	**Proband's sibling Y. (n = 2)**	**Proband Sh.-T (n = 5)**	**Proband's sibling (n = 1)**
	Average ± SE	**Average ± SE**	**Average ± SE**	**Average**	**Range**	
TRP (μM)	23 ± 2	**135** ± 27	**166** ± 17	**180**	23.6–61.8	25
KYN (μM)	1.7 ± 0.2	1.5 ± 0.23	1.8 ± 0.30	2.8	1.2–2.0	1.7
3HOKYN (μM)	1.1 ± 0.1	1.7 ± 0.41	1.5 ± 0.37	3.6	1.2–2.8	0.80
3HOAA (μM)	4.5 ± 0.7	5.0 ± 2.1	**2.4** ± 0.67	**2.3**	1.3–30.0	1.8
KA (μM)	3.3 ± 0.4	4.3 ± 1.2	5.0 ± 0.95	7.1	2.3–4.6	3.6
4PA (μM)	6.0 ± 0.9	**11.1** ± 2.1	5.3 ± 0.49	**14.3**	**0.6–3.5**	**2.1**
IND (μM)	576 ± 53	**182** ± 38	**365** ± 33	660	446–767	74
4PA/TRP	0.29 ± 0.03	**0.136** ± 0.05	**0.04** ± 0.005	**0.087**	**0.02–0.06**	**0.08**
4PA/KYN	4.1 ± 0.5	**8.3** ± 2.1	3.4 ± 0.46	**8.2**	**0.03–2.69**	**1.3**
4PA/3HOKYN	8.42 ± 1.45	9.4 ± 3.4	**4.5** ± 0.81	**4.2**	**0.3–2.3**	**2.6**
4PA/(KYN + 3HOKYN)	2.5 ± 0.35	4.0 ± 0.96	1.7 ± 0.21	2.7	**0.16–0.85**	**0.86**
KYN/TRP	0.08 ± 0.005	**0.016** ± 0.005	**0.01** ± 0.003	**0.014**	**0.02–0.06**	**0.06**
3HOKYN/KYN	0.72 ± 0.08	**1.14** ± 0.21	0.72 ± 0.14	**1.80**	1.0–2.12	0.48
3HOAA/3HOKYN	6.0 ± 1.1	**2.6** ± 0.87	**1.2** ± 0.21	**0.7**	**0.58–2.7**	**2.3**
KA/KYN	2.5 ± 0.4	2.8 ± 0.64	2.9 ± 0.39	2.8	1.5–3.54	2.2
KA/3HOAA	2.2 ± 0.6	1.9 ± 0.63	3.5 ± 1.1	3.0	0.7–2.6	2.0
KYN/(3HOAA/3HOKYN)	1.06 ± 0.27	1.16 ± 0.48	1.48 ± 0.52	5.03	0.46–3.5	0.73
KA/(3HOAA/3HOKYN)	2.0 ± 0.5	**3.8** ± 1.5	**3.9** ± 1.2	**12.4**	0.9–6.5	1.6
TRP/(3HOAA/3HOKYN)	14 ± 3	**65** ± 17	**106** ± 29	**305**	9.1–57.9	11
IND/TRP	29.4 ± 2.8	**1.8** ± 0.60	**2.3** ± 0.29	**3.4**	**7.9–23.2**	**2.9**
IND/KYN	433 ± 50	**128** ± 21	**225** ± 25	**272**	372–432.8	**45**

Parameters similarly altered in family members are shown in bold.

Table 2. Urinary tryptophan metabolites and correlations between them in epileptic families compared to healthy controls.

In both brothers, the values of 3HOAA/3HOKYN ratios were low, reflecting the low kynureninase activity; the value of this ratio in the asymptomatic brother did not exceed one-third of that in healthy controls (**Table 2**). The IND levels, as well as IND/TRP ratios, were also strongly diminished in both siblings, indicating severe disruption of the alternative route of TRP metabolism.

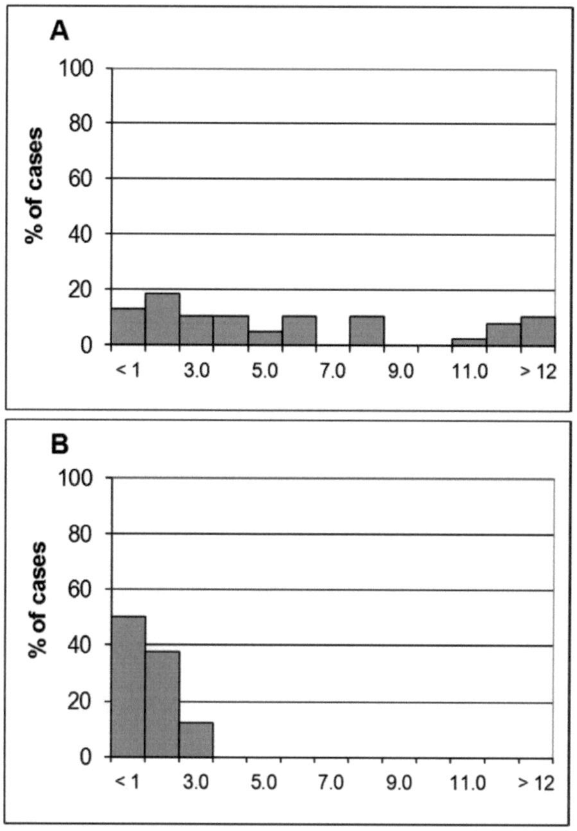

Figure 9. Distribution of 3HOAA/3HOKYN ratios in healthy controls (A) in comparison with epileptic families (B).

2.2. Discussion

Thus, the low activity of kynureninase (mirrored by 3-HOAA/3-HOKYN ratios) and disordered alternative route of TRP metabolism turned out to be the common hidden signs of asymptomatic relatives in both epileptic families, whereas hypertryptophanuria and the elevated level of 4-PA (signifying the increased plasma PLP level) [63] were inherent only in members of the first family (**Table 2**).

Histograms of the distribution of KYN/TRP and 3HOAA/3HOKYN ratios summarized in both families (**Figures 9** and **10**) reveal the reduced activity of both IDO and kynureninase in epileptic families, in comparison with healthy controls.

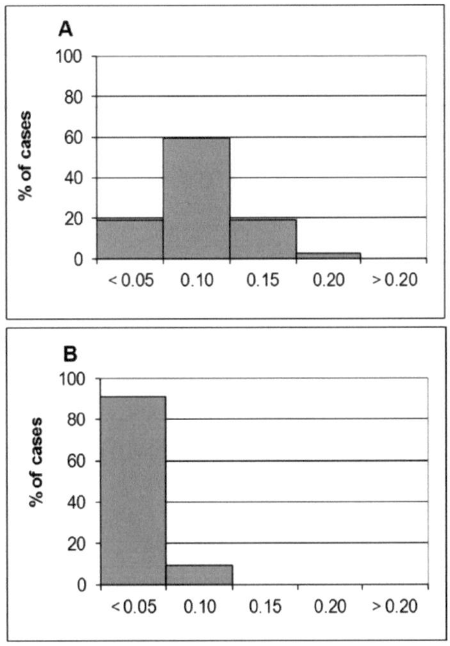

Figure 10. Distribution of the KYN/TRP ratios in healthy controls (A) in comparison with epileptic families (B).

This similarity of studied PLP-dependent disorders in epileptic probands and their asymptomatic first-degree relatives allows considering these disorders as inherent hidden traits of such families. Moreover, in clinically unaffected relatives these disorders are sometimes even more severe than in probands themselves (**Table 2**). The term "endophenotype" [64], as a heritable biochemical sign, which manifests in an individual whether or not illness is active and "co-segregated" with illness within the family, seems the most adequate definition of the state.

Judging by data obtained, *The inherent derangement of pyridoxine metabolism is a part of epilepsy etiology*. Repeated seizure attacks, superimposed on an inherently dysfunctional system of pyridoxine metabolism, may apparently provide extreme diversity of repeated results.

Van Gelder et al. [21–23, 65] were the first to find increased plasma levels of glutamate in first-degree relatives of epileptic patients just as in the patients themselves. The authors, however, considered their finding as a single symptom, rather than the manifestation of pyridoxine metabolism disorders. Later, these results were repeated, and plasma excess of aspartate and glycine along with the reduced level of urinary taurine was found in asymptomatic first-degree relatives of epileptic patients [66, 67], as well as in probands themselves. And again, the combination of biochemical alterations common to epileptic families was not explained, though PLP-dependent metabolism of amino acids pointed to the etiology of these familiar disorders.

We believe that reduced activity of alkaline phosphatase, the enzyme which dephosphorylates PLP and thus provides pyridoxal transport through membranes, may be the main factor of pyridoxine disorders in epileptic patients and their first-degree relatives.

http://dx.doi.org/10.5772/64691

In our experiments carried out in genetically epilepsy-prone and control epilepsy-resistant BALB/c mice (selectively bred from BALB/c strain for susceptibility or resistance to audiogenic seizures) [35, 36, 49], ALP activity in the cortex and hippocampus of seizure-naïve epilepsy-prone mice amounted to only 77.2 ± 6.7 and 74.1± 6.1% of activity inherent in epilepsy-resistant controls (Bresler a. Dolina, unpublished). In agreement with these data, the elevated PLP level was found in the brain of epilepsy-prone DBA/2 mice, in comparison with control epilepsy-resistant animals of the same strain [68].

Recently, it was shown that mice with a splice site mutation in the Akp2 gene for tissue nonspecific isoenzyme of ALP (TNSALP) have approximately 50% of normal plasma ALP activity and possess the elevated PLP plasma level, but do not manifest spontaneous seizures [69]. Unlike them, TNSALP knockout mice have 20-fold elevation of serum PLP level, large reduction in the intracellular brain PLP and lethal convulsions relieved by pyridoxal administration [70, 71].

We believe that disorders of pyridoxine metabolism in epileptic families are the consequences of inborn hypophosphatasia caused by a low activity of TNSALP. Mutations in *ALPL* gene, which encodes TNSALP, are responsible for the reduction of enzymatic activity [71–73]. The clinical spectrum of congenital hypophosphatasia presents a wide variety of phenotypes—from newborn, or infant convulsions controlled by pyridoxine [74–79] to their asymptomatic parents [80–84], whose ALP deficiency may be manifested, for example, by osteoarthropathy and/or odontohypophosphatasia. Diversity of these manifestations may depend on the extent of ALP activity reduction which, in its turn, depends on the variability of mutations in "candidate" ALP genes. Mutations in candidate genes may become the determining factor of pyridoxine metabolism disorders in epileptic families.

In their turn, disruptions of pyridoxine metabolism affect the production of PLP-dependent neurotransmitters. The imbalance of excitatory and inhibitory neurotransmitters becomes the neurochemical background of enhanced familial seizure predisposition.

We believe that *long-term* pyridoxine treatment started at early development (7–10 mg/kg daily) is safe and effective protective replacement therapy for a child born in epileptic families.

3. Conclusion

The pilot clinical trial carried out in children with different forms of epilepsy has confirmed our previous assumption of affected pyridoxine metabolism as an inborn genetic sign in epilepsy [35, 61]. We believe that clinical manifestations of inborn errors of pyridoxine metabolism are a kind of clinical continuum, ranging from severe convulsions resistant to AEDs to more common AEDs correctable forms of epilepsy, and up to remote symptoms in asymptomatic relatives of epileptic probands. This clinical continuum is open to *long-term high dose pyridoxine replacement therapy*. According to our experience, prolonged (over the years) pyridoxine treatment in pharmacological doses (10 mg/kg not exceeding 200 mg/daily) is valuable for different types of epilepsy (excluding—at least at present—absence and atonic forms). Being started at early stages of the disease and targeted at the stable correction of PLP-dependent metabolic disturbances, such a treatment will be effective by itself, and also as a background for AED management. It seems reasonable to suggest the same **long-term** pyridoxine treatment as a safe and effective protective replacement therapy for a child born in epileptic families.

Acknowledgements

The author is indebted to Dr. J. Levin for invaluable editorial corrections and wishes to acknowledge Mr. P. Danichev's excellent technical assistance and graphic presentation. The study was funded by Advance Neuroprotective System (ANS) sources.

Abbreviations

PDE	pyridoxine-dependent epilepsy
PLP	pyridoxal-5-phosphate
AED	antiepileptic drug(s)
GAD	glutamic acid decarboxylase
TRP	tryptophan
KYN	kynurenine
IDO	indoleamine 2, 3-dioxygenase (IDO)
3-HOKYN	3-hydroxykynurenine
3-HOAA	3-hydroxyanthranilic acid
KA	kynurenic acid
IND	indoxyl sulfate
4-PA	4-pyridoxic acid
ALP	alkaline phosphatase
TNSALP	tissue nonspecific isoenzyme of ALP

Author details

Svetlana A. Dolina

Address all correspondence to: dolina.svetlana@gmail.com

Advanced Neuroprotective Systems LTD., Ness-Ziona, Israel

References

[1] Hunt AD, Stokes JM, Crory Jr W, Stroud HH. Pyridoxine-dependency: report of a case of intractable convulsions in an infant controlled by pyridoxine. Paediatrics 1954;13:140–5. DOI:10.1177/088307389200700104.

[2] Surtees RA, Mills PB, Clayton P. Inborn errors affecting vitamin B6 metabolism. Future Neurol 2006;1(5):61520. DOI:10.2217/14796708.1.5.615.

[3] Mills PB, Footitt EJ, Mills KA, et al. Genotypic and phenotypic spectrum of pyridoxine-dependent epilepsy (ALDH7A1 deficiency). Brain 2010;133(7):2148–59. DOI:10.1093/brain/awq143 2148-2159.

[4] Bankier A, Turner M, Hopkins JJ. Pyridoxine-dependent seizures-a wider clinical spectrum. Arch Dis Child 1983;58:415–8. DOI:10.1016/S1570-9639(03)00045-1.

[5] Baxter P. Pyridoxine-dependent seizures: a clinical and biochemical conundrum. Biochim Biophys Acta 2003;1647(1–2):36–41. DOI:10.1016/S1570-9639(03)00045-1.

[6] Albersen M, Bosma M, Jans J, et al. Vitamin B6 in plasma and cerebrospinal fluid of children. PLoS One 2015;10(3):e0120972. DOI:10.1371/journal.pone.0120972.

[7] Gospe Jr SM, Olin KL, Keen CL. Reduced GABA synthesis in pyridoxine-dependent seizures. Lancet 1994;343(8906):7910233. DOI:10.1016/S0140-6736(94)90236-4.

[8] Cormier-Daire V, Dagoneau N, Nabbout R, et al. A gene for pyridoxine-dependent epilepsy maps to chromosome 5q31. Am J Hum Genet 2000;67:991–3. DOI: 10.1086/303087.

[9] Plecko B, Hikel C, Korenke GC, et al. Pipecolic acid as a diagnostic marker of pyridoxine-dependent epilepsy. Neuropediatrics 2005;36(3):200–5. DOI:10.1055/s-2005-865727.

[10] Plecko B, Paul K, Paschke E, et al. Biochemical and molecular characterization of 18 patients with pyridoxine-dependent epilepsy and mutation of the antiquitin (ALDH7A1) gene. Hum Mutat 2007;28(1):19–26. DOI:10.1002/humu.20433.

[11] Bennett CL, Huynh HM, Chance PF. Genetic heterogeneity for autosomal recessive pyridoxine-dependent seizures. Neurogenetics 2005;6:143–9. DOI:10.1007/s10048-005-0221-8.

[12] Walker V, Mills GA, Peters SA, Merton WL. Fits, pyridoxine and hyperprolinemia type two. Arch Dis Child 2000;82(3):236–7.

[13] Scriver CR, Beaudet AL, Sly WS, Valle D, editors. The metabolic and molecular bases of inherited disease. 8th ed. New York, NY: McGraw-Hill; 2001. p. 2863–913.

[14] Clayton PT. B6-responsive disorders: a model of vitamin dependency. J Inherent Metab Dis 2006;29(2–3):317–26. DOI:10.1007/s10545-005-0243-2.

[15] Goutieres F, Aicardi J. Atypical presentations of pyridoxine-dependent seizures: a treatable cause of intractable epilepsy in infants. Ann Neurol 1985;17(2):117–20.

[16] Yamamoto H, Murakami H, Horiguchi K, et al. Studies on the cerebrospinal fluid kynurenic acid concentration in epileptic children. Brain Dev 1995;17(5):327–9. DOI: 10.1016/j.visres.2003.11.003.

[17] Langlais PJ, Wardlow ML, Yamamoto H. Changes in CSF neurotransmitters in infantile spasms. Pediatr Neurol 1991;7(6):440–5.

[18] Yamamoto H, Shindo I, Egawa B, et al. Kynurenic acid is decreased in cerebrospinal fluid of patients with infantile spasms. Pediatr Neurol 1994;10(1):9–12.

[19] Appleton RE. Infantile spasms. Arch Dis Child 1993;69(5):614–8.

[20] Metzler DE. Biochemistry. The chemical reactions of living cells. New York, San Francisco, London: Academic Press; 2003.

[21] Van Gelder NM. Epilepsy and glutamic acid. Union Med Can 1980;109(7):996–1003.

[22] Van Gelder NM, Janjua NA, Metrakos K, et al. Plasma amino acids in 3/sec spike-wave epilepsy. Neurochem Res 1980;5(6):659–71.

[23] Perry TL, Hansen S. Amino acid abnormalities in epileptogenic foci. Neurology 1981;31(7):872–6.

[24] Sherwin AL, Van Gelder NM. Amino acid and catecholamine markers of metabolic abnormalities in human focal epilepsy. Adv Neurol 1986;44:1011–32.

[25] Sherwin A, Robitaille Y, Quesney F, et al. Excitatory amino acids are elevated in human epileptic cerebral cortex. Neurology 1988;38(6):920–3.

[26] Labiner DM, Yan CC, Weinand ME, et al. Disturbances of amino acids from the temporal lobe synaptosomes in human complex partial epilepsy. Neurochem Res 1999;24(11):1379–83.

[27] Ito M. Neurochemical approach to epilepsy. No To Hattatsu 1994;26(2):101–10.

[28] Bonhaus DW, Laird H, Mimaki T, Jamamura HI, Huxtable R. Possible bases for the anticonvulsant action of taurine. Prog Clin Biol Res 1983;125:195–209.

[29] Van Gelder NM. Pathologies of the CNS and associated taurine changes. Adv Exp Med Biol 1992;315:253–61.

[30] Yamamoto M, Takahashi S, Otsuki S, et al. GABA levels in cerebrospinal fluid of patients with epilepsy. Folia Psychiatr Neurol Jpn 1985;39(4):515–9.

[31] Pearl PL, Gibson KM. Clinical aspects of the disorders of GABA metabolism in children. Curr Opin Neurol 2004;17(2):107–113.

[32] Crawford PM, Chadwick DW. GABA and amino acid concentrations in lumbar CSF in patients with treated and untreated epilepsy. Epilepsy Res 1987;1(6):328–38.

[33] Spector R, Johanson CE. Vitamin transport and homeostasis in mammalian brain: focus on vitamins B and E. J Neurochem 2007;103:425–38.

[34] Dolina S. Is pyridoxine dependency an inborn error of metabolism triggering enhanced convulsibility in different animal models of genetic epilepsy? A commentary. Neurosciences 1992;18(Suppl. 2):153–62.

[35] Dolina S, Peeling J, Sutherland G, Pillay N, Greenberg A. Effect of sustained pyridoxine treatment on seizure susceptibility and regional brain amino acid levels in genetically epilepsy-prone BALB/c mice. Epilepsia 1993;34:33–42.

[36] Dolina S, Rabinkov A, Pressman E. Pyridoxal-5-phospate dependent kynurenine pathway in genetic epilepsy. Effect of persistent high dose pyridoxine treatment. In: 10th International Symposium on Vitamin B6 and Carbonyl Catalysis, Santa Fe, New Mexico, USA; 1999. p. 32.

[37] Dailey JW, Mishra PK, Ko KH, Penny JE, Jobe PC. Serotonergic abnormalities in the central nervous system of seizure-naive genetically epilepsy-prone rats. Life Sci 1992;50(4):319–26.

[38] Dalgliesh CE, Tekman S. The excretion of kynurenine and 3-hydroxykynurenine by man. Biochem J 1954;56:458–63.

[39] Hughes PAM, Bower BD, Raine DN, Syed N. Metabolism of tryptophan in childhood epilepsy. Arch Dis Child 1966;4:1642–51.

[40] Hughes PAM, Bower BD, Raine DN, Syed N. Effect of treatment on the metabolism of tryptophan in childhood epilepsy. Arch Dis Child 1967;42:281–8.

[41] Hansson O. Tryptophan loading and pyridoxine treatment in children with epilepsy. Ann NY Acad Sci 1969;166:306–9.

[42] Bender DA. The kynurenine pathway of tryptophan metabolism. In: Stone TW, editor. Quinolinic acid and the kynurenines. Boca Raton, FL: CRC Press, Inc.; 1989. p. 3–39.

[43] Stone TW. Endogenous neurotoxins from tryptophan. Toxicon 2001;39(1):61–73.

[44] Allegri G, Costa C, Baccichetti F, Biasiolo M. Effects of two different loading doses of L-tryptophan on the urinary excretion of tryptophan metabolites in rats, mice and guinea pigs. Correlation with the enzyme activities. Ital J Biochem 1987;36(3):194–203.

[45] Holmes GL. How to evaluate the patient after a first seizure. Postgrad Med 1988;83(2): 199–209.

[46] Holmes GL. Overtreatment in children with epilepsy. Epilepsy Res 2002;52(1):35–42.

[47] Connick JH, Heywood GC, Sills GJ, et al. Nicotinylalanine increases cerebral kynurenic acid content and has anticonvulsant activity. Gen Pharmacol 1992;239(2):235–9.

[48] Herve C, Beyne P, Jamault H, Delacoux E. Determination of tryptophan and its kynurenine pathway metabolites in human serum by high-performance liquid

chromatography with simultaneous ultraviolet and fluorimetric detection. J Chromatogr 1996;675:157–61.

[49] Dolina S, Margalit D, Malitsky S, Pressman E, Rabinkov A. Epilepsy as pyridoxine-dependent condition: Quantified urinary biomarkers for status evaluation and monitoring antiepileptic treatment. Med Hypothes 2012;79:157–64.

[50] Dolina S, Margalit D, Malitsky S, Rabinkov A. Attention-deficit hyperactivity disorder (ADHD) as a pyridoxine-dependent condition: Urinary diagnostic biomarkers. Med Hypothes 2014;82:111–16.

[51] Braunstein AE, Goryachenkova EV, Paskina TS. Enzymatic formation of alanine from l-kynurenine and l-tryptophan, and role of vitamin B6 in this process. Biokhimya (Russ) 1949;14:163–71.

[52] Soda K, Tanazawa K. Kynureninases: enzymological properties and regulation mechanism. Adv Enzymol 1979;49:1–40.

[53] Walsh HA, Bottling NP. Purification and biochemical characterization of some of the properties of recombinant human kynureninase. Eur J Biochem 2002;269:2069–74.

[54] Carpendo R, Chiardi A, Russi P, et al. Inhibitors of kynurenine hydroxylase and kynureninase increase cerebral formation of kynureninate and have sedative and anticonvulsant activities. Neuroscience 1994;61(920):237–43.

[55] Kazamatsuri H. Elevated serum alkaline phosphatase levels in epilepsy during diphenylhydantoin therapy. N Engl J Med 1970;283(25):1411–2.

[56] Kruse K, Bartels H, Gunter H. Serum alkaline phosphatase isoenzymes in epileptic children receiving anticonvulsant drugs. Eur J Pediatr 1977;126(4):237–42.

[57] Vouldris K, Moustaki M, Zies PM, et al. Alkaline phosphatase and its isoenzyme activity for the evaluation of bone metabolism in children receiving anticonvulsant monotherapy. Seizure 2002;11(6):377–80.

[58] Smith D, Defalla BA, Chadwick DW. The misdiagnosis of epilepsy and the management of refractory epilepsy in a specialist clinic. QJM 1999;92(1):15–23.

[59] Schmidt D, Löscher W. Uncontrolled epilepsy following discontinuation of antiepileptic drugs in seizure-free patients: a review of current clinical experience. Acta Neurol Scand 2005;111(5):291–300.

[60] Schmidt D, Schachter SC, editors. Epilepsy problem solving in clinical practice. Martin Dunitz; 2000.

[61] Dolina S. Is pyridoxine dependency an inborn metabolism error in genetic epilepsy? Pediatric epileptology. Cleveland, OH: Book of Abstracts; 1988. p. 35.

[62] Ubbink JB, Vermaak WJ, Delport R, et al. The relationship between vitamin B6 metabolism, asthma, and theophyllin therapy. Ann N Y Acad Sci 1990;585:285–94.

[63] Lumeng L, Aronoff GR, et al. Relationship between body store of vitamin B6 and plasma pyridoxal-P clearance: metabolic balance studies in humans. J Lab Clin Med 1985;106(5):491–7.

[64] Gottesman I, Gould TD. The endophenotype concept in psychiatry: etymology and strategic intentions. Am J Psych 2003;160:636–45.

[65] Janjua NA, Itano T, Kugoh T, et al. Familial increase in plasma glutamic acid in epilepsy. Epilepsy Res 1992;11(1):37–44.

[66] Haines JL, Panter SS, Rich SS, Eaton JW, Tsai MY, Anderson E, Opitz JM. Reduced plasma haptoglobin and urinary taurine in familial seizures identified through the multisib strategy. Am J Med Genet 1986;24(4):723–34.

[67] Monako F, Gianelli M, Scviavell MP, et al. Plasma amino acid alterations in idiopathic generalized epilepsy: an investigation in probands and their first degree relatives. Ital J Neurol Sci 1994;15(3):137–44.

[68] Chung SH, Cox RA. Determination of pyridoxal phosphate levels in the brain of audiogenic and normal mice. Neurochem Res 1983;8(10):1245–59.

[69] Polewski M, Johnson K, et al. Novel mouse model of autonomic semidominant adult hypophosphatasia has a splice site mutation in the tissue nonspecific alkaline phosphatase gene Akp2. J Bone Miner Res 2007;22(9):1397–407.

[70] Waymire KG, Mahuren JD, Jaje JM, et al. Mice lacking tissue non-specific alkaline phosphatase die from seizures due to defective metabolism of vitamin B-6. Nat Genet 1995;11:45–51.

[71] Narisawa S, Wennberg C, Millan JL. Abnormal vitamin B6 metabolism in alkaline phosphatase knock-out mice causes multiple abnormalities, but not the impaired bone mineralization. Pathology. 2001;193(1):125–33.

[72] Bloch-Zupan A. Hypophosphatasia: diagnosis and clinical signs-adental surgeon perspective. Int J Pediatr Dentistry 2016;83(3), 346–8. DOI: 10.1016.

[73] Henthorn PS, Whyte MP. Missense mutations of the tissue-nonspecific alkaline phosphatase gene in hypophosphatasia. Clin Chem 1992;38(12):2501–5.

[74] Baumgartner-Sigl S, Haberlandt E, Mumm S, et al. Pyridoxine-responsible seizures as the first symptom of infantile hypophosphatasia caused by two novel missense mutations (c.677T>C, p.M226T; c.1112C>T, p.T731I) of the tissue-nonspecific alkaline phosphatase gene. Bone 2007;40(6):1655–61.

[75] Nunes ML, Mugnol F, Bica I, et al. Pyridoxine-dependent seizures associated with hypophosphatasia in a newborn. J Child Neurol 2002;17(3):222–4.

[76] Yamamoto H, Sasamoto Y, Miyamoto Y, et al. A successful treatment with pyridoxal phosphate for west syndrome in hypophosphatasia. Pediatr Neurol 2004;30(3):216–8.

[77] Litmanovitz I, Reish O, Dolfin T, et al. Glu274Lys/Gly309Arg mutation of the tissue-nonspecific alkaline phosphatase gene in neonatal hypophosphatasia associated with convulsions. J Inherit Metab Dis 2002;25(1):35–40.

[78] Ozono K, Yamagata M, Michigami T, et al. Identification of novel missense mutations (Phe310Leu and Gly439Arg) in a neonatal case of hypophosphatasia. J Clin Endocrinol Metab 1996;81(12):4458–61.

[79] Smilari P, Romeo DM, Palazzo P, et al. Neonatal hypophosphatasia and seizures. A case report. Minerva Pediatr 2005;57(5):319–23.

[80] Stoll C, Fishbach M, Terzic J, et al. Severe hypophosphatasia due to mutations in the tissue-nonspecific alkaline phosphatase (TNSALP) gene. Genet Couns 2002;13(3):289–95.

[81] Sugimoto N, Iwamoto S, Hoshino Y, et al. A novel missense mutation of the tissue-nonspecific alkaline phosphatase gene detected in a patient with hypophosphatasia. Hum Genet 1998;43(3):160–4.

[82] Taillandier A, Cozien E, Muller F, et al. Fifteen new mutations (-195C>T, L-12X, 298-2A>G, T117N, A159T, R229S, 997+2T>A, E274X, A331T, H364R, D389G, 1256delC, R433H, N461I, C472S) in the tissue-nonspecific alkaline phosphatase (TNSALP) gene in patients with hypophosphatasia. Hum Mutat 2000;15(3):293.

[83] Watanabe H, Takinami H, Goseki-Sone M, et al. Characterization of the mutant (A115V) tissue-nonspecific alkaline phosphatase gene from adult-type hypophosphatasia. Biochem Biophys Res Commun 2005;327(1):124–9.

[84] Khandwala HM, Mumms S, Whyte MP. Low serum alkaline phosphatase activity and pathologic fracture: case report and brief review of hypophosphatasia diagnosed in adulthood. Endocr Pract 2006;12(6):676–81.

Section 2

The Psychiatric Issues in Epilepsy

Chapter 5

Epidemiology and Risk Factors for Suicide Among Adult Patients with Epilepsy

Anna Staniszewska, Marta Dąbrowska-Bender, Marcin Sobiecki, Grzegorz Juszczyk, Dominik Olejniczak, Aleksandra Czerw and Magdalena Bujalska-Zadrożny

Additional information is available at the end of the chapter

http://dx.doi.org/10.5772/64454

Abstract

Suicides constitute a serious public health issue worldwide. The number of suicide victims has been increasing over the years. Susceptibility to suicidal behaviour depends on the interaction of a number of factors. The reasons for taking a decision on committing suicide may objectively seem prosaic, and yet, according to the victim, cannot be resolved in any other way. Very often, it is the disease which is a risk factor for suicide. Suicidal thoughts, suicidal behaviours and suicide attempts as well as committed suicides occur far more frequently in epileptic patients than in the general population. There are many reasons for suicides committed by patients suffering from epilepsy. This paper presents basic data on epidemiology and risk factors of suicide attempts among patients with epilepsy. Risk factors in this group of patients include, inter alia, prior suicide attempts, co-morbidity of epilepsy with depression and other mental disorders, early onset (before 18 years of age), type and frequency of epileptic seizures and the use of anti-epileptic drugs, particularly in polytherapy.

Keywords: epilepsy, epidemiology, risk factors for suicide, suicide, antiepileptic drugs

1. Introduction

The World Health Organization (WHO) estimates that every 40 seconds one person dies as a result of suicide somewhere in the world [1]. Pursuant to data collected by the National Police

Headquarters 8579 suicide attempts have been reported, 6101 of which ended in death in the year 2013. The three main determined reasons for the suicides were family discord (n=999), mental illness (n=797) and chronic disease (n=570), and in the majority of cases investigators failed to determine the reasons behind the suicide attempt (n=3,663) [2]. Available literature suggests that the occurrence of a chronic disease is associated with increased vulnerability to suicidal behaviour [3]. The chronic nature of epilepsy, numerous limitations resulting from the disease, myths regarding the disease itself and persons affected by it as well as stigmatisation of patients all adversely affect the patients' well-being and quality of life [74]. Decreased self-esteem may in turn result in the occurrence of suicidal thoughts [4]. The aim of this paper is to describe epidemiological data and present risk factors for suicidal behaviour in patients with epilepsy. Taking these aspects into account in the treatment and secondary prevention regarding epileptic patients can help reduce that risk.

2. Prevalence of suicide in patients with epilepsy

Estimates from an 8-year observation period of epileptic patients confirm that 30% of patients die in accidents, 23% die suddenly, 16% die as a result of an epileptic seizure and 14% commit suicide [5].

Publication	Country	Observation period (in years)	Number of deaths	Number of suicides	Percentage of suicides
Cockerell et al. [10]	England	8	792	1	0.13%
Currie et al. [11]	England	7	666	3	0.45%
Elwes et al. [12]	England	11	102	1	0.98%
Hennessy et al. [13]	England	20	299	1	0.33%
Lhatoo et al. [14]	England	11.8	792	1	0.13%
Lindsay et al. [15]	England	13	100	1	1.00%
Lip et al. [16]	England	5	1000	3	0.30%
White et al. [17]	England	26	1980	21	1.06%
Bladin [18]	Australia	4	110	1	0.91%
McIntosh et al. [19]	Australia	10	325	4	1.23%
Ding et al. [20]	China	2.5	2455	4	0.16%
Dalby [21]	Denmark	16	346	2	0.58%
Lühdorf et al. [22]	Denmark	4	249	1	0.40%
Olesen et al. [23]	Denmark	10	6780	422	6.22%
Aikiä et al. [24]	Finland	>1	105	1	0.95%
Iivanainen and Lehtinen [25]	Finland	76	1481	13	0.88%

Publication	Country	Observation period (in years)	Number of deaths	Number of suicides	Percentage of suicides
Jutila et al. [26]	Finland	11	140	1	0.71%
Sillanpaa and Shinnar [27]	Finland	20	233	1	0.43%
Loiseau et al. [28]	France	1	804	1	0.12%
Shackleton et al. [29]	Netherlands	28	1355	7	0.52%
Rafnsson et al. [7]	Iceland	5	244	4	1.64%
Fukuchi et al. [5]	Japan	14	1722	6	0.35%
Camfield et al. [30]	Canada	8	692	3	0.43%
Garcia-Flores [31]	Mexico	20	112	5	4.46%
Guldvog et al. [32]	Norway	36	64	2	3.13%
Krohn [33]	Norway	10	107	3	2.80%
Stepien et al. [34]	Poland	9	54	2	3.70%
Zielinski [35]	Poland	2	6710	16	0.24%
Forsgren et al. [36]	Sweden	7	296	1	0.34%
Nilsson et al. [6]	Sweden	9	6880	26	0.38%
Chen et al. [37]	Taiwan	10	263	2	0.76%
Tsai [38]	Taiwan	1	1224	3	0.25%
Blumer et al. [39]	USA	12	10,739	5	0.05%
Day et al. [40]	USA	14	10,030	2	0.02%
Foldvary et al. [41]	USA	22	79	1	1.27%
Freytag and Lindenberg [42]	USA	11	294	9	3.06%
Quigg et al. [43]	USA	7	107	3	2.80%
Hauser et al. [44]	USA	39	618	3	0.49%
Mendez et al. [45]	USA	8	1611	4	0.25%
Salanova et al. [46]	USA	15	215	2	0.93%
Sperling et al. [47]	USA	4.5	583	2	0.34%
Kelemen et al. [48]	Hungary	6	94	1	1.06%
D'Alessandro et al. [49]	Italy	5	161	1	0.62%

Table 1. Frequency of suicides in the deaths of epileptic patients.

The risk of suicide in patients with epilepsy is greater than in the general population. The standardised mortality ratio (SMR) for suicides in patients with epilepsy as compared with the general population ranges from 3.5 to 5.8 [6, 7]. Based on a review of 21 studies, it has been estimated that on average 11.5% (0–67%) deaths of epileptic deaths are due to suicide [8].

Available epidemiological data indicate that the risk of suicides committed among epileptic patients is ca. 3–10 times greater compared to the general population. However, some researchers believe that this risk can be even greater, up to 25 times more in certain types of disease, e.g. in patients diagnosed with temporal lobe epilepsy [9]. **Table 1** summarises the number of deaths resulting from suicide when compared to all deaths among patients diagnosed with epilepsy within studies conducted in different countries.

The epidemiological data presented in **Table 1** differ substantially depending on the country and the area of the world. This results from the observation period and the population of epileptic patients.

3. Risk factors for suicide among epileptic patients

The motives behind suicide attempts in patients with epilepsy include factors characteristic for both the general population and factors typical of this disease.

Risk factors for suicide attempts have been listed by Patterson in the following abbreviation: SAD PERSONS—S, Sex (male); A, Age (elderly or adolescent); D, Depression; P, Previous suicide attempts; E, Ethanol abuse; R, Rational thinking loss, psychosis; S, Social support lacking; O, Organised plan to commit suicide; N, No spouse; S, Somatic sickness [3].

The above-mentioned risk factors for suicide are confirmed by other authors, adding to that list suicide attempts in the family and in the immediate environment, mental disorders, including anxiety apart from depression [8, 50, 51], white race, self-inflicted injury in the interview, and alcohol abuse [52].

Taking into account patients suffering from chronic diseases, the risk factors for suicide attempts include stigmatisation, discrimination, taking medication that possibly induces depression and easy access to toxic drugs [53]. Specific risk factors for suicide in epileptic patients can be grouped into several major categories.

3.1. Type of epileptic seizures

Additional risk factors in epileptic patients are related to the type of epileptic seizures. The risk of suicide attempts increase in the case of simple partial seizures, in primarily and secondarily generalised seizures with regard to partial complex seizures and temporal lobe epileptic seizures in male patients [54]. Furthermore, more frequent seizures, regardless of their type and the age at which the patient was diagnosed with epilepsy, also constitute risk factor for suicide attempts [9]. Additionally, it was found that the risk of suicide is over 5 times higher in patients with a 6-month history of the disease and that this risk decreases with the disease duration [55]. A study conducted in Finland among children below 16 years of age diagnosed with idiopathic or cryptogenic epilepsy reported two cases of suicide (where n = 122), however such self-destructive behaviour was not observed in children with symptomatic epilepsy [56].

3.2. Previous suicide attempts

It was also found that previous suicide attempts among epileptic patients increases the risk of another suicide in the future by ca. 38.4% when compared to the general population [57]. Similar results were obtained in a study conducted in Sweden, where that percentage amounted to 46.2%. Interestingly enough, not only epileptic patients are characterised by increased risk of suicide, but there is also a 5-times greater risk of epilepsy in persons who attempted to commit suicide prior to their diagnosis [58]. It is worth noting that this risk was not associated with the incidence of depressive disorders and alcohol abuse. Deterioration of cognitive functions and personality disorders resulting from the frequency of seizures increase the risk of suicide attempts [59].

3.3. Depression and other mental disorders

Many researchers are convinced that the main risk factor for suicidal thoughts in epileptic patients is co-morbid depression and other mental disorders. A study conducted in Canada demonstrated that during the lifetime of epileptic patients as compared with the general population, the following occur more often: depression (17.4% vs 10.7%), anxiety disorders (22.8% vs 11.2%) and suicidal thoughts (25% vs 13.3%) [60]. This was confirmed by results of a study conducted in Denmark on a group of 492 patients with epilepsy who committed suicide, as compared with the control group. It was proven that the risk of suicide increases over 29 times when an epileptic patient also suffer from a mental illness. In the same study, it was calculated that the risk of suicide in epileptic patients increases almost twofold in the case of a history of a mental illness [55]. It was found that in women suffering from epilepsy and with a history of mental illness, the risk of committing suicide is 23 times greater than in the case of women without these two conditions, and in comparison with men suffering from both epilepsy and a mental disease, that risk is 10 times higher [55].

It was also estimated that the risk of suicide in patients with epilepsy increases almost 14 times in the case of the co-morbidity of mental disorders, including 32 times more in the case of mood disorders and 12 times more in anxiety disorders [55]. Similarly, a study conducted in Sweden showed that co-morbidity of epilepsy with mental disorders is related to 9 times greater increase of suicide risk [6]. The MEPSY study carried out among Korean patients demonstrated that risk factors for suicide among epileptic patients include advanced depression (OR = 6.448; 95% CI = 3.739–11.120; $p < 0.001$), generalised anxiety disorder (OR = 3.561; 95% CI = 1.966–6.452; $p < 0.001$), as well as history of febrile seizures (OR = 2.188; 95% CI = 1.318–3.632; $p = 0.002$) [61]. Kanemoto et al. [62] observed a greater risk of suicide attempts in patients with temporal lope epilepsy who experienced psychotic episodes (7%) than during acute interictal psychosis (2%) or post-stroke confusion (0%).

3.4. Emotional and social disorders

Risk factors for attempted suicide in adult epileptic patients also include emotional disorders [63]. Buljan et al., a study carried out among hospitalised patients, have shown that next to mental disorders, another statistically significant risk factor for suicide attempts in epileptic patients is also a difficult family situation. The authors have estimated that 14.6% patients treated in Croatia attempted to commit suicide for that reason [50]. Results of the Hawton et al. [75] paper indicate a much higher percentage of suicide attempts among patients with epilepsy who have trouble finding employment. A multivariate analysis of logistic regression has confirmed that unemployment (Exp (B) 33.9; $p = 0.007$) is associated with suicidal thoughts in epileptic patients treated in Bosnia and Herzegovina, as is the sense of hopelessness (Exp (B) 14.9; $p = 0.001$) [64].

3.5. The use of antiepileptic drugs

Apart from current or past co-morbidity with psychiatric disorders, other risk factors include the use of anti-psychotics and the first instance of a seizure before 18 years of age [65]. In January 2008, the Food and Drug Administration (FDA) alerted that the use of anti-epileptic drugs (AEDs) is associated with an increased risk of suicide in patients who use them. FDA conducted an analysis of 199 placebo-controlled randomised studies on the risk of suicide attempts in connection with the use of 11 anti-epileptic drugs. The study included 27,863 patients treated with AEDS and 16,029 patients administered with placebo. Each group included at least 20 people treated for at least 7 days. The analysis included 25% of patients diagnosed with epilepsy, 27% of patients with mental disorders and 46% suffering from pain associated with the disease. Committed suicide was reported in four patients taking AEDs vs none patients in the placebo group; a suicide attempt was reported in 30 vs 8 persons, respectively, and suicidal thoughts were reported in 67 vs 29 persons, respectively. Relative risk of suicide for patients treated with AEDs vs placebo was 3.5 for people suffering from epilepsy, 1.5 for people with mental disorders and 1.9 for the remainder of the study group. FDA has concluded that patients using anti-epileptic drugs have a higher risk of suicidal thoughts and behaviour than the population taking a placebo [66].

In another study conducted on a population of 269,937 people aged ≥15 years of age, treated with anti-epileptic drugs, 26 suicides, 801 suicide attempts and 41 sudden deaths were reported. It was estimated that the risk of suicide behaviour was lower in patients using topiramate than in patients using gabapentin, lamotrigine, oxcarbazepine or tiagabine. However, an elevated risk of a sudden death occurred in a group of younger and older patients using gabapentin, in patients with mood disorders and epilepsy as compared with a group taking carbamazepine [67].

A study conducted on a group of 131,178 patients with epilepsy, pain, bipolar disorder, depressive disorder and schizophrenia demonstrated no difference in the risk of suicide for people using gabapentin [68].

Another study conducted in the United Kingdom compared 453 epileptic patients treated with AEDs with 8962 people in a control group matched in terms of age and gender. The anti-epileptic drugs used were classified into four groups: barbiturates, conventional AEDs, new generation AEDs with a low (lamotrigine, gabapentin, pregabalin, oxcarbazepine) or high (levetiracetam, tiagabine, topiramate, vigabatrin) depression-inducing effect. It was found that new generation AEDs with a high depression-inducing effect increased the risk of self-inflicted injuries/suicidal behaviours, it was however obvious only in patients with co-morbid mental disorders [69]. Yet another study shows that the use of barbiturates is associated with inducing depressive symptoms, which may lead to abnormal behaviour, depression and suicidal thoughts, particularly in children [70].

Drug	Mechanism of action	Risk of suicide
Phenobarbital	Effect on GABA No effect on glutamate No effect on serotonin	Proven suicidality risk
Phenytoin	Effect of Na^+ channels No effect on glutamate No effect on serotonin	Proven suicidality risk
Carbamazepine Oxcarbazepine Valproate Lamotrigine	Improve cognitive functions and mood in epileptic patients, and effect on serotonin	Antisuicidal properties
Topiramate Tiagabine Vigabatrin Levetiracetam	Exert negative effects on mood and cognition, and no effect on serotonin	Influence on suicidality has not been proven in evidence-based studies yet
Zonisamide	Exert negative effects on mood and cognition, but effect on serotonin	Influence on suicidality has not been proven in evidence-based studies yet
Gabapentin	Exert positive psychotropic effects on mood and cognition, but no effect on serotonin	Antisuicidal properties

Table 2. Antiepileptic drugs and risk of suicide [71].

A study based on data from the Danish National Prescription Registry concerning 169,725 AEDs (only 2.6% of prescribed for epilepsy treatment) confirmed increased risk of suicide (OR = 1.85; 95% CI = 1.4–2.5), in particular in patients treated with clonazepam, valproic acid, luminal and lamotrigine [23].

Furthermore, it was indicated that the use of anti-epileptic drugs in polytherapy is also a factor in the risk of suicide [65].

On the one hand, some AEDs can cause depression, which itself is the main risk factor for suicidality, but on the other hand, other AEDs have effect similar to antidepressants, and these properties exert antisuicidal effect. The AEDs differ mechanism of action, influence on cognition and mood in epileptic patients and suicidality. Probably, serotonin may play a role in the mechanism of action of some antiepileptic drugs. AEDs with serotonergic properties should reduce the suicidality risk, because they exert effects similar to antidepressants. Perhaps, psychotropic effects of AEDs may be the result of effects on the receptor functions: γ-gamma-aminobutyric acid (GABA) ergic and antiglutamatergic and neurochemical mechanisms [71]. **Table 2** shows the influence of some AED on suicide risk.

Not much data are available on the risk of suicidal attempts in a group of patients subjected to surgical treatment of epilepsy. A study that involved the observation of 396 patients subjected to surgical treatment of epilepsy indicates that 4 of the 27 reported deaths were caused by suicide, despite good control of epileptic seizures [72]. An analysis of the period which lapsed from the surgery indicates that the risk of a suicide attempt is greatest during the first 6 months after the surgical intervention [73].

During the past few years, a number of studies have been published trying to examine the correlation between AEDs and suicide. However, relationships between suicidal behaviour and AEDs are unclear, show a lack of concordance and are affected by a number of limitations (e.g., observational studies, more than one risk factor in patients with epilepsy).

4. Summary

An essential element of addressing this subject is to know all the possible risk factors for suicide attempts resulting both from the disease itself and additional causes in order to prevent suicide in epileptic patients effectively and in a timely manner. When conducting an interview, neurologists should pay special attention to whether the patient or his/her family has additional mental issues or whether any prior suicide attempts had been reported in the patient or his/her family. Additionally, when monitoring the treatment progress, it is necessary to verify the symptoms of depressed mood, in particular if the patient uses new generation anti-epileptic drugs, which can cause depression. A significant preventive factor also includes assessing the patient's social relationships (family, friends and work), in particular emotional problems, which can significantly impact suicide attempts.

Author details

Anna Staniszewska[1*], Marta Dąbrowska-Bender[2], Marcin Sobiecki[1], Grzegorz Juszczyk[2], Dominik Olejniczak[2], Aleksandra Czerw[2] and Magdalena Bujalska-Zadrożny[3]

*Address all correspondence to: anna.staniszewska@wum.edu.pl

1 Department of Experimental and Clinical Pharmacology, Medical University of Warsaw, Warsaw, Poland

2 Department of Public Health, Medical University of Warsaw, Warsaw, Poland

3 Department of Pharmacodynamics, Medical University of Warsaw, Warsaw, Poland

References

[1] Preventing suicide: A global imperative [Internet]. 2014. Available from: http://who.int/mental_health/suicide-prevention/world_report_ 2014/en. [Accessed: 2015-03-25]

[2] Suicide 2013 [Internet]. 2013. Available from: http://statystyka.policja.pl/st/wybrane-statystyki/samobojstwa/100065,Samobojstwa-2013.html [Accessed: 2015-03-25]

[3] Patterson WM, Dohn HH, Bird J, et al. Evaluation of suicidal patients: the SAD PERSONS scale. Psychosomatics. 1983;24(4):343-349. DOI: 10.1016/S0033-3182(83)73213-5

[4] Akiskal HS, Benazzi F. Psychopathologic correlates of suicidal ideation in major depressive outpatients: is it all due to unrecognized (bipolar) depressive mixed states? Psychopathology. 2005;38(5):273-280. DOI: 10.1159/000088445

[5] Fukuchi T, Kanemoto K, Kato M, Ishida S, Yuasa S, Kawasaki J, et al. Death in epilepsy with special attention to suicide cases. Epilepsy Research. 2002;51(3):233-236. DOI: 10.1016/S0920-1211(02)00151-1

[6] Nilsson L, Tomson T, Farahmand BY, Diwan V, Persson PG. Cause-specific mortality in epilepsy: a cohort study of more than 9.000 patients once hospitalized for epilepsy. Epilepsia. 1997;38(10):1062-1068. DOI: 10.1111/j.1528-1157.1997.tb01194.x

[7] Rafnsson V, Olafsson E, Hauser WA, Gudmundsson G. Cause-specific mortality in adults with unprovoked seizures. A population-based incidence cohort study. Neuro-epidemiology 2001;20:232-236. DOI: 10.1159/000054795

[8] Jones JE, Hermann BP, Barry JJ, Gilliam FG, Kanner AM, Meador KJ. Rates and risk factors for suicide. suicidal ideation. and suicidal attempts in chronic epilepsy. Epilepsy & Behavior. 2003;4(3):31-38. DOI: 10.1016/j.yebeh.2003.08.019

[9] Lambert MV, Robertson MM. Depression in epilepsy: etiology, phenomenology and treatment. Epilepsia.1999;40(10):21-47. DOI: doi: 10.1111/j.1528-1157.1999.tb00884.x.

[10] Cockerell OC, Johnson AL, Sander JW, Hart YM, Goodridge DM, Shorvon SD. Mortality from epilepsy: results from a prospective population-based study. Lancet. 1994;344:918-921. DOI: 10.1016/S0140-6736(94)92270-5

[11] Currie S, Heathfield KW, Henson RA, Scott DF. Clinical course and prognosis of temporal lobe epilepsy: a survey of 666 patients. Brain. 1971;94:173-190. DOI: 10.1093/brain/94.1.173

[12] Elwes RD, Dunn G, Binnie CD, Polkey CE. Outcome following resective surgery for temporal lobe epilepsy: a prospective follow up study of 102 consecutive cases. Journal of Neurology, Neurosurgery & Psychiatry 1991;54:949-952. DOI: 10.1136/jnnp.54.11.949

[13] Hennessy MJ, Langan Y, Binnie CD, Polkey CE, Nashef L. A study of mortality after temporal lobe epilepsy surgery. Neurology. 1999;53:1276-1283. DOI: 10.1212/WNL. 53.6.1276: 1526-632X

[14] Lhatoo SD, Johnson AL, Goodridge DM, MacDonald BK, Sander JW, Shorvon SD. Mortality in epilepsy in the first 11 to 14 years after diagnosis: multivariate analysis of a long-term, prospective, population-based cohort. . Annals of Neurology 2001;49(3): 336-344. DOI: DOI: 10.1002/ana.70

[15] Lindsay J, Ounsted C, Richards P. Long-term outcome in children with temporal lobe seizures: I. Social outcome and childhood factors. Developmental Medicine & Child Neurology. 1979;21:285-298. DOI: 10.1111/j.1469-8749.1979.tb01621.x

[16] Lip GYH, Brodie MJ. Sudden death in epilepsy: an avoidable outcome? Journal of the Royal Society of Medicine 1992;85:609-611.

[17] White SJ, McLean AE, Howland C. Anticonvulsant drugs and cancer: a cohort study in patients with severe epilepsy. Lancet. 1979;2:458-461. DOI: 10.1016/ S0140-6736(79)91505-8

[18] Bladin P. Psychosocial difficulties and outcome after temporal lobectomy. Epilepsia. 1992;33(5):898-907. DOI: 10.1111/j.1528-1157.1992.tb02198.x

[19] McIntosh AM, Kalnins RM, Mitchell LA, Fabinyi GC, Briellmann RS, Berkovic SF. Temporal lobectomy: long-term seizure outcome. late recurrence and risks for seizure recurrence. Brain. 2004;127:2018-2030. DOI: 10.1093/brain/awh221

[20] Ding D, Wang W, Wu J, Ma G, Dai X, Yang B, Wang T, Yuan C, Hong Z, De Boer HM, Prilipko L, Sander JW. Premature mortality in people with epilepsy in rural China: a prospective study. The Lancet. Neurology 2006;5:823-827. DOI: 10.1016/ S1474-4422(06)70528-2

[21] Dalby MA. Epilepsy and 3 per second spike and wave rhythms: a clinical electroencephalographic and prognostic analysis of 346 patients. Acta Neurologica Scandinavica. 1969;45(Suppl. 40):1-18. DOI: 10.1111/j.1600-0404.1969.tb02143.x

[22] Lühdorf K, Jensen LK, Plesner AM. Epilepsy in the elderly: life expectancy and causes of death. Acta Neurologica Scandinavica 1987;76:183-190. DOI: 10.1111/j. 1600-0404.1987.tb03565.x

[23] Olesen JB, Hansen PR, Erdal J, Abildstrøm SZ, Weeke P, Fosbøl EL, Poulsen HE, Gunnar H, Gislason GH. Antiepileptic drugs and risk of suicide: a nationwide study. Pharmacoepidemiology and Drug Safety. 2010;19(5):518-524. DOI: 10.1002/pds.1932

[24] Aikiä M, Jutila L, Salmenperä T, Mervaala E, Kälviäinen R. Comparison of the cognitive effects of tiagabine and carbamazepine as monotherapy in newly diagnosed adult patients with partial epilepsy: pooled analysis of two long-term, randomized, follow-up studies. Epilepsia. 2006;47(7):1121-1127. DOI: 10.1111/j.1528-1167.2006.00545.x

[25] Iivanainen M, Lehtinen J, Causes of death in institutionalized epileptics. Epilepsia. 1979;20(5):485-491. DOI: 10.1111/j.1528-1157.1979.tb04830.x

[26] Jutila L, Immonen A, Mervaala E, Partanen J, Partanen K, Puranen M, Kälviäinen R, Alafuzoff I, Hurskainen H, Vapalahti M, Ylinen A. Long term outcome of temporal lobe epilepsy surgery: analyses of 140 consecutive patients. Journal of Neurology, Neurosurgery & Psychiatry 2002;73:486-494. DOI: 10.1136/jnnp.73.5.486

[27] Sillampaa M. Social functioning and seizure status of young adults with onset of epilepsy in childhood: an epidemiological 20- year follow-up study. Acta Neurologica Scandinavica (Suppl.). 1983;96:1-81. DOI: 10.1111/j.1600-0404.1983.tb01529.x

[28] Loiseau J, Picot MC, Loiseau P. Short-term mortality after a first epileptic seizure: a population-based study. Epilepsia. 1999;40(10):1388-1392. DOI: 10.1111/j.1528-1157.1999.tb02010.x

[29] Shackleton DP, Westendorp RG, Trenite DG, Vandenbroucke JP. Mortality in patients with epilepsy: 40 years of follow up in a Dutch cohort study. Journal of Neurology, Neurosurgery & Psychiatry 1999;66:636-640. DOI: 10.1136/jnnp.66.5.636

[30] Camfield CS, Camfield PR, Veugelers PJ. Death in children with epilepsy: a population-based study. Lancet. 2002;359:1891-1895. DOI: 10.1016/S0140-6736(02)08779-2

[31] Garcia-Flores E. Surgical treatment of complex partial seizures: 20 years' experience. Stereotactic and Functional Neurosurgery 1994;62:216-221. DOI: 10.1159/000098622

[32] Guldvog B, Loyning Y, Hauglie-Hanssen E, Flood S, Bjornaes H. Surgical treatment for partial epilepsy among Norwegian children and adolescent. Epilepsia. 1994;35(3): 554-565. DOI: DOI: 10.1111/j.1528-1157.1994.tb02475.x

[33] Krohn W. Causes of death among epileptics. Epilepsia. 1963;4(1-4):315-321. DOI: 10.1111/j.1528-1157.1963.tb05228.x

[34] Stepien L, Bidzinski J, Mazurowski W. The results of surgical treatment of temporal lobe epilepsy. Polish Medical Journal 1969;8:1184-119.

[35] Zielinski J. Epilepsy and mortality rate and cause of death. Epilepsia. 1974;15:191-201. DOI: 10.1111/j.1528-1157.1974.tb04941.x

[36] Forsgren L, Edvinsson SO, Nyström L, Blomquist HK. Influence of epilepsy on mortality in mental retardation: an epidemiologic study. Epilepsia. 1996;37(10):956-963. DOI: 10.1111/j.1528-1157.1996.tb00533.x

[37] Chen RC, Chang YC, Chen TH, Wu HM, Liou HH. Mortality in adult patients with epilepsy in Taiwan. Epileptic Disorders 2005;7:213-219.

[38] Tsai JJ. Mortality of epilepsy from national vital statistics and University Epilepsy Clinic in Taiwan. Epilepsia. 2005;46(Suppl 11):8-10. DOI: 10.1111/j.1528-1167.2005.00400.x

[39] Blumer D, Montouris G, Davies K, Wyler A, Phillips B, Hermann B. Suicide in epilepsy: psychopathology, pathogenesis, and prevention. Epilepsy Behavior. 2002;3:232-241.

[40] Day SM, Wu YW, Strauss DJ, Shavelle RM, Reynolds RJ. Causes of death in remote symptomatic epilepsy. Neurology. 2005;65:216-222. DOI: 10.1212/01.wnl.0000169018.44950.68: 1526-632X

[41] Foldvary N, Nashold B, Mascha E, Thompson EA, Lee N, McNamara JO, Lewis DV, Luther JS, Friedman AH, Radtke RA. Seizure outcome after temporal lobectomy for temporal lobe epilepsy: a Kaplan-Meier survival analysis. Neurology. 2000;54:630-634. DOI: 10.1212/WNL.54.3.630: 1526-632X

[42] Freytag E, Lindenberg R. 294 medicolegal autopsies on epileptics. Archives of Pathology 1964;78:274-286.

[43] Quigg M, Broshek DK, Heidal-Schiltz S, Maedgen JW, Bertram EH. Depression in intractable partial epilepsy varies by laterality of focus and surgery. Epilepsia. 2003;44(3):419-424. DOI: 10.1046/j.1528-1157.2003.18802.x

[44] Hauser WA, Annegers JF, Elveback LR. Mortality in patientswith epilepsy. Epilepsia. 1980;21(4):399-412. DOI: 10.1111/j.1528-1157.1980.tb04088.x

[45] Mendez MF, Doss RC. Ictal and psychiatric aspects of suicide in epileptic patients. The International Journal of Psychiatry in Medicine. 1992;22(3):231-237. DOI: 10.2190/7PD3-C5MM-M0GJ-WJWT

[46] Salanova V, Markand O, Worth R. Temporal lobe epilepsy surgery: outcome. complications, and late mortality rate in 215 patients. Epilepsia. 2002;43(2):170-174. DOI: 10.1046/j.1528-1157.2002.33800.x

[47] Sperling MR, Harris A, Nei M, Liporace JD, O'Connor MJ. Mortality after epilepsy surgery. Epilepsia. 2005;46(Suppl 11):49-53. DOI: 10.1111/j.1528-1167.2005.00410.x

[48] Kelemen A, Barsi P, Eross L, Vajda J, Czirják S, Borbély C, Rásonyi G, Halász P. Long-term outcome after temporal lobe surgery – prediction of late worsening of seizure control. Seizure. 2006;15(1):49-55. DOI: 10.1016/j.seizure.2005.10.007

[49] D'Alessandro R, Guarino M, Greco G, Bassein L. Risk of seizures while awake in pure sleep epilepsies: a prospective study. Neurology.2004;62(2):254-257. DOI: 10.1212/01.WNL.0000103859.26880.6E: 1526-632X

[50] Buljan R, Santić AM. Suicide attempts in hospital-treated epilepsy patients. Acta Clinica Croatica. 2011;50(4):485-490.

[51] Mainio A, Alamäki K, Karvonen K, Hakko H, Särkioja T, Räsänen P. Depression and suicide in epileptic victims: a population-based study of suicide victims during the years 1988-2002 in northern Finland. Epilepsy Behavior 2007;11:389-393. DOI: 10.1016/j.yebeh.2007.05.012

[52] Grzywa A, Kucmin A, Kucmin T. Suicide problems – epidemiology, factors, motivesand prevention. Part I. Polish Medical Journal. 2009;161:432–436.

[53] Grabowska-Grzyb A. Psychiatric disorders in epilepsy. Polish Neurological Review. 2005;1(2):53–59.

[54] Kalinin VV, Polyanskiy DA. Gender and suicidality prediction in epilepsy. Epilepsy Behavior 2005;7:657-663. DOI: 10.1016/j.yebeh.2005.06.007

[55] Christensen J, Vestergaard M, Mortensen PB, Sidenius P, Agerbo E. Epilepsy and risk of suicide: a population-based case-control study. The Lancet. Neurology 2007;6:693-698. DOI: 10.1016/S1474-4422(07)70175-8

[56] Sillanpaa M, Shinnar S. Long-term mortality in childhood-onset epilepsy. The New England Journal of Medicine. 2010;363(26):2522-2529. DOI: 10.1056/NEJMoa0911610

[57] Harris EC, Barraclough B. Suicide as an outcome for mental disorders. A meta-analysis.. Archives of Neurology 1989;46:1065-1068. DOI: 10.1001/archneur.1989.00520460041011

[58] Hesdorffer DC, Hauser WA, Ludvigsson P, Olafsson E, Kjartansson O. Depression and attempted suicide as risk factors for incident unprovoked seizures and epilepsy. Annals of Neurology. 2006;59(1):35-41. DOI: 10.1002/ana.20685

[59] Ritaccio A, Devinsky O. Personality disorders in epilepsy. In: Ettinger AB, Kanner AM, editors. Psychiatric issues in epilepsy: a practical guide to diagnose and treatment. 2nd ed. Philadelphia: Lippincott Williams and Wilkins; 2007. p. 147-161.

[60] Tellez-Zenteno JF, Patten SB, Jetté N, Williams J, Wiebe S. Psychiatric comorbidity in epilepsy: a population-based analysis. Epilepsia. 2007;48(12):2336-2344. DOI: 10.1111/j.1528-1167.2007.01222.x

[61] Seo JG, Lee JJ, Cho YW, et al. Suicidality and its risk factors in Korean people with epilepsy: A MEPSY Study. Journal of Clinical Neurology 2015;11(1):32-41. DOI: 10.3988/jcn.2015.11.1.32

[62] Kanemoto K, Kawasaki J, Mori E. Violence and epilepsy: a close relation between violence and postictal psychosis. Epilepsia.1999;40:107-109. DOI: 10.1111/j.1528-1157.1999.tb01996.x

[63] Nuhu FT, Lasisi MD, Yusuf AJ, Aremu SB. Suicide risk among adults with epilepsy in Kaduna, Nigeria. General Hospital Psychiatry. 2013;35(5):517-520. DOI: 10.1016/j.genhosppsych.2013.04.012

[64] Andrijić NL, Alajbegović A, Zec SL, Loga S. Suicidal ideation and thoughts of death in epilepsy patients. Psychiatria Danubina. 2014;26(1):52-55.

[65] Nilsson L, Ahlbom A, Farahmand BY, Asberg M, Tomson T. Risk factors for suicide in epilepsy: a case control study. Epilepsia. 2002;43(6):644-651. DOI: 10.1046/j.1528-1157.2002.40001.x

[66] Information for Healthcare Professionals on Suicidality and Antiepileptic Drugs. [Internet]. 2008. Available from: http://www.fda.gov/cder/drug/InfoSheets/HCP/antiepilepticsHCP.htm. [Accessed: 2016-02-21]

[67] Patoro E, Bohn RL, Wahl PM, et al. Anticonvulsant medications and the risk of suicide, attempted suicide, or violent death. JAMA. 2010;303(14):1401-1409. DOI: 10.1001/jama.2010.410

[68] Gibbons RD, Hur K, Brown CH, et al. Gabapentin and suicide attempts. Pharmacoepidemiology and Drug Safety. 2010;19(12):1241-1247. DOI: 10.1002/pds.2036

[69] Andersohn F, Schade R, Willich SN, et al. Use of antiepileptic drugs in epilepsy and the risk of self-harm or suicidal behavior. Neurology. 2010;75(4):335-340. DOI: 10.1212/WNL.0b013e3181ea157e

[70] Brent DA, Crumrine PK, Varma RR, et al. Phenobarbital treatment and major depressive disorder in children with epilepsy. Pediatrics. 1987;80:909.

[71] Kalinin VV. Suicidality and antiepileptic drugs. Is there a link? Drug Safety.2007;30(2): 123-142. DOI:10.2165/00002018-20073002 0-00003

[72] Hamid H, Devinsky O, Vickrey BG, Berg AT, Bazil CW, Langfitt JT, et al. Suicide outcomes after resective epilepsy surgery. Epilepsy Behavior. 2011;20(3):462-464. DOI: 10.1016/j.yebeh.2010.12.031

[73] Bagary M. Epilepsy, antiepileptic drugs and suicidality. Current Opinion in Neurology. 2011;24(2):177-182. DOI: 10.1097/WCO.0b013e328344533e

[74] Zachwieja J. Effect of selected factors on the quality of life of people with epilepsy. The Journal of Neurological and Neurosurgical Nursing. 2013;2(3):117–124.

[75] Hawton K, Fagg J, Marsack P. Association between epilepsy and attempted suicide. Journal of Neurology, Neurosurgery & Psychiatry. 1980;43(2):168-170. DOI: 10.1136/jnnp.43.2.168

Chapter 6

Focus Laterality and Interface Between Depression and Anxiety in Patients with Temporal Lobe Epilepsy

Vladimir V. Kalinin, Elena V. Zheleznova,
Lyudmila V. Sokolova, Anna A. Zemlyanaya and
Kirill Subbotin

Additional information is available at the end of the chapter

http://dx.doi.org/10.5772/63562

Abstract

The aim of the current study was to evaluate an interaction between anxiety and depression in persons with temporal lobe epilepsy (TLE) in relation to foci lateralization. Ninety-four patients with temporal lobe epilepsy were included in the study (25 cases with left-sided focus activity, 25 cases with right-sided focus activity, and 44 patients with bilateral foci activity). The Hopkins Symptoms Check List (SCL-90) scale was used for psychopathological assessment. Pearson product moment correlations between nine constructs of SCL-90 were calculated separately for left-sided, right-sided, and bilateral foci groups. On the final stage, forward stepwise regression analysis was used for left-sided, right-sided, and bilateral foci groups separately. As dependent variables, the SCL-90 constructs of depression and anxiety were used. The obtained findings have shown the existence of close correlation between constructs of depression and anxiety in the right-sided focus and bilateral foci TLE patients, whereas the correlation was less expressed in the left-sided focus group. Regression analysis revealed the dependence of depression on anxiety and vice versa dependence of anxiety on depression in the right-sided focus group, but not the left-sided focus group. Depression and anxiety seem to represent one more solid syndrome in TLE patients with right-sided focus activity and rather two independent syndromes in TLE patients with the left-sided focus activity.

Keywords: temporal lobe epilepsy, focus laterality, affective disorder, anxiety disorder, SCL-90 constructs

1. Introduction

The concomitant psychopathological disorders, i.e., organic affective disorder and organic anxiety disorder are thought to be the most frequent co-morbid pathology in patients with temporal lobe epilepsy (TLE). Their frequency seems to achieve about 10–50% in TLE [1–6]. Nonetheless, the data on psychopathology of these states are scarce and rather controversial. It concerns the issue of possible relation between focus laterality and kind of prevailed affective symptoms in TLE. Thus, if some authors draw attention to the principal role of left temporal foci coupled with decreased functional state of frontal lobes in the genesis of depression, other researchers stress that the focus lateralization has no relation to the consequent affective disorder development [1–5].

Data on verified association between depression, anxiety and other concomitant symptoms and their interaction in TLE patients in relation with focus laterality are rather absent, although they could shed light on pathogenesis of affective and anxiety syndromes in terms of neuropsychiatry and evolution.

Here should be stressed that variables connected with right hemisphere are believed to be older and appear on earlier stage of phylogeny and ontogenesis, whereas the left hemisphere variables are much younger and appear on later stage of evolution [7]. If any discrepancies in certain signs and symptoms between both hemispheres existed, then probable evolutionary sequence of these variables could be suggested and their different role in mental disorders in terms of course and prognosis might be predicted.

In our previous study [8], we have shown that the diagnosis of organic affective disorder was observed more frequently in patients with right-sided foci, whereas the diagnosis of organic anxiety disorder in patients with left-sided foci ($\chi^2 = 7.0$ $p = 0.0081$; Fisher's exact test $p = 0.018$). In other words, the right-sided focus determines the symptoms of depression, whereas the left-sided focus causes the symptoms of anxiety in interictal period in TLE. In evolutionary terms, it implies that depression is older disorder than anxiety. Nevertheless, the certain co-morbidity between anxiety and depression exists in TLE patients with left-sided focus, and in lesser degree in patients with right-sided focus, and co-morbid anxiety and depression states usually appear more frequently in patients with left-sided focus activity [9, 10].

Principally, the similar association is true for patients with stroke, and persons with left hemisphere stroke are characterized by mixed anxiety and depressive symptoms in the form of the so-called catastrophic reaction (term proposed by Kurt Goldstein) compared with patients with right hemisphere stroke in whom the depression with prominent indifference usually appears [11–13].

2. Objective

The main aim of the current study was to evaluate an interaction between different psychopathological constructs (with principal emphasis on anxiety and depression) in persons with TLE in relation to focus lateralization.

3. Material and methods

The study has been carried out on 94 patients with TLE. Among all, studied patients were 38 men and 56 women. The focus laterality was detected strictly by visual EEG method, and data on ictal semiotics have not been used for this purpose. The left-sided foci were detected in 25 (11 men, 14 women) patients, the right-sided foci in 25 (11 men, 14 women) patients, and the bilateral foci in 44 (16 men and 28 women). The symptomatic form of TLE was diagnosed in 40 patients, and cryptogenic form in 54 patients.

All patients were evaluated by psychiatrists in order to set a psychiatric diagnosis. ICD-10 criteria were used for these purposes. In line with these criteria, the next disorders were diagnosed: (1) organic affective disorder (F06.3) (24 patients) and (2) organic anxiety disorder (F06.4) (48 patients).

Along with above-mentioned ICD-10 criteria, the diagnosis of "Interictal dysphoric disorder" also was used (22 patients), although it was not represented in ICD-10.

The rating of psychopathological symptoms of Hopkins Symptoms Check List (SCL-90) scale has been performed by patients themselves [14, 15]. Raw data of SCL-90 were then transformed into nine constructs that have been included in the final analysis of interaction between affective and anxiety syndromes. In accordance with SCL-90 design, the next nine constructs have been created: "somatization", "obsessive-compulsive", "interpersonal sensitivity" "depression", "anxiety", "hostility", "phobic anxiety", "paranoid ideation", and "psychoticism" [14, 15].

AED	Left-sided focus Mean daily dose and number of patients	Right-sided focus Mean daily dose and number of patients	Bilateral Foci Mean daily dose and number of patients
Topiramate	115.63±39.93 (n=8)	116.67±35.36 (n=8)	133.93±33.41 (n=14)
Valproates	1133.33±321.45 (n=5)	1105±520.42 (n=4)	1051.25±329.92 (n=13)
Carbamazepine	962.50±320.43 (n=8)	800.0±244.95 (n=8)	700.0±229.98 (n=10)
Phenobarbital	100.0±70.71 (n=4)	150.0±70.71 (n=5)	115.71±77.05 (n=7)

Table 1. Used antiepileptic drugs and their daily doses in studied patients.

All patients continued to intake antiepileptic drugs (AEDs) as monotherapy. The principal data on AEDs are listed in **Table 1**.

4. Statistics

All data were statistically processed by Statistica program (6th version) on personal computer. Student's *t*-test was performed on the first step for comparison of means of SCL-90 constructs in left-, right-sided foci, and bilateral foci groups.

The correlation analysis was chosen for purpose of evaluation of associations between the different psychopathological syndromes, and the product moment correlation (Pearson correlations) between all SCL-90 constructs was obtained separately within group with left-sided and right-sided foci activity for this purpose. The ratings of correlation between SCL-90 constructs have been compared between studied groups for purpose to find any possible discrepancies between them. A suggestion has been made that the closer correlation between two variables, the more common mechanism in their origin they have.

On the final stage, the multiple regression analysis (forward stepwise regression) was used for left-sided, right-sided, and bilateral foci groups separately. Multiple regression analysis has been selected as optimal for study of joint effect of a number of different factors on outcome variable [16, 17]. As dependent variables, the SCL-90 constructs of depression and anxiety subsequently were used.

5. Results

The principal results are depicted in **Tables 1–7**. In **Table 1**, the mean daily doses of AEDs are shown, and no statistically significant differences between compared groups are observed. In **Table 2**, the mean values of SCL-90 constructs are listed. No significant discrepancies between left-sided-, right-sided-, and bilateral foci groups on SCL-90 constructs have been obtained. It implies that focus lateralization has no influence on the expression of each SCL-90 construct, and their rates in both groups were practically equal.

SCL-90 construct	Left-sided focus	Right-sided focus	Bilateral foci
Somatization	8.78±5.64	6.43±5.24	7.07±6.38
Obsessive-compulsive	8.82±5.56	9.17±9.9	7.63±6.57
Interpersonal sensitivity	7.26±6.21	6.65±4.94	7.68±6.17
Depression	8.43±7.11	7.78±6.87	7.39±6.52
Anxiety	6.26±4.27	6.73±6.98	5.66±5.49
Aggressiveness & Hostility	3.65±2.87	4.52±4.25	4.20±3.52
Phobia	3.35±3.78	2.78±2.58	3.07±3.25
Paranoid ideations	3.48±3.88	4.00±4.34	3.70±3.34
Psychoticism	3.22±3.84	3.65±4.87	3.36±4.23

No statistically significant discrepancies were obtained.

Table 2. Values of SCL-90 constructs (Mean± Std.Dev.) in TLE patients with left-right-sided and bilateral activity.

	Somatization	Obsessions	Sensitivity	Depression	Anxiety	Hostiliy	Phobia	Paranoid ideations	Psychoticism
Somatization	-	**0.68**	0.40	0.39	**0.78**	**0.51**	**0.44**	**0.49**	**0.62**
Obsessions		-	**0.81**	**0.84**	**0.78**	**0.74**	**0.71**	**0.68**	**0.65**
Sensitivity			-	**0.80**	**0.67**	**0.62**	**0.72**	**0.77**	0.43
Depression				-	**0.60***	**0.79**	**0.53***	**0.52**	**0.65**
Anxiety					-	**0.74**	**0.62**	**0.77**	**0.68**
Hostility						-	0.34	**0.64**	**0.78**
Phobia							-	**0.55**	0.34
Paranoid ideations								-	**0.51***
Psychoticism									-

Note: significant Pearson product moment correlation (p <0.05) are marked by bold.

Table 3. Correlation matrix of SCL-90 constructs in TLE patients with left-sided focus.

	Somat	Obses	Sensit	Depres	Anxiety	Hostility	Phobia	Paranoid	Psychot
Somat	-	**0.80**	**0.73**	**0.77***	**0.85**	**0.62**	**0.58**	**0.73**	**0.86***
Obses		-	**0.69**	**0.69**	**0.77**	**0.59**	**0.65**	**0.83**	**0.93***
Sensit			-	**0.75**	**0.58**	**0.55**	**0.49**	**0.68**	**0.75***
Depres				-	**0.85**	**0.80**	0.28	**0.80**	**0.66**
Anxiety					-	**0.78**	**0.51**	**0.87**	**0.80**
Hostility						-	0.22	**0.71**	**0.60**
Phobia							-	**0.59**	**0.73***
Paranoid								-	**0,79***
Psychot									-

Note: significant Pearson product moment correlation (p<0.05) are marked by bold.
* - statistically significant differences in Pearson correlation between patients with left-sided focus and right-sided focus activity.

Table 4. Correlation matrix of SCL-90 constructs in TLE patients with right-sided focus.

	Somat	Obses	Sensit	Depres	Anxiety	Hostility	Phobia	Paranoid	Psychot
Somat	-	**0,46***	**0.58**	**0.72§**	**0.78**	**0.52**	**0.61**	**0.30***	**0.53***
Obses		-	**0.58§**	**0.54§**	**0.47§***	**0.41§**	**0.47**	**0.41***	**0.50***
Sensit			-	**0.77**	**0.73**	**0.79**	**0.77**	**0.66**	**0.75**
Depres				-	**0.82**	**0.71**	**0.75**	**0.59**	**0.83**

	Somat	Obses	Sensit	Depres	Anxiety	Hostility	Phobia	Paranoid	Psychot
Anxiety					-	**0.64**	**0.74**	**0.46***	**0.64**
Hostility						-	**0.85**	**0.71**	**0.83**
Phobia							-	**0.74**	**0.77**
Paranoid								-	**0.76**
Psychot									-

Note: significant Pearson product moment correlation (p<0.05) are marked by bold.
*- statistically significant differences in correlations between bilateral foci group and right-sided focus group.
§- statistically significant differences in correlations between bilateral foci group and left-sided focus group.

Table 5. Correlation matrix of SCL-90 constructs in TLE patients with bilateral foci.

In **Tables 3–5**, the correlation matrixes are shown for all SCL-90 constructs separately for groups with left-sided (**Table 3**), right-sided (**Table 4**), and bilateral focus activity (**Table 5**).

As can be seen in patients with right-sided focus, as a whole, the values of Pearson product moment correlation were higher than in the left-sided and bilateral group. Comparison between right-sided and left-sided groups revealed that the correlations between depression and other constructs, such as somatization ($r = 0.77$ versus $r = 0.39$), anxiety ($r = 0.84$ versus $r = 0.61$), and paranoid ideations (r = 0,78 versus $r = 0.54$) were higher in patients with the right-sided focus. Comparison of the right-sided focus patients with patients with bilateral foci also revealed higher correlations between somatization on the one hand, and obsessions ($r = 0.80$; $p < 0.01$), paranoid ideations ($r = 0.73$; $p < 0.01$), and psychoticism ($r = 0.86$; $p < 0.01$), on the other hand, in the right-sided focus group. Similarly, the correlation between anxiety and paranoid ideations was higher in the right-sided focus group ($r = 0.87$; $p < 0.001$) than in the bilateral foci group ($r = 0.46$; $p < 0.01$).

On the contrary, the correlation between depression and phobia was higher in the bilateral foci patients ($r = 0.75$; $p < 0.01$), than in the right-sided focus group ($r = 0.28$; n.s.) and left-sided focus group ($r = 0.53$; $p < 0.01$). In the right-sided focus patients, the associations of depression seem to be higher with somatization, anxiety, and paranoid ideations and less with phobia in comparison with the left-sided focus patients.

Data on the multiple regression analysis are listed in **Tables 6** and **7**. In **Table 6**, the results of multiple regression analysis for depression as dependent variable for three compared groups are presented. As can be seen, certain discrepancies between groups exist. In TLE patients with right-sided foci, the depression score was determined by rate of anxiety, obsessions, and interpersonal sensitivity, whereas the psychoticism reduced the final score of depression.

Similarly in the group with left-sided focus, the level of depression was determined by rate of obsessions and interpersonal sensitivity. Nonetheless, unlike the persons with right-sided focus, in patients with left-sided focus anxiety has not been interrelated with depression. In addition, a high level of paranoid ideations finally reduced score of depression. In other words, in patients with the left-sided foci depression and anxiety seem to be independent variables, whereas in the right-sided foci patients these constructs are interconnected.

Item	TLE patients with left-sided focus	TLE patients with right-sided focus	TLE patients with bilateral foci
Intercept	-0.324	-0.808	1.123
Somatization SCL-90	-0.240	-	0.158
Obsessions SCL-90	**+0.476**	**+0.438**	-
Interpersonal Sensitivity SCL-90	**+0.520**	**+0.592**	-
Anxiety SCL-90	-	**+0.839**	**+0.366**
Hostility and Aggression SCL-90	+0.320	-	-
Phobic anxiety SCL-90	-	-0.210	-
Paranoid Ideations SCL-90	**-0.370**	-	-
Psychoticism SCL-90	+0.216	**-0.710**	**+0.513**

Table 6. Forward stepwise regression analysis (values of beta coefficients) for the depression (SCL-90), as dependent variable in group with left-, right-sided and bilateral foci.

Item	TLE patients with left-sided focus	TLE patients with right-sided focus	TLE patients with bilateral foci
Intercept	+0.345	+1.268	-0.610
Somatization SCL-90	**+0.466**	+0.246	**+0.314**
Obsessions SCL-90	-0.220	**-0.460**	-
Interpersonal Sensitivity SCL-90	-	**-0.500**	+0.174
Depression SCL-90	-	**+0.545**	**+0.478**
Hostility and Aggression SCL-90	**+0.400**	-	-
Phobic anxiety SCL-90	**+0.292**	-	+0.243
Paranoid Ideations SCL-90	**+0.271**	**+0.448**	-
Psychoticism SCL-90	-	**+0.701**	-0.240

Note: Statistically significant values of beta coefficients are marked by bold.

Table 7. Forward stepwise regression analysis (values of beta coefficients) for the anxiety (SCL-90), as dependent variable in group with left-, right-sided and bilateral foci.

In the bilateral foci group, the rate of depression was determined by level of anxiety and psychoticism, and this implies that all these constructs are interconnected.

Similar findings on interaction between depression and anxiety were obtained based on regression analysis data when the anxiety was selected as dependent variable (**Table 7**). In the right-sided foci TLE patients, the final rate of anxiety was determined by the level of depression, and in addition by paranoid ideations and psychoticism, whereas the interpersonal sensitivity and obsessions reduced the final score of anxiety.

In the bilateral foci group, the rate of anxiety depends on the level of depression and somatization, whereas in the group with the left-sided foci, the level of anxiety was independent on depression, but was determined by constructs of somatization, hostility, aggression, phobic anxiety, and paranoid ideations.

6. Discussion

The current study was designed in order to analyze the influence of foci laterality in patients with temporal lobe epilepsy on psychopathological variables of SCL-90 with special emphasis on interaction between depression and anxiety. The study has certain limitations, and may be criticized for the lack of special psychometric scales, i.e., Hamilton rating scales for depression and anxiety. The psychometric quantified scales and the psychometric data have not been taken into account in the present study, since the controversial rate for their use exists, and some authors argue against their expansive use in psychiatry [18–20].

To our knowledge, this is the first attempt to analyze the effect of foci laterality on interaction between anxiety and depression in patients with TLE.

The main findings have shown that the right and left foci have an unequal effect on linkage between depression and anxiety in patients with TLE, although there has not been observed any effect of foci on mean average of any SCL-90 constructs. Moreover, as has been observed, the mean daily doses of used antiepileptic drugs had no statistically significant influence on the left-sided, the right-sided, and bilateral foci patients. It implies that obtained findings could not been caused by AEDs effect itself.

The principal results have shown that in patients with TLE with the right-sided focus and bilateral foci the closer association between symptoms of anxiety and depression exist, whereas in patients with left-sided foci this correlation is much less expressed. Moreover, multiple regression analysis could not reveal any statistically significant influence of anxiety on depression and vice versa in patients with left-sided foci, although the stable constellation of constructs including depression, interpersonal sensitivity, and obsessions was revealed in each hemisphere irrespective of focus laterality. It concerns strictly patients with unilateral foci, but not with bilateral foci. It implies the stable cluster pattern of depression, obsessions, and interpersonal sensitivity both in the right-sided- and in the left-sided focus patients can exist. Taking these data together, suggestion can be made that in the right-sided foci patients the more solid syndrome of depression with anxiety develops, whereas in the left-sided focus cases the looser associations between both disorders exist. In other words, in the cases of right-sided foci we may suggest the development of single poor differentiated syndrome, consisting of both depression and anxiety. On the contrary, in the patients with left-sided foci rather two independent syndromes (depression and anxiety) usually originate, and the so-called co-morbidity of depressive-anxiety disorders exists.

Despite the outer similarity in psychopathological symptoms in TLE patients with left-sided- and right-sided focus activity, the definite inner discrepancies in origin mechanisms of studied psychiatric disorders exist in relation to focus laterality. Probably, these discrepancies could explain the variability of drug responses in cases with externally similar affective and anxiety disorders, since their hemispheric origin is not usually taken into account. Psychiatric disorders with right hemisphere origin (in TLE patients with right focus activity) hypothetically are thought to be more favorable for antidepressant treatment, than disorders with left hemisphere origin (TLE patients with left focus activity), since the existence of two or more independent syndromes with different pathogenesis in the left-sided focus patients could be suggested, although this should be proven in a special study.

Data on correlation analysis in TLE patients with bilateral foci activity seem to be similar to findings on TLE patients with right-sided focus, and practically similar correlations between constructs of depression and anxiety in these groups exist. Obviously, the right-sided focus in patients with bilateral foci continues to have impact on syndrome genesis in manner similar to patients with definite right-sided- but not left-sided foci, although it concerns strictly constructs of depression and anxiety.

In our previous study, the preponderance of depression in patients with right-sided foci was observed. On the other hand, the higher frequency of anxiety disorder in patients with left-sided foci was obtained [8]. At the first glance, the certain contradiction with the findings of the current study exists. This contradiction seems to be explained by different methods used in these studies. Thus, in previous work [8], the diagnosis was made exclusively based on psychiatrists observations and data by Hamilton's rating scales for depression and anxiety were also used supplementary to physician decisions. In the present study, the subjective data of patients on the SCL-90 questionnaire were the corner stone of trial design. The more solid right-sided syndrome in the present study could be regarded by physicians as depressive one, although it may have as depressive, as anxiety symptoms. On the other hand, the left-sided syndrome due its more definite anxiety symptoms, independent of depression could be considered by psychiatrists as anxiety disorder, although it remains as pure speculative suggestion.

The rule, proposed Geodakian asserts, that signs and symptoms, associated with right hemisphere are older, than signs linked with left hemisphere [7]. In accordance with this paradigm, we may suggest that more monolithic depressive-anxiety syndrome revealed in cases with right-sided foci in evolutionary terms is older, than independent depression and anxiety, attributed to left hemisphere. Taking all these data, conclusion can be made on evolutionary direction of some psychopathological syndromes. The evolution of psychopathological signs goes from right hemisphere with less differentiated syndromes through bilateral foci to the left hemisphere with more differentiated signs, although this suggestion is thought to remain purely speculative. The independent anxiety and depression syndromes seem to be a prerogative of the left hemisphere. The current study should be continued in order to shed light on evolution of other psychopathological syndromes. Obtained findings stress the role of foci laterality in interaction between of depressive and anxiety syndromes in TLE, and may be presumably extrapolated on brain mechanisms of affective and anxiety disorders irrespective of epilepsy. If the proposed hypothesis was true, the right hemisphere involvement in the mechanisms of less differentiated symptoms of depression and anxiety and the left hemisphere involvement in the genesis of two separate syndromes of anxiety and depression should be suggested, although that speculative assumption should be proved in special studies.

Author details

Vladimir V. Kalinin*, Elena V. Zheleznova, Lyudmila V. Sokolova, Anna A. Zemlyanaya and Kirill Subbotin

*Address all correspondence to: doct.kalinin@mail.ru; research-kalinin@yandex.ru

Department of Brain Organic Disorders, Epilepsy of Moscow Research Institute of Psychiatry of Ministry of Health and Social Development, Moscow, Russia

References

[1] Hermann B.P., Seidenberg M., Woodard A. et al. Psychiatric comorbidity in chronic epilepsy: identification, consequence, and treatment of major depression. Epilepsia 2000; 41: S31–S41.

[2] Mendez M.F., Cummings J.L., Benson D.F. Depression in epilepsy. Significance and phenomenology. Arch Neurol 1986; 43: 766–770.

[3] Gilliam F.G., Santos J., Vahle V. et al. Depression in epilepsy: ignoring clinical expression of neuronal network dysfunction? Epilepsia 2004; 45(Suppl): 28–33.

[4] Kanner A., Nieto J. Depressive disorders in epilepsy. Neurology 1999; 53(Suppl 2): S26–S32.

[5] Kanner A. Depression in neurological disorders. Lundbeck Institute, Cambridge Medical Communication Ltd, 2005, 161 pp.

[6] Barry J.J., Ettinger A.B., Friel P. et al. Consensus statement: The evaluation and treatment of people with epilepsy and affective disorders. Epilepsy Behav 2008; 13(Suppl 1): S1–S29

[7] Geodakian V.A. Asynchronous asymmetry (sexual and lateral differentiation as a consequence of asynchronous evolution). J Higher Nervous Activity 1993, 43: 543–561 (in Russian).

[8] Kalinin V.V., Polyanskiy D.A. Focus laterality and interictal psychiatric disorder in temporal lobe epilepsy. Seizure 2009; 18(3): p. 176–179.

[9] Marsh L., Rao V. Psychiatric complications in patients with epilepsy: a review. Epilepsy Res 2002; 49: 11–33.

[10] Robinson R.G., Fiedorowicz J.G. Anxiety. In Coffey C.E., McAllister T.W., Silver J.M. (Eds.), Guide to neuropsychiatric therapeutics. Philadelphia, LWW, 2007, pp.138–169.

[11] Dam H., Pedersen H.E., Ahlgren P. Depression among patients with stroke. Acta Psychiatr Scand 1989; 80: 118–124.

[12] Kirshner H.S. Behavioral neurology. Practical science of mind and brain. Boston, Butterworth-Heinemann, 2002, 474 pp.

[13] Goldstein K. Language and language disturbances. Aphasic symptom complexes and their significance for medicine and theory of language. New York, Grune & Stratton, 1948, pp. 10–13.

[14] Derogatis L.R., Lipman R., Covi L. SCL-90: an outpatient psychiatric rating scale: preliminary report. Psychopharmacol Bull 1973; 9: 13–28.

[15] Derogatis L.R., Cleary P.A. Confirmation of the dimensional structure of SCL-90: a study of construct validation. J Clin Psychol 1977; 33: 981–989.

[16] Matthews D.E., Farewell V.T. Using and understanding medical statistics, 3rd ed., revised. Karger, Basel, 1996, 246 pp.

[17] Feinstein A.R. Principles of medical statistics. Boca Raton, Chapman & Hall/CRC, 2002, 701 pp.

[18] Nierenberg A., Sonino N. From clinical observations to clinimetrics: a tribute to Alvan R. Feinstein, M.D. Psychother Psychosomat 2004; 73: 131–133.

[19] Faravelli C. Assessment of psychopathology. Psychother Psychosomat 2004; 73: 139–141.

[20] Fava G.A., Ruini C., Rafanelli C. Psychometric theory is an obstacle to the progress of clinical research. Psychother Psychosomat 2004; 73: 145–148.

Chapter 7

Psychiatric Comorbidities and Quality of Life in Epilepsy

Ayşe Kutlu and Serap Mülayim

Additional information is available at the end of the chapter

http://dx.doi.org/10.5772/64880

Abstract

Epilepsy is a chronic disorder characterized by a spontaneous tendency to recurrent seizures which affects patients' cognitive, behavioral, psychological, and social functioning. Epileptic patients face various problems that result in a lower quality of life. Seizure frequency, drug side effects, psychological comorbidity, and stigma are the major factors affecting the quality of lives of patients with epilepsy. Depression, anxiety, psychosis, and cognitive impairment are some of the comorbid psychiatric problems accompanying the clinical picture in epilepsy. Also the role of antiepileptic drugs (AEDs) in psychopathology of epilepsy should not be underestimated. One of the most important reasons why health-related quality of life (HRQOL) has become important for epileptic patients is related with well-known characteristics of this disorder. Its chronic nature, presence of unexpected, intractable and frequent seizures, and stigma are some of these characteristics among others. With the review of the current literature, it can be concluded that there is still a need for further scientific research to find out more clear relation between epilepsy, comorbidities, and HRQOL.

Keywords: epilepsy, psychiatric comorbidities, quality of life

1. Introduction

Epilepsy is a chronic disorder characterized by recurrent seizures which impairs patient's quality of life through cognitive, behavioral, psychological, and social functioning [1]. It has been reported that the total lifetime risk for epilepsy and for any unprovoked seizure are 3.1 and 4.1%, respectively in industrialized countries. The estimation of annual incidence of epilepsy is reported as high as 43 cases per 100,000 of the population in so-called developed countries, and is almost double this figure in the developing world [2]. Another estimation points out that there are 50 million people who have epilepsy in the world [3, 4]. It was suggested that more than 80% of people with epilepsy live in developing countries, where the condition remains largely untreated [5, 6].

The science of health-related quality of life (HRQOL) measurements rapidly evolved during the 1980s and 1990s within general health and in all medicine disciplines [7]. HRQOL has become so important for patients with epilepsy (PWE) because of well-known characteristics of this disorder. Among these characteristics, chronic nature, unexpectability, intractable and/ or frequent seizures, stigma, and side effects of the antiepileptic drugs are acknowledged. Also, neurobiological, cognitive, psychological, and social consequences of epilepsy are very important [8].

Patients with epilepsy (PWE) encounter various problems due to this disorder which conduce a lower quality of life (QOL). Seizure frequency, side effects of the antiepileptic drugs, psychological problems, and stigma are the major factors determining severity of the disease and these factors may cause an important impact on life quality of PWE. Therefore, identifying the factors which mostly affect are important for improving epileptic patients' quality of lives [9].

2. Psychiatric comorbidities

2.1. Depression

Psychiatric disorders are frequent in epilepsy and they have a marked effect in QOL, morbidity, and mortality. Mood and anxiety disorders are the most frequent problems [10]. Depression is the most frequent psychiatric comorbidity in epilepsy, affecting one of every three patients with epilepsy in clinical studies [11] and lifetime prevalence rates of depression range between 30 and 35% in patients with epilepsy [10].

The International League Against Epilepsy (ILAE) has recognized the importance of comorbidities in the management of PWE. But, these comorbidities are usually ignored, unless they lead to a major disability. This may be related to several factors, such as patients not giving enough information about their psychiatric state or neurologists may not be specifically trained for these comorbidities [12]. In a recent study reported by Kanner et al., it was demonstrated that comorbid psychiatric problems affect the quality of life, so patients with subsyndromic depressive episodes (SSDEs), major depressive episodes (MDEs), anxiety disorders, and mixed MDEs (or SSDEs) with anxiety disorders have a significantly worse QOL than asymptomatic patients [13]. Authors also demonstrated that occurrence of mixed disorders resulted with unfavorable HRQOL than the occurrence of anxiety disorders alone. Another important finding of this study was that the comorbid occurrence of depression and anxiety disorders accompanied to epilepsy cause to important clinical results beyond their impact on HRQOL which include:

1. An increased suicidal risk.
2. A worse course and poorer response to treatment of a depressive disorder.

http://dx.doi.org/10.5772/64880

3. An increased risk of MDE recurrence; types of anxiety increased the probability of a new depressive episode.

4. Pharmacoresistant temporal lobe epilepsy patients encountered unsatisfied results including increased risk of failure to achieve seizure-free state after anterotemporal lobectomy [13].

Literature survey reveals enough evidence regarding the negative impact of mood disorders and anxiety symptoms on the quality of life of PWEs [14–20]. Symptoms of depression and anxiety are independently associated with reduced HRQOL; psychiatric comorbidity explains more variance in HRQOL than the combined groups of clinical seizure or demographic variables [18]. A study with a large sample included 435 PWEs aiming to investigate the relative impact of mood and anxiety symptoms as well as social- and seizure-related variables on HRQOL [21]; the presence of depressive symptoms was the strongest predictor of the composite and subscales of the Quality of Life in Epilepsy instrument used (QOLIE-31). In other studies conducted on patients with pharmacoresistant temporal lobe epilepsy (TLE), symptoms of depression were found to be the strongest independent predictors of poor QOL but (unexpectedly) not the seizure frequency or severity [14, 15, 17].

Kim et al. studied impact of depression and anxiety on adverse event profiles in Korean people with epilepsy. Consecutively, 453 patients who took antiepileptic drugs for at least 1 year completed self-reported questionnaires. They used Liverpool adverse events profile (LAEP), Beck Depression Inventory (BDI), and Beck Anxiety Inventory (BAI). In this study, it was reported that BAI, BDI scores, and the duration of antiepileptic drug treatment were significant predictors [22].

Another important point is the women with epilepsy of childbearing age. Increased risk of depression is a considerable problem for these patients. Lack of occupation, the presence of an underlying disabling condition (with treatment), and the severity of epilepsy are the significant properties accompanied to depression. Compared with the general population depressed women with epilepsy display greater impairment of HRQOL with epilepsy also images the physical, social, and emotional aspects of the disease [23].

Depressive disorders are associated with a worse response of seizures to antiepileptic drug treatment [24]. Hitiris et al. [25] retrospectively searched 780 patients with new onset epilepsy. Epileptic patients with a history of depression had two times more risk in developing refractory epilepsy.

Endocrine, neurotransmitter, and immunologic disturbances were found to be related with depression in patients with epilepsy. Especially, serotonin, glutamate, and GABA have an important role in epileptic seizures. Fluoxetine, a selective serotonin reuptake inhibitor (SSRI), has been shown to be effective in seizure prevention in a focal epilepsy model in rats [26]. Mazarati et al. studied an animal model of status epilepticus demonstrated abnormal 5-HT secretion in the raphe-hippocampal serotonergic pathway, lower serotonin concentrations in the hippocampus, and decreased serotonin release from the hippocampus following raphe stimulation [27]. Also, fluoxetine administration reversed the cortical hyperexcitability following status epilepticus. In animal models of depression, dysfunction of glutamate transporter proteins was shown, causing neuronal hyperexcitability and neuronal death [28]. In humans with depression, reduced expression of several glutamate transporter proteins was found in the frontal cortex and striatum in postmortem brain tissue that resulted in elevated synaptic glutamate concentrations [29]. By depression decreased cerebrospinal fluid concentration of GABA [30] and intracortical GABA signal on MR spectroscopy (MRS) [21, 28, 31–34] arises as a result of decreased GABAergic activity. For example, Rajkowska et al. [35] determined a significant decrease in GABAergic interneurons in the dorsolateral prefrontal cortex of the brains of the major depressive disorder patients (MDD) in a postmortem study which included 14 MDD patients (nine of whom died because of suicide) and nine controls [36]. Studies designed with transcranial magnetic stimulation (TMS), as a treatment modality for resistant MDD, also display decreased GABAergic activity in patients with depression [24].

2.2. Anxiety

Clinical studies found that 11–25% of PWE suffered from anxiety, which are higher proportions than healthy people [37]. These rates of depression and anxiety were close to that of drug-refractory epilepsy in a long-term population-based study [38]. The prevalence of depression or anxiety is higher in refractory epilepsy, and especially temporal lobe epilepsy (TLE), than in the general population of PWE [39–41]. The amygdala is important for the fear sensation. The avoidance behavior associated with fear is related to the output of the amygdala to the peri-aqueductal gray matter. Symptoms of anxiety disorders image the activation of the fear circuit involving structures of the hippocampus which is related with re-experiencing fear [42, 43]. Both in anxiety and epilepsy neurons discharging excitatory currents are associated with similar mechanisms [44]. Therefore, the amygdala and hippocampus play a critical pathophysiological role in both anxiety and epilepsy. The orbitofrontal cortex, insula, and cingulate gyrus are also essential in the central mediation of anxiety [45]. Inhibition of γ-aminobutyric acid (GABA)is an important factor in the pathogenesis of anxiety [44]. The $GABA_A$ receptor has an important role in controlling fear. Drugs affecting on $GABA_A$ receptors (like benzodiazepines and barbiturates) may increase the seizure threshold and also control anxiety symptoms by reducing neuronal excitability [46].

Tellez-Zentano et al. studied anxiety disorders in PWE; they found that people without epilepsy reported a lifetime incidence of 11.2% for any anxiety disorder compared with 22.8% in the group with epilepsy [10]. Rai et al. reported increased prevalence of depressive and anxiety disorders in people with epilepsy [47, 48].

We may think that the prevalence of anxiety disorders should be higher in refractory patients than in well-controlled patients. Brandt and Mula displayed a prevalence of 19.6% in patients with refractory epilepsy which is not different than the ratios reported in general epilepsy population [47]. Another important point stated was that the people with shorter epilepsy duration and younger age were more likely to have an anxiety disorder. This could show that the PWE can learn how to cope with the disease as getting older or with increasing duration of the disease. Also, it has been shown that patients in younger age and shorter duration of epilepsy are more likely to have anxiety disorders. This may be explained by patients acquiring coping strategies as years go by Brandt and Mula [47].

Depression and anxiety increase suicide risk, suicidal ideation, and stigmatization in PWE [37, 39]. Recent studies performed with newly diagnosed epileptic patients, identified depression, and anxiety as risk factors of drug-refractory epilepsy [13, 25]. These risk factors have also been associated with worse outcomes of epileptic surgery [49, 50]. In addition, depression and anxiety have been associated with increased adverse events in response to antiepileptic drugs (AEDs)in PWE [51]. Ultimately, the psychiatric and clinical effects of depression and anxiety can impair the quality of life (QOL)of PWE. Therefore, early detection and management of depression and anxiety are critical for the management of PWE.

2.3. Psychosis

There is a higher incidence of psychosis (9%) in PWE, when compared to the general population (1%) [52]. Psychoses in epilepsy have a complex psychopathology that is similar to the positive symptoms of schizophrenia and usually without negative symptoms [53]. Psychoses with seizure disorders can be classified as ictal, postictal, and interictal, depending on the onset of symptoms. Postictal psychosis most commonly appears within a week of the last seizure, whereas psychosis in forced normalization continues to manifest after normalization and with a clear state of consciousness [54]. Forced normalization can be defined by the emergence of psychosis after the control of seizures. The mechanism is unknown, but it can occur whether convulsions are controlled by medication, surgery, or neurostimulation [55]. Hilger et al. retrospectively analyzed 1434 patients with epilepsy, evaluated with prolonged EEG monitoring in order to estimate the prevalence of postictal psychosis (PP) and interictal psychosis (IP) [56]. They found that the overall prevalence of psychosis was 5.9%; prevalence of PP; and IP was 3.7 and 2.2%, respectively. They showed that the 97.6% of the patients with psychosis had localization-related epilepsy. Prevalence of psychosis was highest (9.3%) in patients with temporal lobe epilepsy [56].

2.4. Cognitive impairment

Cognitive impairment is a very important problem for PWE and their families. Memory impairment in epilepsy has been shown in neuropsychological studies and temporal lobe epilepsy (TLE) is an important risk factor. Brain training exercises in the form of activities such as reading, doing crosswords, and sudoku have been shown to improve memory function. Thompson et al. studied patients with temporal lobe epilepsy who had memory impairments. They showed that the traditional memory rehabilitation techniques can help to reduce the burden of memory impairment in temporal lobe epilepsy [57, 58].

Regarding the psychiatric comorbidities of epilepsy, Kanner highlighted some important points. First, he stated that the psychiatric disorders and epilepsy had a bidirectional relationship. The PWE have an increased risk of developing psychiatric comorbidities, but also patients with a primary psychiatric disorder have a greater risk of developing epilepsy. Second, he reported that the PWE with psychiatric comorbidities are less likely to become seizure-free with antiepileptic drugs (AEDs) and with epilepsy surgery. In addition, they are more likely to develop adverse events to AEDs. Finally, Kanner pointed out the importance of psychiatric evaluation of the patients with epilepsy especially who are being considered for surgery.

Because after epilepsy surgery, presurgical comorbid disorders may remit, recur, or be exacerbated [59].

2.5. Stigma

Stigma is associated with feared or perceived discrimination and an important psychosocial burden in people with epilepsy. Stigma among people with epilepsy brings out impairment in quality of life. Also, stigma is associated with aggravation of psychosocial burden like anxiety and depression for people with epilepsy [60]. Generally, prevention of seizures is not adequate in order to relieve the burden of epilepsy, also attenuating of perception of stigma matters for quality of life of individual with epilepsy [61]. Beside impact of stigma on quality of life of individual with epilepsy is frequently underestimated whereas stigma affects quality of life more than frequency of seizure and adverse effects of antiepileptic drugs.

Fisher demonstrated psychosocial symptoms like depression were quite important as initial reaction to the diagnosis of epilepsy and perceived stigma was associated with psychosocial symptoms [62]. A study which was intended to obtain certain demographic, clinical, and psychosocial traits associated with perceived stigma indicated that; being single, having poor quality of life, having difficulty in understanding the written information, and use of behavioral disengagement as a coping mechanism were enhancing factors for perceived stigma [63]. Previous studies demonstrated that low socioeconomic status compared with high socioeconomic status worsens the perception of stigma among PWE [61, 64]. Baker et al. published the largest population-based study to evaluate the stigma of epilepsy in 15 European countries [65]. Stigma data were collected from over 5000 PWE. Perception of stigma was correlated with anxiety, long-term health problems, injuries, and adverse effect of antiepileptic drugs [65]. Another study performed which the epilepsy-related stigma percentages were obtained from the previous largest population-based study. Results of the study suggested overall quality of health system, the health expenditure per capita, and the perceived quality of life have little effect on perceived stigma among individuals with epilepsy. Mentioned trail indicated the role of the public health system invests on awareness programs to increase public knowledge and reduce stigma [60]. Increasing the level of contact between PWE and people without epilepsy may lead changing negative public attitudes [66]. A trial aimed to investigate the relation between the level of knowledge about epilepsy and perception of stigma in adolescents and their mothers was performed. This trial demonstrated that the level of knowledge about epilepsy among adolescents with epilepsy was significantly related to their perception of stigma. As a result, knowledge of epilepsy can minimize the impact of perceived stigma, depressive feelings, and anxiety. This trial indicated also that correlation between the level of the maternal concealment behavior and adolescent with epilepsy's perception of stigma was more significant than maternal knowledge of epilepsy or maternal perception of stigma [67].

Stigma can be categorized into enacted stigma and perceived stigma [63]. Actual disapprobation and discrimination determined against individual with epilepsy is accepted as enacted stigma. However, perceived stigma is characterized as fear of encountering enacted stigma, feeling guilty, and shame about epilepsy. Epilepsy is not the only highly stigmatized illness but one of the most important of them like tuberculosis, leprosy, or HIV/AIDS [61].

In conclusion, epilepsy is a disease with many complications which lowers quality of life of PWE. Stigma, seizure frequency, drugs' adverse reactions, and neuropsychiatric issues are the major factors which are associated with the quality of lives of PWE.

2.6. Self-esteem

Self-esteem has been shown as the most important part of the ego and a major factor effecting psychosocial well-being [68]. The most important determinants of self-esteem are what we think of ourselves, how we assess ourselves when compared to others [68]. Literature analysis shows different results in the correlation between epilepsy and self-esteem [69–70]. Gauffin et al. studied self-esteem in young PWE and compared it with the earlier results [71]. They found that there was a decline in both sense of coherence and self-esteem overtime in young adults with epilepsy. On the other hand, Lee et al. reported that epilepsy in general has little impact on overall self-esteem in adolescents [71].

3. Antiepileptic drugs and suicidality

The pathogenesis of AED induced depressive symptoms is probably multifactorial. In which some of the factors are associated with the drug and other factors may be related to the patient. GABAergic properties, rapid titration of the drug, interaction with folate metabolism may be the drug-related factors. Whereas, poorly controlled seizures, structural abnormalities in the limbic system like small hippocampal volumes may be the patient-related factors [72].

May be the result of effects on the function of two types of receptor GABAergic and antiglutamatergic receptors are considered to be the two main receptors responsible from the psychotropic effects of AEDs but there may also be other possible mechanisms. Presumably, other neurochemical pathways especially a serotonergic mechanism should be considered in psychotropic effects of AEDs [73].

People with epilepsy seemed to have an increased risk for suicide. The risk increases with a history of a psychiatric illness. The AEDs may increase the risk of suicide in PWE, but it is not certain. Some AEDs shown to have negative effects on mood. Especially, barbiturates, vigabatrin, tiagabine, and topiramate were associated with depressive symptoms. In 2008, the Food and Drug Administration (FDA) drew attention on an increased risk of suicidality in people taking AEDs [74] and pharmaceutical companies had been asked to submit data from placebo-controlled trials of AEDs. Suicide-related adverse events occurring during double-blind treatment with an AED (concerning 11 AEDs) were searched. In this study, nearly 28,000 people taking AEDs and more than 16,000 people taking placebo were analyzed. In this analysis, the odds ratios for suicidality were increased for topiramate, but neither barbiturates nor vigabatrin were included in the analysis, and there were few suicidality events reported in the tiagabine trials. Carbamazepine, lamotrigine, and valproate are used as mood stabilizers. In the FDA analysis, carbamazepine and valproate were shown to have a nonsignificant protective effect against suicidality, whereas odds ratios of lamotrigine were significantly increased.

Further clinical prospective studies are needed to evaluate the relation between AEDs and suicidality because FDA analysis may have methodological concerns [72, 74].

Mood disorders, family history of a psychiatric illness, and risk of suicide must be carefully monitored in PWE. Psychiatry consultation must be organized for patients with such symptoms and it is very important to choose the AEDs according to both seizure type and the risk of possible drug induced depressive symptoms [72].

4. Quality of life in PWE

Previous researches regarding quality of life (QOL) in epilepsy showed many different results [75, 76]. Although most studies highlighted the negative effects of epilepsy on patients' quality of lives, there are still some other reports which showed minor or no effect [75, 76]. Some authors suggested that the impact of epilepsy might be minimal if the disease is stabile [75, 76]. On the other hand, epileptic patients living in Europe and North America were reported to have important impairment in HRQOL [77, 78]. The different results reported may be associated with the methodological and/or cultural factors. However, it can be easily noticed that especially in studies with larger samples, HRQOL is decreased in PWE [79, 80].

Baker et al. reported that epilepsy has the potential to negatively affect different aspects of quality of life [79]. They collected data from 3889 PWE from 10 different countries. In this multicenter study, it was shown that nervousness, headaches, and tiredness were the most frequent factors affecting the daily activities.

Short Form-36 (SF-36) was used in Baker et al.'s study and patients scored significantly lower in domains such as physical and social functioning, energy, and vitality [76]. In another multicenter study conducted by Baker et al., data from more than 5000 patients were analyzed and reported that epilepsy had a negative effect on patients' social and psychological well-being [80].

Kutlu et al. investigated the HRQOL, anxiety, and depression states of patients with epilepsy (PWE) [81]. The SF-36 scores were significantly lower in all subscales in PWE compared with the control group. Total scores for Beck Depression Inventory (BDI) were significantly higher in epilepsy patients. Hamilton anxiety scale was also significantly increased in PWE. It was concluded that epilepsy significantly effects with QOL of patients. In the patient group relationship between the seizure frequency and vitality was found to be statistically significant [81]. Birbeck et al. in their study evaluating ability of HRQOL measures to detect change overtime in people with epilepsy, suggested that SF-36 yielded responsiveness indices comparable to those of the epilepsy targeted measures [82].

Recently, Chen et al. studied factors affecting QOL in 260 PWE in Taiwan in a cross-sectional, correlational study. They used the Quality of Life in Epilepsy-31 (QOLIE-31) questionnaire for evaluating HRQOL [9]. In this study, scores for the QOLIE-31 were correlated with the demographic characteristics, sleep quality, symptoms of anxiety and depression, epilepsy-specific variables such as, seizure frequency; types, number, and frequency of AEDs; and adverse events of AED and social support. They reported that seven factors were predictive for quality of life: anxiety, depression, adverse events of AEDs, social support, seizure frequency of at least once in 3 months, household income of male gender. Another recent study was conducted by Mutluay et al., which they investigated the HRQOL in 124 PWE in Turkey [83]. This study measured the QOL in epilepsy and determined associated demographic and clinical factors by means of the Short Form-36 health survey. They found that patients with epilepsy do not perceive impaired physical health status. However, their mental health appears vulnerable, especially in women. In this study, the major burden was in the mental health category. They also reported that a positive treatment response is an important determinant of the HRQOL in PWE. Temporal lobe epilepsy (TLE) is the most common type of medically intractable epilepsy and is accepted as a prototype for a surgically remediable epilepsy when hippocampal sclerosis is the pathological substrate [84]. A reduction in seizure frequency and an improvement in the HRQOL are expected for patients with intractable epilepsy after epilepsy surgery [85]. Several studies indicate that complete seizure freedom is a strongly associated with psychosocial adjustment [86]. However, others show a poor correlation with postoperative seizure freedom. After surgery even if the seizures are completely lost, patients may still suffer from comorbidities such as depression, anxiety, and stigma. This can be explained by the "burden of normality" concept [84]. Patients' status changes from chronically ill to cured state in which the patient has to face the responsibilities of a normal life like finding a job and learn to continue and adjust life without the "advantages" of a chronic illness. Aydemir et al. studied 20 patients with intractable temporal lobe epilepsy who were waiting for surgery and 21 patients who had surgery. They used SF-36, Beck Depression Inventory, State Trait Anxiety Inventory, stigma and impact of epilepsy inventories, and a form asking their own perspectives about epilepsy and surgery. They found that QOL of patients after surgery was found to be better than before surgery. They also reported that seizure frequency, comorbidity, and AEDs affected HRQOL negatively. Impact of epilepsy levels was found to be higher among the preoperative patients [84]. A very important study was conducted by Taft et al. [87]. In this prospective study, HRQOL, mood, and patient satisfaction in epilepsy surgery candidates before and 2 years after epilepsy surgery was studied. They used Short Form Health Survey (SF-36), the Hospital Anxiety and Depression scale (HAD) at baseline and after 2-year follow-ups and also operated patients answered patient satisfaction questions. In patients who were seizure-free after epilepsy surgery HRQOL improved and anxiety decreased. Operated patients found surgery beneficial. But a very important point noticed in this study was that only about half of the seizure-free patients showed HRQOL improvements, in which that seizure freedom does not always improve patients' quality of lives.

5. Conclusion

Psychologically, PWE may have feelings of worthlessness, fear, stigma, anger, and hopelessness, and may exhibit passive behavior [88]. Stigmatization leads to discrimination, and PWE have been the target of prejudicial behavior in many aspects of life, over many centuries and in many cultures [89]. These factors decrease their psychosocial function, self-efficacy, and quality of life [90, 91] and even increase the suicide rate [90–92].

Recognition of the past and current comorbid psychiatric disorders needs to be incorporated into the evaluation of every PWE, including those with a newly diagnosed seizure disorder. Future research will need to determine whether an early remission of psychiatric disorders reverses the worse course of the seizure disorder. Finally, presurgical psychiatric evaluations must be conducted in all patients undergoing a presurgical evaluation.

Epilepsy, with its rich clinical features, is particularly important for HRQOL research. Epileptic patients may experience various problems which will result in a lower quality of life. Seizure frequency, side effects of the antiepileptic drugs, psychological comorbidity, and stigma are important factors associated with the severity of the disease and these factors may cause an important impact on life quality of epileptic patients. Stemming from a thorough review of the current literature, we can conclude that there is still a need for further scientific research with further validated instruments to find out more clear relation between epilepsy and HRQOL.

Author details

Ayşe Kutlu* and Serap Mülayim

*Address all correspondence to: draysekutlu@yahoo.com

Department of Neurology, Faculty of Medicine, Kocaeli University, Kocaeli, Turkey

References

[1] Foldwary N, Wyllie E. Epilepsy. In: Goetz GC, Pappert EJ, eds. Textbook of Clinical Neurology. Philedelphia: W.B. Saunders Company; 1999:1059–1088.

[2] McHugh JC, Delanty N. Epidemiology and classification of epilepsy. Int Rev Neurobiol. 2008;83:11–26.

[3] World Health Organization. International Classification of Functioning Disability and Health: ICF. Geneva: WHO; 2001.

[4] Leonardi M, Ustun TB. The global burden of epilepsy. Epilepsia. 2002;43(Suppl. 6):21–5.

[5] ILAE/IBE/WHO. "Out of the shadows": global campaign against epilepsy. ILAE/IBE/WHO Annual Report. Geneva: WHO; 1999.

[6] Meinardi H, Scott RA, Reis R, Sander JW. The treatment gap in epilepsy: the current situation and ways forward. Epilepsia. 2001;42:136–49.

[7] Tulsky DS, Rosenthal M. Quality of life measurement in rehabilitation medicine: building an agenda for the future. Arch Phys Med Rehabil. 2002;83(Suppl. 2):1–3.

[8] Mula M, Cock HR. More than seizures: improving the lives of people with refractory epilepsy. Eur J Neurol. 2015;22:24–30.

[9] Chen HF, Tsai YF, Mo-Song Hsi MS, Chen J. Factors affecting quality of life in adults with epilepsy in Taiwan: a cross-sectional, correlational study. Epilepsy Behav. 2016;58(26–32).

[10] Tellez-Zenteno JF, Patten SB, Jette N, Williams J, Wiebe S. Psychiatric comorbidity in epilepsy: a population-based analysis. Epilepsia. 2007;48:2336–2344.

[11] Kanner AM, Schachter SC, Barry JJ, Hersdorffer DC, Mula M, Trimble M, et al. Depression and epilepsy: epidemiologic and neurobiologic perspectives that may explain their high comorbid occurrence. Epilepsy Behav. 2012;24(156–168).

[12] Mula M, Kanner AM. Introduction—treatment of psychiatric disorders in adults with epilepsy: what every epileptologist should know. Epilepsia. 2013;54(Suppl. 1):1–2.

[13] Kanner AM, Barry JJ, Gilliam F, Hermann B, Meador KJ. Anxiety disorders, subsyndromic depressive episodes, and major depressive episodes: do they differ on their impact on the quality of life of patients with epilepsy? Epilepsia. 2010;51(7):1152–1158.

[14] Perrine K, Hermann BP, Meador KJ, Vickrey BG, Cramer JA, Hays RD, Devinsky O. The relationship of neuropsychological functioning to quality of life in epilepsy. Arch Neurol. 1995;52:997–1003.

[15] Gilliam FG. Optimizing health outcomes in active epilepsy. Neurology. 2002;58(Suppl. 5):9–19.

[16] Cramer JA, Blum M, Reed M, Fanning K, Epilepsy Impact Project. The influence of comorbid depression on quality of life for people with epilepsy. Epilepsy Behav. 2003;4:515–521.

[17] Boylan LS, Flint LA, Labovitz DL, Jackson SC, Starner K, Devinsky O. Depression but not seizure frequency predicts quality of life in treatment-resistant epilepsy. Neurology. 2004;62:258–261.

[18] Johnson EK, Jones JE, Seidenberg M, Hermann BP. The relative impact of anxiety, depression, and clinical seizure features on health related quality of life in epilepsy. Epilepsia. 2004;45:544–550.

[19] Loring DW, Meador KJ, Lee GP. Determinants of quality of life in epilepsy. Epilepsy Behav. 2004;5:976–980.

[20] Tracy JI, Dechant V, Sperling MR, Cho R, Glosser D. The association of mood with quality of life ratings in epilepsy. Neurology. 2007;68:1101–1107.

[21] Tracy JI, Dechant V, Sperling MR, Cho R, Glosser D. The association of mood with quality of life ratings in epilepsy. Neurology 2007; 68:1101–1107.

[22] Kim SK, Park SP, Kwon O. Impact of depression and anxiety on adverse event profiles in Korean people with epilepsy. Epilepsy Behav. 2015;46:185–191.

[23] Beghi E, Roncolato M, and Visona G. Depression and altered quality of life in women with epilepsy of childbearing age. Epilepsia. 2004;45(1):64–70.

[24] Kanner AM. Is depression associated with an increased risk of treatment-resistant epilepsy? Research strategies to investigate this question. Epilepsy Behav. 2014;38:3–7.

[25] Hitiris N, Mohanraj R, Norrie J, et al. Predictors of pharmacoresistant epilepsy. Epilepsy Res. 2007;75:192–6.

[26] Prendiville S, Gale K. Anticonvulsant effect of fluoxetine on focally evoked limbic motor seizures in rats. Epilepsia. 1993;34(2):381–4.

[27] Mazarati AM, Siddarth P, Baldwin RA, Sankar R. Depression after status epilepticus: behavioural and biochemical deficits and effects of fluoxetine. Brain. 2008;131:2071–83.

[28] Sanacora G, Mason GF, Rothman DL, Krystal JH. Increased occipital cortex GABA concentrations in depressed patients after therapy with selective serotonin reuptake inhibitors. Am J Psychiatry 2002;159:663–5.

[29] Zink M, Vollmayr B, Gebicke-Haerter PJ, Henn FA. Reduced expression of glutamate transporters vGluT1, EAAT2 and EAAT4 in learned helpless rats, an animal model of depression. Neuropharmacology. 2010;58:465–73.

[30] Bonanno G, Giambelli R, Raiteri L, et al. Chronic antidepressants reduce depolarization-evoked glutamate release and protein interactions favoring formation of SNARE complex in hippocampus. J Neurosci. 2005;25:3270–9.

[31] Gerner RH, Hare TA. CSF GABA in normal subjects and patients with depression, schizophrenia, mania, and anorexia nervosa. Am J Psychiatry. 1981;138:1098–101.

[32] Sanacora G, Gueorguieva R, Epperson, et al. Subtype-specific alterations of gamma-aminobutyric acid and glutamate in patients with major depression. Arch Gen Psychiatry. 2004;61:705–13.

[33] Bhagwagar Z, Wylezinska M, Jezzard, et al. Reduction in occipital cortex gamma-aminobutyric acid concentrations in medication-free recovered unipolar depressed and bipolar subjects. Biol Psychiatry. 2007;61:806–12.

[34] Sanacora G, Mason GF, Rothman DL, et al. Increased cortical GABA concentrations in depressed patients receiving ECT. Am J Psychiatry. 2003;160:577–9.

[35] Rajkowska G, O'Dwyer G Zsofia Teleki Z, Stockmeier CA, Miguel-Hidalgo JJ. GABAergic Neurons Immunoreactive for Calcium Binding Proteins are Reduced in the Prefrontal Cortex in Major Depression. Neuropsychopharmacology 2007 ;32(2):471–82.

[36] Price RB, Shungu DC, Mao X, Nestadt P, Kelly C, Collins KA, et al. Amino acid neurotransmitters assessed by proton magnetic resonance spectroscopy: relationship to treatment resistance in major depressive disorder. Biol Psychiatry. 2009;65:792–800.

[37] Kwon O, Park S-P. Depression and anxiety in people with epilepsy. J Clin Neurol 2014;10(3):175–88.

[38] Sillanpää M, Schmidt D. Natural history of treated childhood-onset epilepsy: prospective, long-term population-based study. Brain. 2006;129(Pt 3):617–24.

[39] Jacoby A, Baker GA, Steen N, Potts P, Chadwick DW. The clinical course of epilepsy and its psychosocial correlates: findings from a U.K. Community study. Epilepsia. 1996;37:148–161.

[40] Gaitatzis A, Trimble MR, Sander JW. The psychiatric comorbidity of epilepsy. Acta Neurol Scand. 2004;110:207–220.

[41] Perini GI, Tosin C, Carraro C, Bernasconi G, Canevini MP, Canger R, et al. Interictal mood and personality disorders in temporal lobe epilepsy and juvenile myoclonic epilepsy. J Neurol Neurosurg Psychiatry. 1996;61:601–5.

[42] Stahl SM. Brainstorms: symptoms and circuits, part 2: anxiety disorders. J Clin Psychiatry. 2003;64:1408–9.

[43] Rogawski MA, Löscher W. The neurobiology of antiepileptic drugs for the treatment of nonepileptic conditions. Nat Med. 2004;10:685–692.

[44] Mula M, Pini S, Cassano GB. The role of anticonvulsant drugs in anxiety disorders: a critical review of the evidence. J Clin Psychopharmacol. 2007;27:263–72.

[45] Rauch SL, Savage CR, Alpert NM, Miguel EC, Baer L, Breiter HC, et al. A positron emission tomographic study of simple phobic symptom provocation. Arch Gen Psychiatry. 1995;52:20–28.

[46] Mula M, Monaco F. Antiepileptic drugs and psychopathology of epilepsy: an update. Epileptic Disord. 2009;11:1–9.

[47] Brandt C, Mula M. Anxiety disorders in people with epilepsy. Epilepsy Behav. 2016;59:87–91.

[48] Rai D, Kerr MP, McManus S, Jordanova V, Lewis G, Brugha TS. Epilepsy and psychiatric comorbidity: a nationally representative population-based study. Epilepsia. 2012;53:1095–103.

[49] Cleary RA, Thompson PJ, Fox Z, Foong J. Predictors of psychiatric and seizure outcome following temporal lobe epilepsy surgery. Epilepsia. 2012;53:1705–12.

[50] de Araújo Filho GM, Gomes FL, Mazetto L, Marinho MM, Tavares IM, Caboclo LO, et al. Major depressive disorder as a predictor of a worse seizure outcome one year after

surgery in patients with temporal lobe epilepsy and mesial temporal sclerosis. Seizure. 2012;21:619–23.

[51] Liik M, Vahter L, Gross-Paju K, Haldre S. Subjective complaints compared to the results of neuropsychological assessment in patients with epilepsy: The influence of comorbid depression. Epilepsy Res. 2009;84:194–200.

[52] Kanner AM, Palac S. Neuropsychiatric complications of epilepsy. Curr Neurol Neurosci Rep. 2002;2(4):365–72.

[53] Hasija D, Jadapalle SLK, Badr A. Status epilepticus and psychosis of epilepsy. Psychiatr Ann. 2012;42(1):11–13.

[54] Schachter SC, Holmes GL, Trenité DK. Behavioral Aspects of Epilepsy: Principles and Practice. New York: Demos Medical Publishing; 2008:489–495.

[55] Loganathan MA, Enja M, Steven Lippmann S. Epilepsy and psychosis interaction. Innov Clin Neurosci. 2015;12(5–6):38–41.

[56] Hilger E, Zimprich F, Pataraia E, Aull-Watschinger S, Jung R, Baumgartner C, Bonelli S. Psychoses in epilepsy: a comparison of postictal and interictal psychoses. Epilepsy Behav. 2016;60:58–62.

[57] Thompson PJ, Duncan JS. Cognitive decline in severe intractable epilepsy. Epilepsia. 2005;46(11):1780–7.

[58] Thompson PJ, Baxendale SA, McEvoy AW, Duncan JS. Cognitive outcomes of temporal lobe epilepsysurgery in older patients. Seizure. 2015;29:41–5.

[59] Andres M. Kanner AM. Do psychiatric comorbidities have a negative impact on the course and treatment of seizure disorders? Curr Opin Neurol. 2013;26:2.

[60] Brigo F, Igwe SC, Ausserer H, Tezzon F, Nardone R, Otte WM. Epilepsy-related stigma in European people with epilepsy: correlations with health system performance and overall quality of life. Epilepsy Behav. 2015;42:18–21.

[61] Leaffer EB, Hesdorffer DC, Begley C. Psychosocial and sociodemographic associates of felt stigma in epilepsy. Epilepsy Behav. 2014;37:104–9.

[62] Fisher RS. Epilepsy from the patient's perspective: review of results of a community-based survey. Epilepsy Behav. 2000;1(4):9–14.

[63] Bautista RED, Shapovalov D, Shoraka AR. Factors associated with increased felt stigma among individuals with epilepsy. Seizure. 2015;30:106–112.

[64] Begley CE, Shegog R, Iyagba B, Chen V, Talluri K, Dubinsky S, et al. Socioeconomic status and self-management in epilepsy: comparison of diverse clinical populations in Houston, Texas. Epilepsy Behav. 2010;19:232–8.

[65] Baker GA, Brooks J, Buck D, Jacoby A. The stigma of epilepsy: a European perspective. Epilepsia. 2000;41:98–104.

[66] De Boer HM, Mula M, Sander JW. The global burden and stigma of epilepsy. Epilepsy Behav. 2008;12:240–6.

[67] Ryu HU, Lee SA, Eom S, Kim HD. Perceived stigma in Korean adolescents with epilepsy: effects of knowledge about epilepsy and maternal perception of stigma. Seizure. 2015;24:38–43.

[68] Winter DG. Personality, Analysis and Interpretations of Lives. New York: McGraw-Hill; 1996.

[69] Baker GA, Spector S, McGrath Y, Soteriou H. Impact of epilepsy in adolescence: a UK controlled study. Epilepsy Behav. 2005;6:556–62.

[70] Reeve DK, Lincoln NB. Coping with the challenge of transition in older adolescents with epilepsy. Seizure. 2002;11:33–9.

[71] Gauffin H, Landtblom AM, Räty L. Self-esteem and sense of coherence in young people with uncomplicated epilepsy: A 5-year follow-up. Epilepsy & Behavior 2010;17:520–524.

[72] Marco Mula M, Gail S. Bell GS, Sander JW. Suicidality in epilepsy and possible effects of antiepileptic drugs. Curr Neurol Neurosci Rep. 2010;10:327–32.

[73] Kalinin VV. Suicidality and antiepileptic drugs: is there a link? Drug Saf. 2007;30(2): 123–42.

[74] US Food and Drug Administration. Antiepileptic drugs and suicidality; 2008 May 23. Available at http://www.fda.gov/ohrms/dockets/ac/08/briefing/2008-4372b1-01-FDA.pdf. Accessed June 2008.

[75] Jacoby A. Felt versus inacted stigma: a concept revisited. Soc Sci Med. 1994;38:269–74.

[76] Leidy NK, Elizhauser A, Vickrey B, et al. Seizure frequency and health-related quality of life in adults with epilepsy. Neurology. 1999;53:162–6.

[77] Stavem K, Loge JH, Kaasa S. Health status of people with epilepsy compared with a general reference population. Epilepsia. 2000;41:85–90.

[78] Buck D, Jacoby A, Baker GA, et al. Cross-cultural differences in health-related quality of life of people with epilepsy: findings from a European study. Quality Life Res 1999;8:675–85.

[79] Baker GA, Jacoby A, Gorry J, Doughty J, Ellina V; on Behalf of the SIGN Group. Quality of life of people with epilepsy in Iran, the Gulf, and Near East. Epilepsia. 2005;46(1): 132–40.

[80] Baker GA, Jacoby A, Buck D, Stalgis C, Monnet D. Quality of life in people with epilepsy: a European study. Epilepsia. 1997;38(3):353–62.

[81] Kutlu A, Başaran S, Altun NS, Unalan H, Komsuoğlu SS. Quality of life, depression and anxiety in patients with epilepsy: controlled study with Short Form 36 Question-

naire, Beck Depression Inventory and Hamilton Anxiety Scale. Neurosurg Q. 2010;20(2):95–99.

[82] Birbeck GL, Kim S, Hays RD, Wickrey BG. Quality of life measures in epilepsy: how well can they detect change overtime? Neurology. 2000;54:1822–7.

[83] Mutluay FK, Gunduz A, Tekeoglu A, Oguz S, Yeni SN. Health related quality of life in patients with epilepsy in Turkey. J Phys Ther Sci. 2016 Jan;28(1):240–5.

[84] Aydemir N, Ozkara C, Canbeyli R, Tekcan A. Changes in quality of life and self-perspective related to surgery in patients with temporal lobe epilepsy. Epilepsy Behav. 2004;5(5):735–42.

[85] Kellett MW, Smith DF, Chadwick DW. Quality of life after epilepsy surgery. J Neurol Neurosurg Psychiatry. 1997;63:52–8.

[86] Selai CE, Elstner K, Trimble MR. Quality of life pre and post epilepsy surgery. Epilepsy Res. 1999;38:67–74.

[87] Taft C, Magnusson ES, Ekstedt G, and Malmgren K. Health-related quality of life, mood, and patient satisfaction after epilepsy surgery in Sweden—a prospective controlled observational study. Epilepsia. 2014;55(6):878–85.

[88] Chen HF, Tsai YF, Lin YP, Mo-Song Shih MS, Chen JC . The relationships among medicine symptom distress, self-efficacy, patient–provider relationship, and medication compliance in patients with epilepsy. Epilepsy Behav. 2010;19:43–9.

[89] Pahl K, de Boer HM. Epilepsy and rights. In: Atlas: epilepsy care in the world. Geneva: WHO; 2005. p. 72–3.

[90] Pramuka M, Hendrickson R, Zinski A, Van Cott AC. A psychosocial self-management program for epilepsy: a randomized pilot study in adults. Epilepsy Behav. 2007;11:533–45.

[91] Bell GS, Gaitatzis A, Bell CL, Johnson AL, Sander JW. Suicide in people with epilepsy: how great is the risk? Epilepsia. 2009;50:1933–42.

[92] Chen HF, Tsai YF. The psychosocial responses and coping strategies in the epilepsy. Chang Gung Nursing 2003;14:21–30.

Section 3

Antiepileptic Drugs: From Modes of Action to Clinical Efficacy and Side Effects

Chapter 8

Antiepileptic Drug Targets: An Update on Ion Channels

Ben A. Chindo, Bulus Adzu and

Karniyus S. Gamaniel

Additional information is available at the end of the chapter

http://dx.doi.org/10.5772/64456

Abstract

Different mechanisms of action have been proposed to explain the effects of antiepileptic drugs (AEDs) including modulation of voltage-dependent sodium calcium and potassium channels, enhancement of γ-aminobutyric acid (GABA)-mediated neuronal inhibition, and reduction in glutamate-mediated excitatory transmission. Recent advances in understanding the physiology of ion channels and genetics basis of epilepsies have given insight into various molecular targets for AEDs. Conventional AEDs predominantly target voltage- and ligand-gated ion channels including the α subunits of voltage-gated Na^+ channels, T-type, and α_2-δ subunits of the voltage-gated Ca^{2+} channels, A- or M-type voltage-gated K^+ channels, the γ-aminobutyric acid (GABA) receptor channel complex, and ionotropic glutamatergic receptors. Molecular cloning of ion channel subunit proteins and studies in epilepsy models suggest additional targets including hyperpolarization-activated cyclic nucleotide-gated cation (HCN) channel subunits, responsible for hyperpolarization-activated current (I_h), voltage-gated chloride channels, and acid-sensing ion channels. This chapter gives an update on voltage- and ligand-gated ion channels, discussing their structures, functions, and relevance as potential targets for AEDs.

Keywords: epilepsy, antiepileptics, voltage-gated ion channels, ligand-gated ion channels

1. Introduction

Epilepsy is one of the most common neurological disorders characterized by recurrent and repeated seizures that vary from the briefest lapses of attention or muscle jerks to severe and prolonged convulsions. Between 1 and 3% of the World's population suffers from epilepsy [1], making it the most prevalence neurological disorder. This debilitating neurological disorder may either be symptomatic of various disorders (e.g., malformative, vascular, infectious, traumatic, metabolic, or tumoral conditions) or idiopathic, which is unrelated to any underlying cause other than a possible hereditary predisposition [2].

The etiology of epilepsy is not fully understood; however, an abnormality of potassium conductance, a defect in the voltage-sensitive ion channels, or deficiency in the membrane ATPase likened to ion transport has been implicated in neuronal membrane instability and seizures [3]. Selective neurotransmitters such as glutamate, aspartate, acetylcholine, noradrenaline, histamine, corticotrophin-releasing factor, purines, peptides, cytokines, and steroid hormones enhance the excitability and propagation of neuronal activity, whereas γ-aminobutyric acid (GABA) and dopamine inhibit neuronal activity and propagation [3]. A relative deficiency of inhibitory neurotransmitters such as GABA or an increase in excitatory neurotransmitters such as glutamate would promote abnormal neuronal activity.

The control of abnormal neuronal activity with antiepileptic drugs (AEDs) is accomplished by elevating the threshold of neurons to electrical or chemical stimuli or by limiting the propagation of seizures discharged from its origin. The AEDs may attenuate or prevent seizures through effects on pathologically altered neurons of seizure foci or alternatively by reducing the spread of excitation from seizure foci to additional brain regions. Raising the threshold involves stabilization of neuronal membranes, whereas limiting the propagation involves reduction of nerve conduction and depression of synaptic transmission. Different mechanisms of action have been proposed to explain the clinical effects of AEDs including the modulation of voltage-dependent sodium channels, modulation of voltage-dependent calcium channels, enhancement of GABA-mediated neuronal inhibition, and reduction in glutamate-mediated excitatory transmission.

Ion channels play an important role in the pathophysiology of all forms of epilepsy, making them obvious targets for AEDs. Aberrant excitability associated with an epileptic discharge is mediated by voltage-gated and/or ligand-gated ion channels, which may be the result of defects in the function of these channels. Modern cellular neurophysiological and biochemical approaches have made it possible to identify these likely molecular targets of AEDs. This chapter gives an update on voltage- and ligand-gated ion channels, discussing their structures, functions, and relevance as potential targets for AEDs.

2. Voltage gated ion channels

This ion channels superfamily, which include the voltage-gated sodium, calcium, and potassium channels, represents the critical sites of action for AEDs. They comprise of 143 genes and encompass the S4 family in which the pore-forming subunits are built on six transmembrane segments (S1–S6), and the fourth segment (S4) contains a voltage-sensing element (**Figure 1**). The voltage-gated ion channels are primarily gated by changes in membrane potential, which cause movement of gating charges across the membrane and drive conformational changes that open and close the pore [4]. The detailed mechanism of voltage-dependent gating is not

http://dx.doi.org/10.5772/64456

well understood, but the positively charged S4 segments are thought to undergo outward and rotational movement through the protein structure during the gating process, as proposed in the sliding helix and helical screw models of gating [4].

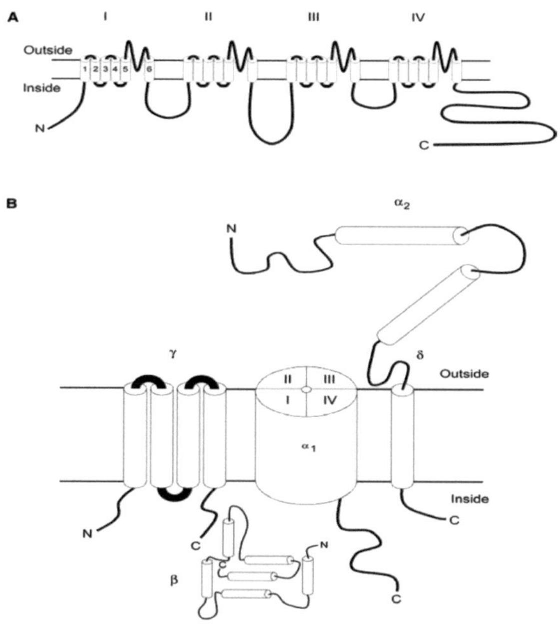

Figure 1. (A) The α subunit of voltage-gated ion channels consisting of four homologous repeats (I–IV), each with six transmembrane domains (1–6). The fourth transmembrane voltage sensor domain (4) has positively charged segments. (B) An assembled calcium channel with auxiliary (β, α-2δ and γ) subunits. The four homologous repeats (I–IV) a1 subunit form the channel pore. The sodium channels are similar, but only has auxiliary β subunits [5].

In voltage-gated Na^+ and Ca^{2+} channels, four domains referred to as I–IV or D1–D4 are expressed around a central pore that conducts the ionic current, while in voltage-gated K^+ channels, the channel is a tetramer of four individual subunits, each containing a single S1–S6 domain, which is also present in calcium-activated K^+ channels, cyclic-nucleotide-gated and the hyperpolarization-activated cyclic nucleotide modulated cation channels [4]. Voltage-gated ion channels also control excitability in the peripheral autonomic nervous system, the cardiovascular system and the digestive system as well as control all secretory functions including the release of hormones [6]. The voltage-gated Na^+, Ca^{2+}, and K^+ channels expressed in the heart are often distinct from, but closely homologous to, those expressed in the brain.

2.1. Voltage gated sodium channels (VGSCs)

The VGSCs are responsible for action potential initiation and propagation in excitable cells, including nerve, muscle and neuroendocrine cell types [7]. They are also expressed at low levels in nonexcitable cells where their physiological role is unclear [8]. VGSCs are heteromers composed of α and β subunits [9]. Four β subunits (β1–β4) have been described, and each α subunit is associated with one or more β subunits [10].

Nine mammalian VGSCs α subunits, designated $Na_v1.1$ to $Na_v1.9$, have been functionally characterized [11]. Four of these including $Na_v1.1$ (*SCN1A*), $Na_v1.2$ (*SCN2A*), $Na_v1.3$ (*SCN3A*) and $Na_v1.6$ (*SCN8A*) are predominantly expressed in the central nervous system and two—$Na_v1.7$ (*SCN9A*) and $Na_v1.8$ (*SCN10A*)—are expressed in the peripheral nervous system and dorsal root ganglia [11]. $Na_v1.4$ (*SCN4A*) and $Na_v1.5$ (*SCN5A*) are expressed in skeletal muscle and cardiac muscle, respectively, but the later is also found in some limbic neurons in the rat brain, including the peri-form cortex. $Na_v1.3$ is significantly expressed in the brain only early in development. $Na_v1.9$ (*SCN11A*) is expressed widely in the brain and spinal cord. There are four auxiliary (β) subunits ($Na_v\beta1$–$Na_v\beta4$; genes *SCN1B–SCN4B*) that can be found in association with the α-units expressed in the brain and have an intramembrane segment and an immunoglobulin-like extracellular element [11]. Fast, transient Na^+ currents that generate action potentials in the mammalian brain are mediated by $Na_v1.1$, $Na_v1.2$, and $Na_v1.6$ isoforms.

VGSCs are key mediators of intrinsic neuronal and muscle excitability making the abnormal VGSCs activity central to the pathophysiology of epileptic seizures. Mutations of neuronal voltage-gated Na^+ channel genes are the most common known cause of familial epilepsy including generalized epilepsy with febrile seizures plus (GEFS+) type 1 and 2, severe myoclonic epilepsy of infancy, intractable childhood epilepsy with generalized tonic-clonic seizures, simple febrile seizures (FS), benign familial neonatal-infantile seizures, and benign familial infantile seizures [12].

VGSCs mediate the persistent, resurgent, or late Na^+ currents that may play a significant role in epilepsy and in the action of AEDs [13]. Many of the most widely used antiepileptic drugs including phenytoin, carbamazepine, and lamotrigine are inhibitors of VGSC function. AEDs produce a voltage- and use-dependent block of the channels by binding predominantly to the inactivated state of the channels, thus suppressing high-frequency, repetitive action potential firing [14]. The downstream effect may reduce action potential-dependent synaptic neurotransmitter release during the high-frequency firing that occurs with epileptic discharges [15]. Some Na^+ channel blocking AEDs may preferentially inhibit glutamate release as a result of selective interactions with Na^+ channels that are located on presynaptic glutamatergic terminals [16]. Voltage-dependent Na^+ channel block may also reduce the propagation of action potentials from the soma into the dendrites and the dendritic amplification of synaptic potentials [17].

Several marketed AEDs including felbamate, topiramate, and zonisamide interact with other ion channel targets [18]. The combination of actions may contribute to the unique clinical efficacies of each of these drugs, suggesting that it may be possible to optimize the activity of drugs that target Na^+ channels with minimal adverse effects [4].

2.2. Voltage gated calcium channels (VGCCs)

The VGCCs are mediators of calcium entry into neurons in response to membrane depolarization [19], which results to a number of essential neuronal responses, such as the activation of calcium-dependent enzymes gene expression, the release of neurotransmitters from presynaptic sites, and the regulation of neuronal excitability [20].

VGCCs are classified into two major categories: the low voltage-activated (LVA) calcium channels (i.e., T-type channels) and the high voltage-activated (HVA) channels [18]. Some of the HVA channel subtypes can be activated at relatively negative voltages under certain circumstances. The LVA channels are activated by small depolarization near typical neuronal resting membrane potentials and are key contributors to neuronal excitability [4]. The HVA channels, which require larger membrane depolarization to open, are further subdivided into L-, N-, R-, P-, and Q-types [4]. The L-type channels are found on cell bodies where they participate, among other functions, in the activation of calcium-dependent enzymes and in calcium-dependent gene transcription events [21]. P- and Q-type channels, like N-type channels, are concentrated at presynaptic nerve terminals where they are linked to the release of neurotransmitters [22]. In the context of neurotransmitter release, N-type channels tend to support inhibitory neurotransmission, whereas the P/Q-type channels have more frequently been linked to the release of excitatory neurotransmitters but can also support inhibitory release [23]. R-type channels are distributed in proximal dendrites and presynaptic nerve termini [24]. Their precise physiological function remains enigmatic; however, there is evidence that these channels may mediate neurotransmitter release at select synapses [25].

HVA calcium channels are heteromultimers that are formed through association of α_1, β, α_2-δ, and γ subunits. Conversely, the LVA channels may contain only the $\alpha 1$ subunit. The $\alpha 1$ subunit is the pore-forming subunit of both LVA and HVA calcium channels that are sufficient to form a voltage-gated calcium-selective pore by itself and it is the sole determinant of the calcium channel subtype [18]. The $\alpha 1$ subunit is associated with auxiliary subunits including the intracellular β subunits ($\beta 1$–$\beta 4$), the largely intramembranal γ subunits ($\gamma 1$–$\gamma 8$), and the intramembranal/extracellular $\alpha 2$-δ subunits (types 1–4) that are unrelated to the sodium channel auxiliary subunits [18].

Ten functional calcium channel $\alpha 1$ subunits are known in vertebrates, which fall into three major classes (Ca_v1, Ca_v2, and Ca_v3) according to their physiological functions and regulations [26]. The Ca_v1 subfamily ($Ca_v1.1$ to $Ca_v1.4$) conducts L-type calcium currents [27], while the Ca_v2 subfamily ($Ca_v2.1$ to $Ca_v2.3$) conducts N-, P/Q- and R-type calcium currents that initiate fast synaptic transmission at synapses in the central and peripheral nervous systems [28]. Among the Ca_v2 family, alternate splice isoforms of $Ca_v2.1$ encode P- and Q-type channels, $Ca_v2.2$ represents N-type channels, and $Ca_v2.3$ corresponds to R-type channels [28]. The Ca_v3 family represents three different types of T-type channels (i.e., $Ca_v3.1$, $Ca_v3.2$, and $Ca_v3.3$) with distinct kinetic properties.

A variety of mutations involving voltage-gated Ca^{2+} channels have been identified in mice that exhibit absence-like seizures [29]. Three recessive mutations in *Cacna1a* ($Ca_v2.1$) that produce absence-like syndromes in *tottering*, *leaner* and *rocker* mice impair channel function, reducing P/Q-type Ca^{2+} currents. L-type channels have not been associated with epilepsy syndromes in mice or humans and are not considered to be targets for AEDs.

AEDs have been reported to inhibit Ca^{2+} currents with the T-type Ca^{2+} channels being the primary target for seizure protection. The T-type Ca^{2+} channels are believed to be the targets of antiabsence agents such as ethosuximide that weakly block native and recombinant T-type Ca^{2+} channel currents [30]. The anticonvulsant action of the barbiturate phenobarbital may be due, in part, to inhibition of Ca^{2+} current as well as an action on $GABA_A$ receptors [31]. Lamotrigine that is widely believed to act primarily on voltage-gated Na^+ channels also inhibits high voltage-activated N- and P/Q-type Ca^{2+} channels and inhibits R-type minimally [32].

The molecular targets for gabapentin and pregabalin are α2-δ proteins, particularly the α2-δ-1 and α2-δ-2 proteins [33, 34]. The exact mechanism by which binding to these proteins protects against seizures is not fully understood. Studies have shown inhibitory effects on voltage-gated Ca^{2+} currents that can selectively block either P/Q- or N-type Ca^{2+} channels [35]. Other studies have shown inhibition of the release of neurotransmitters [36]. Gabapentin and pregabalin inhibit neurotransmitter release in many systems mainly by interaction of α2-δ with synaptic proteins that are involved in the release or trafficking of synaptic vesicles rather than inhibition of calcium influx [4]. The variability in the effects on Ca^{2+} current may relate to differences in expression of the α2-δ subunit in different cell types or in response to different conditions.

2.3. Voltage gated potassium channels (K_V)

Voltage-gated potassium channels are the most diverse group of ion channels that play a key role in setting the resting membrane potential and serve to limit excitability in neural cells. They are activated by depolarization and the outward movement of potassium ions through these channels repolarizes the membrane to end action potentials and hyperpolarizes the membrane potential immediately following action potentials [6].

A typical K^+ channel is a tetramer of α subunits that can assemble into homo- and hetero-tetramers, leading to a wide diversity of different channel complexes including the six transmembrane helix voltage-gated (K_v) channels, the two transmembrane-helix inward-rectifier (K_{ir}) channels, the Ca^{2+}-activated K^+ channels (K_{Ca}), and the tandem-pore domain (K_{2P}) channels [37]. The K_v and K_{Ca} families are of particular relevance in epilepsy.

The K_v channels are involved in diverse physiological processes ranging from repolarization of neuronal or cardiac action potentials, overregulating calcium signaling and cell volume to driving cellular proliferation and migration. The K_v family has more than 40 members that are classified into 12 distinct subfamilies based on their amino acid sequence homology (K_v1 to K_v12) [37]. They conduct voltage-gated K^+ currents that have diverse functions in neurons, including the K_v1 (delayed rectifier and A-current), K_v2 (delayed rectifier), K_v3 (high-voltage-activated, fast kinetics), K_v4 (somatodendritic A-current), and K_v7 (M-current) [37]. A-currents and M-currents play important roles in regulating the excitability of neurons in brain regions relevant to epilepsy such as the neocortex and the hippocampus [38].

Several K^+ channel genes have been associated with different forms of epilepsy including *KCNA1* (encodes K_v1.1), auxiliary β2 subunit *KCNAB2* (encodes K_v1), *KCNQ2* (encodes K_v7.2), *KCNQ3* (encodes K_v7.3), *KCNMA1* gene that encodes the αsubunit of K_{Ca}1.1, *KCNJ3* (encodes K_{ir}3.1), *KCNJ6* (encodes K_{ir}3.2), *KCNJ10* (encodes K_{ir}4.1), *KCNJ11* (K_{ir}6.2), *KCNK9* (TASK3) [6].

K_v channels are valid molecular targets for both convulsant and anticonvulsant agents. Classical pharmacological antagonists of K_v channels include 4-aminopyridine (4-AP) commonly used to induce seizures in rodent models and brain slices [39], which is a blocker of

K_v1, K_v3, and K_v4 channels. Several classes of compounds identified as K^+ channel openers could potentially have anticonvulsant activity. K_{ATP} ($K_{ir}6.x$) channel openers, such as cromakalim and diazoxide, were reported to inhibit epileptic discharges in brain slices [40].

Actions of several established AEDs on various K^+ currents have been reported. Ethosuximide reduces sustained K^+ currents in thalamic neurons by blocking Ca^{2+}-activated K^+ current [41]. Pregabalin opens ATP-sensitive K^+ channels [42], while lamotrigine reduces the amplitude of A-type K^+ currents in cultured hippocampal neurons and levetiracetam inhibits delayed rectifier in isolated hippocampal neurons [4]. These inhibitory actions enhance excitability and unlikely contribute to anticonvulsant activity.

A broad range of K^+ channels offers many unexploited molecular targets, particularly the channels generating the A-type and M-type currents. Other members of the voltage-gated ion channel superfamily, including inwardly rectifying, Ca^{2+}-activated K^+ channels, are also potential targets that have not been validated.

2.4. Voltage-gated chloride channels (ClCs)

ClCs are expressed in the hippocampus where they mediate chloride currents in pyramidal cells of the hippocampus. They are involved in regulating chloride homeostasis [43], excitability [44], and acidification of synaptic vesicles [45]. One of the ClCs expressed in neurons is ClC-2, which is a widely expressed chloride channel of the CLC family of chloride channels and transporters. ClC-2 is activated by hyperpolarization, cell swelling, a rise in intracellular chloride concentration, or mild extracellular acidification [46, 47].

Genes encoding nine voltage-gated chlorides channels ($ClCs^-$) with diverse functions in plasma membranes and intracellular organelles have been identified by molecular studies. One of these channels, ClC-2, a homodimeric channel found in neurons and glia (encoded by the *CLCN2* gene), has been implicated in epilepsy [48]. Over the past years, several mutations in the gene encoding for ClC-2 have been described [49], but whether mutations in ClC-2 cause epilepsy or not has been controversial. However, functional studies in transfected cells suggest that the mutations cause a loss of function [50]. Although ClC-2 knockout mice do not have epilepsy [51], ClC-2 mutations cosegregated in three families with various idiopathic generalized epilepsy syndromes, including juvenile myoclonic epilepsy (JME), juvenile absence epilepsy, childhood absence epilepsy (CAE), and epilepsy with grand mal seizures on awakening (EGMA) [52]. Epilepsy-associated ClC-2 mutations may lead to impairment of $GABA_A$-mediated inhibition or may even become excitatory [4]. Strategies that attempt to influence Cl^- gradients by altering the activity of the transporters that determine Cl^- gradients (NKCC1 and KCC2) are an attractive area of research, given the widespread expression of ClC-2 in many tissues.

2.5. Hyperpolarization-activated cyclic nucleotide-gated cation (HCN) channels

Hyperpolarization-activated cyclic nucleotide-gated (HCN) channels activation mechanism, their modulation *in vivo*, their cellular and subcellular distribution and their interaction with agonists or antagonists remain unclear [53]. HCN channels, members of the superfamily of voltage-gated cation channels that open upon hyperpolarization and close at positive potential [54], represent the molecular αsubunits of native "funny" channels found in the heart (where they are referred to as "pacemaker" channels) and the brain. Although the first complete functional description of the funny current was made in the cardiac sino-atrial node (SAN), an equivalent current (termed I_h for hyperpolarization-activated current) was also reported and its properties were investigated in a large variety of neuronal cells, where they contribute to a set of functions such as working memory, motor learning, generation of rhythmic activity, control of the membrane resting potential, regulation of cell excitability, dendritic integration, and synaptic transmission [55].

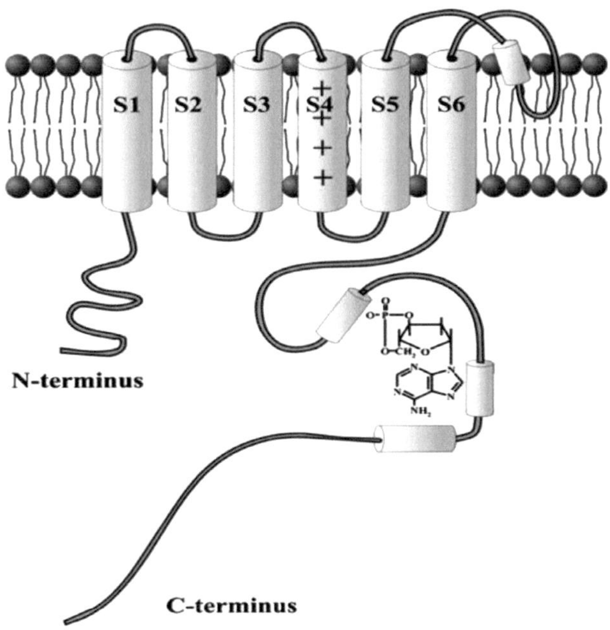

Figure 2. HCN channel topology consisting of six transmembrane domains (S1–S6). S4, the putative voltage sensor characterized by the presence of 11 basic amino acids (two lysines, seven arginines, and two histidines) within its domain, is present in all the four HCN subunits. Here, the domains involved in cyclic nucleotide binding (CNBD) in the C-terminus and the cAMP molecule are also shown [57].

HCN channels form macromolecular complexes that consist of the principal ion-conducting channel core and auxiliary subunits that are either permanently assembled with the channel core or can bind and unbind in a regulated fashion [38]. HCN channels (h-channels) are a family of six transmembrane domains (**Figure 2**), single pore-loop, hyperpolarization-activated, nonselective cation channels, which are key regulators of neuronal excitation and inhibition, and have a rich diversity of subunit composition, distribution, modulation, and function. Genes coding for four distinct channel isoforms have been cloned (HCN1–4), and HCN channel transcripts and proteins are widely and variably distributed throughout the mammalian central nervous system [56]. Each of the four identified subunits (HCN1–4) has six transmembrane segments. HCN2 is generally considered to be widely distributed in the nervous system, and HCN3 is generally poorly expressed except for the olfactory bulb, hypothalamus and retinal cones pedicles [53]. HCN1 has been detected specifically in the neocortex, hippocampus, cerebellar cortex, and brainstem [56], whereas HCN4 channels are highly expressed in particular in thalamic nuclei, basal ganglia, and olfactory bulb [56].

At the cellular level, several basic functions including control of the membrane resting potential and dendritic integration have been attributed to these channels. It was therefore hypothesized that the dysfunction and/or inadequate expression of HCN channels may be a disease-causing factor. Dysregulation of HCN channel expression and aberrant HCN channel function have been implicated in various types of idiopathic and acquired epilepsies. HCN2 deficiencies are pathological hallmarks of absence epilepsy [58]. Deletion of HCN1 is associated with increased seizure severity and risk of seizure-related death in different limbic seizure induction models [59]. Genetic studies suggest that the suppression of HCN channels in neurons is involved in generation of neuronal hyperexcitability, which have been reported in temporal lobe epilepsy, the most common and severe form of epilepsy in adults [60].

The reciprocal interactions between neuronal activity and h-channels indicate that these ion channels could be promising novel targets for antiepileptic therapies. I_h is an attractive potential AED target for different types of epilepsy. However, the complexity and diversity of the mechanisms connecting impaired HCN channel activity with epilepsy make it very challenging to develop a generally applicable rationale for the design of anticonvulsant drugs based on HCN channels. Drugs targeting HCN1 might be relevant for limbic seizures, whereas those affecting HCN2 may be more relevant to absence epilepsy. ZD-7288, a blocker of HCN channels, inhibits spontaneous epileptiform bursting in the hippocampal slice, confirming the potential of I_h inhibition as an anticonvulsant approach [61]. Lamotrigine and gabapentin upregulate the activity of HCN channels [62, 63]. It may be speculated that the action of both drugs is directed primarily at HCN1, which is the main HCN subtype in the cortex and hippocampus. In rat hippocampal pyramidal neurons, lamotrigine has also been reported to decrease dendritic excitability by increasing I_h [64].

3. Ligand-gated ion channels

Ligand-gated ion channels in the mammalian brain include the Cys-loop receptors comprising the $GABA_A$, glycine, nicotinic cholinergic and 5-HT_3 receptors (**Figure 3**), and the ionotropic glutamate receptors comprising the (±)-*α*-amino-3-hydroxy-5-methyl-4-isoxazolepropionic acid (AMPA), kainate, and *N*-methyl-D-aspartate (NMDA) receptors besides the adenosine triphosphate (ATP)-gated P2X channels and the transient receptor potential (TRP) channels. $GABA_A$ receptors are permeable to Cl^- and HCO_3^-, while the ionotropic glutamate receptors are cation permeable, with significant variation in the extent of Ca^{2+} permeability. The majority of known convulsant compounds act via the ligand-gated ion channels to diminish GABA-mediated transmission either by direct action on $GABA_A$ receptors or by other effects on GABAergic function.

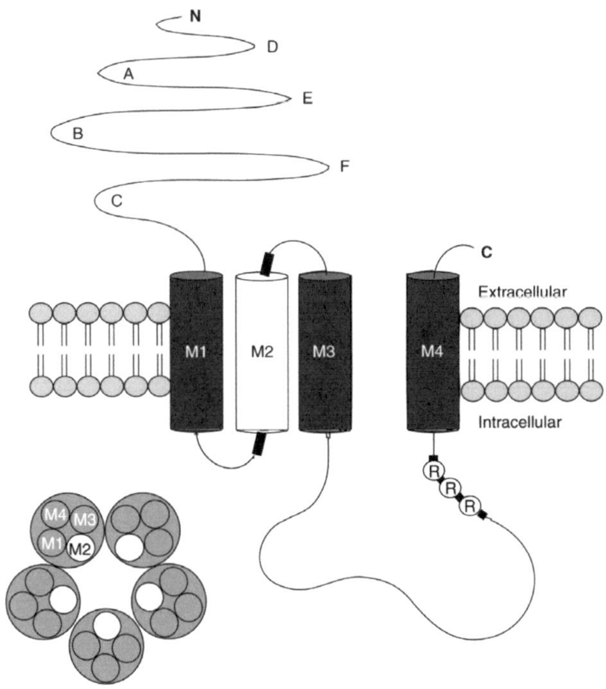

Figure 3. A typical Cys-loop receptor subunit. A cross section of the transmembrane region at the lower left shows five subunits that form a central ion-conducting pore. Six loops form the ligand binding site (A–F) and the region that influences ion conductivity (R-R-R) [65].

3.1. GABA$_A$ receptors

γ-Aminobutyric acid (GABA) is a major inhibitory neurotransmitter in the vertebrate central nervous system (CNS) that activates GABA$_A$, GABA$_B$, and GABA$_C$ receptors. GABA$_A$ receptors are pentameric structures composed of different combinations of subunits arranged around a central Cl^--selective pore [66]. Studies have indentified 19 subunits (α1–6, β1–3, γ1–3, δ, ε, θ, π, ρ1–3) encoded by 19 distinct genes that form ligand-gated ion channel complexes [67]. The inclusion of a ρ subunit (ρ1–ρ3) distinguishes the bicuculline-insensitive GABA$_C$ receptor family [68]. The subunit composition determines the biophysical properties, pharmacological characteristics [most notably the sensitivity to benzodiazepines (BZ)], and subcellular localization of the GABA$_A$ receptors [67]. Their modulatory domains include binding sites for benzodiazepines (BZ site), GABA, barbiturates, nonbarbiturate anesthetics and ethanol, neurosteroids, picrotoxin, penicillin, and zinc.

Genetic studies in humans reveal a range of idiopathic generalized epilepsy syndromes linked to mutations in the GABA$_A$ receptor [69]. A mutation in the GABA$_A$ receptor α1 subunit is associated with autosomal dominant juvenile myoclonic epilepsy [70]. Mutations involving the γ2 subunit in two cases are associated with GEFS+ and in two cases associated with childhood absence epilepsy with febrile convulsions [69]. Studies revealed spontaneous

http://dx.doi.org/10.5772/64456

seizures in β3 knockout mice [71], supporting that seizures that are prominent feature of the Angelman syndrome are due specifically to defects in $GABA_A$ receptors.

$GABA_A$ receptors are acknowledged targets of many available anticonvulsants including drugs enhancing $GABA_A$ receptor action through a direct interaction with the receptor (benzodiazepines, barbiturates, propofol, stiripentol, topiramate, carbamazepine, phenytoin, felbamate) or indirectly by increasing the available GABA (tiagabine, vigabatrine, gabapentin, valproate) [68]. Furthermore, anticonvulsants can reduce the depolarizing effects of $GABA_A$ receptors by inhibiting carbonic anhydrase (topiramate, zonisamide, acetazolamide) [68]. Studies in genetically modified mice have helped establish the role played by subunit composition in the antiepileptic and other pharmacological actions of drugs acting on the $GABA_A$ receptor [72].

Majority of drugs that act on $GABA_A$ receptors do so at modulatory sites distinct from the GABA recognition site. The anticonvulsant actions of benzodiazepines result in large part from their ability to enhance GABA-induced increase in the conductance of chloride ions [73]. A therapeutically relevant concentration of benzodiazepines acts at subsets of $GABA_A$ receptor channel complex and increases the frequency, but not duration of opening of GABA-activated chloride channels [74]. The mechanisms underlying the actions of barbiturates on $GABA_A$ receptors appear to be distinct from those of either GABA or the benzodiazepines. Barbiturates potentiate GABA-induced chloride currents by prolonging periods during which bursts of channel opening occur rather than by increasing the frequency of these bursts [74].

Substantial effort has been devoted to obtaining $GABA_A$ receptor positive allosteric modulators with reduced activity on $GABA_A$ receptors containing $\alpha 1$ subunits, to avoid the sedation mediated by these receptors. Nonbenzodiazepines that bind to the benzodiazepine site have been developed; some are partial agonists with reduced efficacy. These subtype-selective agents could potentially be superior to benzodiazepines for chronic epilepsy therapy, but have not been demonstrated that they are less sedative or more importantly less susceptible to tolerance [4].

3.2. Ionotropic glutamate receptors

The ionotropic glutamate receptors consist of three receptor superfamilies of ligand-gated cation channels including AMPA, kainate, and NMDA that mediate most of the fast excitatory transmission in the CNS and are thus involved in all brain functions. They are tetrameric structures with four subunits for the AMPA receptors, five subunits for the kainite receptors and seven subunits for the NMDA receptors [75].

Little evidence for spontaneous mutations involving glutamate receptors has been demonstrated in epilepsy syndromes in human or mouse. Juvenile absence epilepsy has been associated with a nine-repeat allele of a tetranucleotide repeat polymorphism in a noncoding region of the GluR5 receptor gene (*GRIK1*) [76]. Studies have shown that alterations in GluR2 editing that cause AMPA receptors to be Ca^{2+} permeable lead to seizures.

Substantial effort has been devoted toward the development of ionotropic glutamate receptor antagonists for epilepsy therapy because of the role of glutamate in the pathophysiology of seizures and the empirical evidence that these antagonists are protective in various animal seizure models [77]. Competitive and noncompetitive NMDA receptor antagonists demonstrated the ability to block seizures in rodent epilepsy and possess protective activity in some rodent models [78, 79]. Competitive NMDA antagonists appeared the most promising in models of generalized seizures.

AMPA receptor antagonists, which are anticonvulsant in a broad range of rodent animal models, have been identified and may have greater potential clinical utility than do the NMDA antagonists [15]. AMPA receptor antagonists have the potential to stop seizures more effectively and may confer neuroprotection by blocking glutamate-induced excitotoxicity, which could diminish the brain damage and neurological morbidity typically associated with status epilepticus.

Three marketed AEDs have been shown to interact with glutamate receptors. Phenobarbital decreases the depolarizing or excitotoxic action of AMPA and kainate at concentrations similar to those at which it potentiates GABA [80]. Topiramate has been reported to block kainate-induced currents in cultured hippocampal neurons [81] by acting specifically on GluR5 kainate receptors and with lower potency on AMPA receptors [82]. Felbamate has several different pharmacological actions including specific inhibitory effect on NMDA receptors that have been proposed as contributing to its clinical efficacy [83].

3.3. Acid-sensing ion channels (ASICs)

Acid-sensing ion channels (ASICs) are superfamily of ligand-gated cation channels that are widely distributed in the mammalian brain, the spinal cord and the peripheral sensory organs. ASICs belong to the degenerin/epithelial Na^+ channels that are activated by external protons. Increase in extracellular proton concentrations, which is associated with physiological conditions such as synaptic signaling and pathological conditions such as tissue inflammation, ischemic stroke, traumatic brain injury, and epileptic seizure, activates this unique family of membrane ion channels. The ASICs rapidly respond to a reduction in extracellular pH with an inward cation current that is quickly inactivated despite the continuous presence of protons in the medium. Abundant experimental evidence shows that ASICs play important roles in physiological/pathological conditions, such as sensory transduction, learning/memory, retinal function, seizure, and ischemia [84].

Seven different ASICs subunits of ASICs (1a, 1b1, 1b2, 2a, 2b, 3, and 4) encoded by four genes have been identified [85, 86]. The 1a, 2a, 2b, and 4 subunits are expressed in the CNS neurons, while all other ASICs subunits with the exception of ASIC4 are expressed in peripheral sensory neurons. ASIC genes are also expressed in non-neuronal tissue such as vascular smooth muscle cells [87] and bone [88].

ASICs are involved in nociception in sensory neurons when injury or inflammation causes acidification. Protons released during high-frequency stimulation of excitatory synapses in the brain activate ASICs to cause postsynaptic depolarization [4], resulting in a reduction in the Mg^{2+} block of NMDA receptors, which promotes epileptic activity. The inhibition of ASICs might therefore reduce excitatory synaptic neurotransmission resulting to anticonvulsant

http://dx.doi.org/10.5772/64456

actions [4]. Acidification that occurs during intense seizure activity could activate ASICs and contribute to seizure-induced brain damage because of Ca^{2+} permeability in many ASICs [89]. ASIC antagonists might minimize these adverse consequences of seizures. There are no selective ASIC antagonists available to test the role of ASICs as anticonvulsant targets; however, the potassium-sparing diuretic amiloride does act as an ASIC antagonist and appears to have anticonvulsant properties [90].

Author details

Ben A. Chindo[1,2*], Bulus Adzu[2] and Karniyus S. Gamaniel[2]

*Address all correspondence to: bachindo@yahoo.com

1 Department of Pharmacology and Toxicology, Faculty of Pharmaceutical Sciences, Kaduna State University, Kaduna, Nigeria

2 Department of Pharmacology and Toxicology, National Institute for Pharmaceutical Research and Development, Abuja, Nigeria

References

[1] Löscher W. Current status and future directions in the pharmacotherapy of epilepsy. Trends Pharmcol Sci 2002; 23: 113–118.

[2] Engel J.A. Proposed diagnostic scheme for people with epileptic seizures and with epilepsy: report of the ILAE task force on classification and terminology. Epilepsia 2001; 42: 796–803.

[3] Rogers S.J., Cavazos J.E. Epilepsy. In: Pharmacotherapy: A Pathophysiologic Approach, (DiPiro, J.T., Talbert, R.L., Yee, G.C., Matzke, G.R., Wells, B.G., Posey, L.M., eds.), 7th edn, McGraw-Hill Co. Inc., New York, 2008; 927–951.

[4] Meldrum B.S., Rogawski M.A. Molecular targets for antiepileptic drug development. Neurotherapeutics 2007; 4: 18–61.

[5] Graves T.D. Ion channels and epilepsy. Q J Med 2006; 99: 201–217

[6] Catterall W.A. The voltage-gated ion channel superfamily. In: Voltage-Gated Ion Channels as Drug Targets. (Triggle, D., eds), Weinheim: WILEY-VCH Verlag GmbH & Co. KGaA, 2006; 7–18.

[7] Stafstrom C.E. Persistent sodium current and its role in epilepsy. Epilepsy Curr 2007; 7: 15–22.

[8] Black J.A., Waxman S.G. Noncanonical roles of voltage-gated sodium channels. Neuron, 2013; 80: 280–291.

[9] Brackenbury W.J., Isom L.L. Na Channel β Subunits: overachievers of the ion channel family. Front Pharmacol 2011; 2: 53.

[10] Meisler M.H., Kearney J.A. Sodium channel mutations in epilepsy and other neurological disorders. J Clin Invest 2005; 115: 2010–2017.

[11] Catterall W.A. Ion channel voltage sensors: structure, function, and pathophysiology. Neuron 2010; 67: 915–928.

[12] Avanzini G., Franceschetti S., Mantegazza M. Epileptogenic channelopathies: experimental models of human pathologies. Epilepsia 2007; 48: 51–64.

[13] Catterall W.A. Sodium channels, inherited epilepsy, and antiepileptic drugs. Annu Rev Pharmacol Toxicol 2014; 54: 317–338.

[14] Errington A.C., Stöhr T., Heers C., Lees G. The investigational anticonvulsant lacosamide selectively enhances slow inactivation of voltage-gated sodium channels. Mol Pharmacol 2008; 73: 157–169.

[15] Rogawski M.A., Taylor C.P. Ion channels. In: Löscher W, Schmidt D. New horizons in the development of antiepileptic drugs: innovative strategies. Epilepsy Res 2006; 69: 183–272.

[16] Prakriya M., Mennerick S. Selective depression of low-release probability excitatory synapses by sodium channel blockers. Neuron 2000; 26: 671–682.

[17] Colbert C.M., Magee J.C., Hoffman D.A., Johnston D. Slow recovery from inactivation of Na+ channels underlies the activity-dependent attenuation of dendritic action potentials in hippocampal CA1 pyramidal neurons. J Neurosci 1997; 17: 6512–6521.

[18] Catterall W.A., Swanson T.M. Structural basis for pharmacology of voltage-gated sodium and calcium channels. Mol Pharmacol 2015; 88: 141–150.

[19] Khosravani H., Zamponi G.W. Voltage-gated calcium channels and idiopathic generalized epilepsies. Physiol Rev 2006; 86: 941–966.

[20] Lopez J.J., Albarran L., Gómez L.J., Smani T., Salido G.M., Rosado J.A. Molecular modulators of store-operated calcium entry. Biochim Biophys Acta 2016; [Epub ahead of print].

[21] Weick J.P., Groth R.D., Isaksen A.L., Mermelstein P.G. Interactions with PDZ proteins are required for L-type calcium channels to activate cAMP response element-binding protein-dependent gene expression. J Neurosci 2003; 23: 3446–3456.

[22] Westenbroek R.E., Sakurai T., Elliott E.M., Hell J.W., Starr T.V., Snutch T.P., Catterall W.A. Immunochemical identification and subcellular distribution of the alpha 1A subunits of brain calcium channels. J Neurosci 1995; 15: 6403–6418.

[23] Leenders AG, van den Maagdenberg AM, Lopes da Silva FH, Sheng ZH, Molenaar PC, and Ghijsen WE. Neurotransmitter release from tottering mice nerve terminals with reduced expression of mutated P- and Q-type Ca^{2+}-channels. Eur J Neurosci 2002; 15: 13–18.

[24] Yokoyama C.T., Westenbroek R.E., Hell J.W., Soong T.W., Snutch T.P., Catterall W.A. Biochemical properties and subcellular distribution of the neuronal class E calcium channel alpha 1 subunit. J Neurosci 1995; 15: 6419–6432.

[25] Wang G., Dayanithi G., Newcomb R., Lemos J.R. An R-type $Ca(2^-)$ current in neurohypophysial terminals preferentially regulates oxytocin secretion. J Neurosci 1999; 19: 9235–9241.

[26] Pietrobon D. Calcium channels and channelopathies of the central nervous system. Mol Neurobiol 2002; 25: 31–50.

[27] Hofmann F., Biel M., Flockerzi V. Molecular basis for Ca^{2+} channel diversity. Annu Rev Neurosci 1994; 17: 399–418.

[28] Snutch T.P., Peloquin J., Mathews E., McRory J.E. Molecular properties of voltage-gated calcium channels. In: Voltage-Gated Calcium Channels. (Zamponi GW ed) New York: Plenum, 2005; 1: 61–94.

[29] Pietrobon D. Function and dysfunction of synaptic calcium channels: insights from mouse models. Curr Opin Neurobiol 2005; 15: 257–265.

[30] Crunelli V., Leresche N. Block of thalamic T-type Ca^{2+} channels by ethosuximide is not the whole story. Epilepsy Curr 2002; 2: 53–56.

[31] Ffrench-Mullen J.M., Barker J.L., Rogawski M.A. Calcium current block by (-)-pentobarbital, phenobarbital, and CHEB but not (+)-pentobarbital in acutely isolated hippocampal CA1 neurons: comparison with effects on GABA-activated Cl^- current. J. Neurosci 1993; 13: 3211–3221.

[32] Pisani, A., Bonsi, P., Martella, G., De Persis, C., Costa, C., Pisani, F.R., Bernardi, G., Calabresi, P. Intracellular calcium increase in epileptiform activity: modulation by levetiracetam and lamotrigine. Epilepsia 2004; 45: 719–728.

[33] Belliotti T.R., Capiris T., Ekhato I.V., Kinsora J.J., Field M.J., Heffner T.G. Structure–activity relationships of pregabalin and analogues that target the $\alpha 2\delta$ protein. J Med Chem 2005; 48: 2294–2307.

[34] Gee N.S., Brown J.P., Dissanayake V.U.K., Offord J., Thurlow R., Woodruff G.N. The novel anticonvulsant drug, gabapentin (neurontin) binds to the $\alpha 2\delta 2$ subunit of a calcium channel. J Biol Chem 1996; 271: 5768–5776.

[35] Fink K., Dooley D.J., Meder W.P., Suman-Chauhan N., Duffy S., Clusmann H., Gothert M. Inhibition of neuronal Ca2+ influx by gabapentin and pregabalin in the human neocortex. Neuropharmacology 2002; 42: 229–236.

[36] Cunningham M.O., Woodhall G.L., Thompson S.E., Dooley D.J., Jones R.S. Dual effects of gabapentin and pregabalin on glutamate release at rat entorhinal synapses *in vitro*. Eur. J Neurosci 2004; 20: 1566–1576.

[37] Gutman G.A., Chandy K.G., Grissmer S., Lazdunski M., McKinnon D., Pardo L.A., Robertson G.A., Rudy B., Sanguinetti M.C., Stühmer W., Wang X. International Union of Pharmacology. LIII. Nomenclature and molecular relationships of voltage-gated potassium channels. Pharmacol Rev 2005; 57: 473–508.

[38] Postea O., Biel M. Exploring HCN channels as novel drug targets. Nat Rev Drug Discov 2011; 10::903–914.

[39] Perreault P., Avoli M. Physiology and pharmacology of epileptiform activity induced by 4-aminopyridine in rat hippocampal slices. J Neurophysiol 1991; 65: 771–785.

[40] Wickenden A.D. Potassium channels as anti-epileptic drug targets. Neuropharmacology 2002; 43: 1055–1060.

[41] Leresche N., Parri H.R., Erdemli G., Guyon A., Turner J.P., Williams S.R., Asprodini E., Crunelli V. On the action of the anti-absence drug ethosuximide in the rat and cat thalamus. J Neurosci 1998; 18: 4842–4853.

[42] Huang C.W., Huang C.C., Wu S.N. The opening effect of pregabalin on ATP-sensitive potassium channels in differentiated hippocampal neuron-derived H19-7 cells. Epilepsia 2006; 47: 720–726.

[43] Staley K., Smith R., Schaack J., Wilcox C., Jentsch T.J. Alteration of $GABA_A$ receptor function following gene transfer of the CLC-2 chloride channel. Neuron, 1996; 17: 543–551.

[44] Madison D.V., Malenka R.C., Nicoll R.A. Phorbol esters block a voltage- sensitive chloride current in hippocampal pyramidal cells. Nature 1986; 321: 695–697.

[45] Stobrawa S.M., Breiderhoff T., Takamori S., Engel D., Schweizer M., Zdebik A.A., Bösl M.R., Ruether K., Jahn H., Draguhn, A., Jahn, R., Jentsch, T.J. Disruption of ClC-3, a chloride channel expressed on synaptic vesicles, leads to a loss of the hippocampus. Neuron 2001; 29: 185–196.

[46] Grunder S., Thiemann A., Pusch M., Jentsch T.J. Regions involved in the opening of CIC-2 chloride channel by voltage and cell volume. Nature 1992; 360: 759–762.

[47] Zúñïga L., Niemeyer M.I., Varela D., Catalán M., Cid L.P., Sepúlveda F.V. The voltage-dependent ClC-2 chloride channel has a dual gating mechanism. J Physiol 2004; 555: 671–682.

[48] Jentsch T.J., Neagoe I., Scheel O. CLC chloride channels and transporters. Curr Opin Neurobiol 2005; 15: 319–325.

[49] Saint-Martin C., Gauvain G., Teodorescu G., Gourfinkel-An I., Fedirko E., Weber Y.G., Maljevic S., Ernst J.P., Garcia-Olivares J., Fahlke C., Nabbout R., LeGuern E., Lerche H.,

Poncer J.C., Depienne C. Two novel CLCN2 mutations accelerating chloride channel deactivation are associated with idiopathic generalized epilepsy. Hum Mutat 2009; 30: 397–405.

[50] Niemeyer M.I., Yusef Y.R., Cornejo I., Flores C.A., Sepulveda F.V., Cid L.P. Functional evaluation of human ClC-2 chloride channel mutations associated with idiopathic generalized epilepsies. Physiol Genomics 2004; 19: 74–83.

[51] Bösl M.R., Stein V., Hubner C., Zdebik A.A., Jordt S.E., Mukhopadhyay A.K., Davidoff M.S., Holstein A.F., Jentsch T.J. Male germ cells and photo-receptors, both dependent on close cell-cell interactions, degenerate upon ClC-2 Cl^- channel disruption. EMBO J 2001; 20: 1289–1299.

[52] Heils A. *CLCN2* and idiopathic generalized epilepsy. Adv Neurol 2005; 95: 265–271.

[53] Biel M., Wahl-Schott C., Michalakis S., Zong X. Hyperpolarization-activated cation channels: from genes to function. Physiol Rev 2009; 89: 847–885

[54] Biel, M., Ludwig, A., Zong, X., Hofmann, F. Hyperpolarization-activated cation channels: a multigene family. Rev Physiol Biochem Pharmacol 1999; 136: 165–181.

[55] Wahl-Schott C., Biel M. HCN channels: structure, cellular regulation and physiological function. Cell Mol. Life Sci 2009; 66: 470–494.

[56] Notomi T., Shigemoto R. Immunohistochemical localization of I_h channel subunits, HCN1–4, in the rat brain. J Comp Neurol 2004; 471: 241–276.

[57] Baruscotti M., Bottelli G., Milanesi R., DiFrancesco J.C., DiFrancesco, D. HCN-related channelopathies. Arch Eur J Physiol 2010; 460: 405–415.

[58] Cho H.J., Furness J.B., Jennings E.A. Post-natal maturation of the hyperpolarisation-activated cation current, Ih, in trigeminal sensory neurons. J Neurophysiol 2011; 106: 2045–2056.

[59] Santoro B., Lee J.Y. Englot D.J., Gildersleeve S., Piskorowski R.A., Siegelbaum S.A., Winawer M.R., Blumenfeld H. Increased seizure severity and seizure-related death in mice lacking HCN1 channels. Epilepsia 2010; 51: 1624–1627.

[60] Shin M., Brager D., Jaramillo T.C., Johnston D., Chetkovich D.M. Mislocalization of h channel subunits underlies h channelopathy in temporal lobe epilepsy. Neurobiol Dis 2008; 32: 26–36.

[61] Arias RL, Bowlby MR. Pharmacological characterization of antiepileptic drugs and experimental analgesics on low magnesium-induced hyperexcitability in rat hippocampal slices. Brain Res 2005; 1047: 233–244.

[62] Poolos N.P., Migliore M., Johnston D. Pharmacological upregulation of h-channels reduces the excitability of pyramidal neuron dendrites. Nat Neurosci 2002; 5: 767–774.

[63] Surges R., Freiman T.M., Feuerstein T.J. Gabapentin increases the hyperpolarization-activated cation current Ih in rat CA1 pyramidal cells. Epilepsia 2003; 44: 150–156.

[64] Peng B.W., Justice J.A., Zhang K., He X.H., Sanchez R.M. Increased basal synaptic inhibition of hippocampal area CA1 pyramidal neurons by an antiepileptic drug that enhances I(H). Neuropsychopharmacology 2010; 35: 464–472.

[65] Thompson A.J., Lummis S.C.R. The 5-HT3 receptor as a therapeutic target. Expert Opin Ther Targets 2007; 11: 527–540.

[66] Barnard E.A. The molecular architecture of $GABA_A$ receptors pharmacology of GABA and glycine neurotransmission. In: Handbook of Experimental Pharmacology. (Möhler, H., eds), Vol. 150, Berlin: Springer; 2001; 94–100.

[67] Möhler H. $GABA_A$ receptor diversity and pharmacology. Cell Tissue Res 2006; 326: 505–516.

[68] Galanopoulou A.S. $GABA_A$ receptors in normal development and seizures: friends or foes? Curr Neuropharmacol 2008; 6: 1–20.

[69] Macdonald R.L., Gallagher M.J., Feng H.J., Kong J. $GABA_A$ receptor epilepsy mutations. Biochem Pharmacol 2004; 68: 1497–1506.

[70] Cossette P., Liu L., Brisebois K., Dong H., Lortie A., Vanasse M., Saint-Hilaire J.M., Carmant L., Verner A., Lu W.Y., Wang Y.T., Rouleau G.A. Mutation of *GABARA1* in an autosomal dominant form of juvenile myoclonic epilepsy. Nat Genet 2002; 31: 184–189.

[71] DeLorey T.M., Handforth A., Anagnostaras S.G., Homanics G.E., Minassian B.A., Asatourian A., Fanselow M.S., Delgado-Escueta A., Ellison G.D., Olsen R.W. Mice lacking the β3 subunit of the GABAA receptor have the epilepsy phenotype and many of the behavioural characteristics of Angelman syndrome. J Neurosci 1998; 18: 8505–8514.

[72] Rudolph U., Möhler H. GABA-based therapeutic approaches: $GABA_A$ receptor subtype functions. Curr Opin Pharmacol 2006; 6: 18–23.

[73] Mennini R., Caccia S., Garattini S. Mechanism of action of anxiolytic drugs. Prog Drug Res 1987; 31: 315–347.

[74] Twyman R.E., Rogers C.J., Macdonald R.L. Differential regulation of gama-aminobutyric acid receptor channels by diazepam and phenobarbital. Ann Rev Neurosci 1989; 25: 213–220.

[75] Mayer M.L., Armstrong N. Structure and function of glutamate receptor ion channels. Annu Rev Physiol 2004; 66: 161–181.

[76] Sander T., Hildmann T., Kretz R., Furst R., Sailer U., Bauer G., Schmitz B., Beck-Mannagetta G., Wienker T.F., Janz D. Allelic association of juvenile absence epilepsy with a GluR5 kainate receptor gene (*GRIK1*) polymorphism. Am J Med Genet 1997; 74: 416–421.

http://dx.doi.org/10.5772/64456

[77] Löscher W. Animal models of epilepsy and epileptic seizures. Handb Exp Pharmacol 1999; 138: 19–62.

[78] Croucher M.J., Collins J.F., Meldrum B.S. Anticonvulsant action of excitatory amino acid antagonists. Science 1982; 216: 899–901.

[79] Meldrum B.S. Excitatory amino acids in epilepsy and potential novel therapies. Epilepsy Res 1992; 12: 189–196.

[80] Ko G.Y., Brown-Croyts L.M., Teyler T.J. The effects of anticonvulsant drugs on NMDA-EPSP, AMPA-EPSP and GABA-IPSP in the rat hippocampus. Brain Res Bull 1997; 42: 297–302.

[81] Gibbs J.W 3rd, Sombati S., DeLorenzo R.J., Coulter D.A. Cellular actions of topiramate: blockade of kainate-evoked inward currents in cultured hippocampal neurons. Epilepsia 2000; 41(suppl 1): S10–S16.

[82] Kaminski R.M., Banerjee M., Rogawski M.A. Topiramate selectively protects against seizures induced by ATPA, a GluR5 kainate receptor agonist. Neuropharmacology 2004; 46: 1097–1104.

[83] Rho J.M., Donevan S.D., Rogawski M.A. Mechanism of action of the anticonvulsant felbamate: opposing effects on *N*-methyl-d aspartate and γ-aminobutyric acid A receptors. Ann Neurol 1994; 35: 229–234.

[84] Zhang M., Gong N., Lu Y.G., Jia N.L., Xu T.L., Chen L. Functional characterization of acid-sensing ion channels in cultured neurons of rat inferior colliculus. Neuroscience 2008; 154: 461–472.

[85] Krishtal O. The ASICs: signaling molecules? Modulators? Trends Neurosci 2003; 26: 477–483.

[86] Waldmann R., Lazdunski M. H(+)-gated cation channels: neuronal acid sensors in the ENaC/DEG family of ion channels. Curr Opin Neurobiol 1998; 8: 418–424.

[87] Grifoni S.C., Jernigan N.L., Hamilton G., Drummond H.A. ASIC proteins regulate smooth muscle cell migration. Microvasc Res 2008; 75: 202–210.

[88] Jahr H., van Driel M., van Osch G.J., Weinans H., van Leeuwen J.P. Identification of acid sensing ion channels in bone. Biochem Biophys Res Commun 2005; 337: 349–354.

[89] Xiong Z.G., Zhu X.M., Chu X.P., Minami M., Hey J., Wei W.L., MacDonald J.F., Wemmie J.A., Price M.P., Welsh M.J., Simon R.P. Neuroprotection in ischemia: blocking calcium-permeable acidsensing ion channels. Cell 2004; 118: 687–698.

[90] Ali A., Pillai K.K., Ahmad F.J., Dua Y., Khan Z.I., Vohora D. Comparative efficacy of liposome-entrapped amiloride and free amiloride in animal models of seizures and serum potassium in mice. Eur Neuropsychopharmacol 2007; 17: 227–229.

Chapter 9

Antiepileptic Drugs and Risk Factors of Vascular Diseases

Jolanta Dorszewska, Urszula Lagan-Jedrzejczyk, Marta Kowalska, Katarzyna Wize and Wojciech Kozubski

Additional information is available at the end of the chapter

http://dx.doi.org/10.5772/64445

Abstract

Epilepsy is one of the most common neurological diseases, affecting approximately 1% of the population. It is a chronic disease and increased incidence falls in the period up to 1 year and 65 years of age. Most patients require long-term antiepileptic drugs (AEDs) therapy. In addition, approximately 30% of patients with epilepsy do not obtain satisfactory seizure control, which is defined as drug-resistant epilepsy. It is postulated that one of the causes of drug resistance can be polymorphisms of *ABCB1/MDR1* gene, tested particularly in tumors. It is believed that the old generation of AEDs, e.g. CBZ, VPA, may change plasma Hcy, asymmetric dimethylarginine (ADMA) levels, disturb lipid levels, C-reactive protein, vitamins, markers of oxidative stress, which are risk factors for vascular and neurodegenerative diseases. Changes in the level of risk factors for vascular disease caused by enzymes inducing AEDs, CBZ, PB, and PHT lead to a small increase in the risk of myocardial infarction. Alteration of Hcy and ADMA levels are also linked to genetic factors, e.g. genetic variants of *MTHFR, MTR, MTHFD1, CBS, DDAH1, eNOS* genes. Individualization of treatment with AEDs and prevention against cardiovascular disease in patients with epilepsy may bring the best therapeutic effects in these patients.

Keywords: AEDs, side effects, epilepsy

1. Introduction

Epilepsy is one of the most common neurological diseases. It is estimated that approximately 50 million people worldwide suffer from epilepsy. The most common treatment of epilepsy is based on long-term use of antiepileptic drugs (AEDs).

AEDs are a very heterogeneous group and exhibit different mechanisms of action. It is divided broadly into two generations: older and newer AEDs. It is believed that the new AEDs are characterized by greater specificity of the mechanism of action, a proper clinical assessment of the first trial and less side effects. New generation (NG) drugs are also rarely caused interactions with other drugs and lesser extent affect mood and cognitive function. On the other hand, the old AEDs should be applied carefully with consideration of drug interactions and potential side effects, e.g., increase homocysteine (Hcy) level [1].

Currently, many studies on hyperhomocysteinemia (HHcy) in epileptic patients treated with AEDs have been performed. The literature indicates that carbamazepine (CBZ) therapy in epileptics leads to an increase of Hcy [2–5]. Treatment with valproic acid (VPA), however, has variable effects; in some cases, Hcy is decreased [6], in others, it is increased [2–4, 7, 8], and in yet others, VPA has no effect on Hcy levels [9–11]. However, lamotrigine (LTG) treatment of epileptic patients has not been shown to lead to an increase in Hcy [6, 12].

It is believed that AEDs increase Hcy level by lowering the level of folate (FA), cofactor remethylation of Hcy to methionine, as a result of impaired the intestinal absorption, increased demand of FA for the hydroxylation processes of AEDs, the activation of hepatic enzymes leading to a final reduction of the FA level or AEDs direct effect on the metabolism of Hcy and renal function [13]. It is believed that only CBZ, phenytoin (PHT), phenobarbital (PB) and primidone reduce the level of FA by an increased activity of liver enzymes [3, 10]. However, VPA does not induce hepatic microsomal enzyme, but may lead to a decrease [2], as well as an increase [3] in the FA level. The VPA may reduce the FA level by inhibiting the enzyme intermediate in biosynthesis of FA and its derivatives. It has been shown that VPA is indeed associated with a lower risk of deficit of FA.

Elevated concentrations of Hcy in epileptic patients treated with AEDs may be associated with a number of clinical complications. It has been shown that increased Hcy level may lead to vascular disease [14], neuropsychiatric [13] and is considered to be a risk factor for seizure and resistance to treatment with AEDs [15].

Literature data have shown that there is a link between HHcy and asymmetric dimethylarginine (ADMA) level in epilepsy [16, 17]. ADMA is considered to be a risk factor for cardiovascular disease [18]. It has been shown that ADMA may mediate atherogenic action of Hcy [14]. ADMA levels in the plasma of patients with atherosclerosis correlate with both endothelial dysfunction and the progression of atherosclerosis [19, 20]. ADMA is a known marker of atherosclerosis [21, 22].

Recent data have also shown that epilepsy patient treated with AEDs may exhibit increased risk of the myocardial infarction, stroke and cardiovascular death [23, 24]. This may be triggered by influencing the serum Hcy and ADMA concentration [16], the serum lipid levels [25], C-reactive protein (CRP), body weight, as well as other atherosclerotic factors by AEDs [1].

2. Epilepsy and antiepileptic drugs

Epilepsy is not a disease in itself but rather a collection of somatic, vegetative or mental symptoms, which may be the result of a morphological or metabolic change in the brain. The etiology of the disease is varied, and among the most common causes are genetic factors, head trauma, tumors, as well as vascular, degenerative, demyelinating, inflammatory and toxic brain diseases. However, in 60% of the patients the causes of the illness remain still unknown. Traditionally, the patient could have been diagnosed of epilepsy after at least two unprovoked seizures occurring greater than 24 h apart. It has changed recently when the International League Against Epilepsy (ILAE) established the new operational (practical) clinical definition. In some cases these new criteria enable the doctors to speed up the diagnosis and apply the AEDs even after first seizure, when there is a high probability of having another attack [26].

AEDs are among the most common medications used in neurology. Nevertheless, treatment of epilepsy despite over 20 antiseizure drugs is still a challenge, even for an experienced neurologist/epileptologist. Unfortunately, the seizure control in almost 20–40% of the patients remains unsatisfactory. The reasons for refractory epilepsy are not fully clear, however, some literature data have shown that polymorphisms of a few genes, e.g., *ABCB1/MDR1* may influence the good or poor therapeutic response [27, 28].

The older generation of AEDs consists of CBZ, VPA, PHT, PB, ethosuximide (ESM) and benzodiazepines (BZDs). The new generation (NG) include LTG, topiramate (TPM), gabapentin (GBP), oxcarbazepine (OXCBZ), levetiracetam (LEV), pregabalin (PGB), tiagabine (TGB), vigabatrin (VGB), lacosamide (LCM), and perampanel (PMP). Very important characteristic of AEDs is their ability to induce liver cytochrome P450 (CBZ, PHT, PB) or to block its activity (VPA), which plays an essential role in drug interactions [16, 29]. AEDs act against different targets and have distinguishing pharmacokinetics, efficacy, tolerability and side effects [30]. Although for some AEDs the precise mechanism of action remains still unknown and most of them seem to exhibit more than one mechanism, especially VPA, TPM, and PB, they may be categorized by their principal goal. CBZ, PHE, LTG, OXCBZ, and ZNS act by blocking the activity of voltage-gated sodium channels, while ESM, GBP and PG modulate calcium ones [31]. Increase in gamma-aminobutyric (GABA)ergic transmission by affecting $GABA_A$ receptors, GABA synthesis reuptake or degradation is known for VGB, TGB and BDP. Inhibition of glutamatergic excitation is distinctive for one of the newest drug—PMP [32]. Another mechanism of action is selectively enhancing slow inactivation of voltage-gated sodium channels which has been proved for LCM. Finally, LEV and BRV have an ability to bind to synaptic vesicle SV2A protein [33].

It is known that the use of AEDs, especially for many years induces many adverse effects. The most common side effects of AEDs are sedation, dizziness, ataxia, headache, joint pain, fever, vomiting, eating disorders, clotting disorders, hair loss, gingival hyperplasia, and allergic reactions [29]. It is believed that the AEDs in pregnant women with epilepsy are the most common causes of fetal defects [34, 35].

3. Polymorphism of the *ABCB1/MDR1* genes and antiepileptic drugs

The *ABCB1/MDR1* gene encodes the P-glycoprotein (P-gp), a transmembrane transporter located at the endothelial cells of the blood-brain barrier (BBB). It is known that overexpression of P-gp by reducing concentration of AEDs in affected brain regions is associated with epilepsy pharmacoresistance. The *ABCB1/MDR1* gene is highly polymorphic therefore it has great variability in the level of P-gp expression and activity among epileptic patients [36]. It is postulated that one of the causes of losing effectiveness of epilepsy treatment may be just polymorphisms of this gene, which has been mostly studied in the context of drug resistant in human cancer cells. There have been described three single nucleotide polymorphisms in the *ABCB1/MDR1* gene C3435T, C1236T and G2677 (A/T) related to epilepsy.

The first, *ABCB1/MDR1* C3435T is located in exon 26. It has been showed that patients with drug-resistant epilepsy were more likely to have the CC than the TT genotype and it is associated with increased expression of the protein that influences the response to AED treatment [37]. These results have not been confirmed by other studies conducted in Indian population [38].

Moreover, the literature data indicate that there is an association between C3435T polymorphism and CBZ doses. The study of Sterjev et al. [39] indicated that patients with the TT genotype require a higher dose of CBZ in comparison with patients with the CT and CC genotypes. No differences in allele frequency and genotype distribution between patient resistance and response on CBZ were observed. Nevertheless, the authors suggest that the genetic variant is not the major responsiveness factor to CBZ treatment. However, in the case of the other hepatic enzyme-inducing AEDs, PB, Basic et al. [40] showed that epileptic patients with CC homozygote had a significantly lower concentration of PB in the cerebrospinal fluid (CSF) than CT heterozygotes and TT homozygotes and they have had also reduced penetration of PB into the brain. Moreover, these patients had a higher seizure frequency than the others.

The other polymorphisms of *ABCB1/MDR1* C1236T and G2677 (A/T) are located in 12 and 21 exons, respectively. It has been showed that both and C3435T polymorphisms have an influence on the AEDs treatment and may be useful in predicting drug-resistant epilepsy [41]. However, the study of Haerian et al. [42] did not demonstrate association between C1236T, C3435T, and G2677 (A/T) and response to VPA treatment in patient with epilepsy. It was found that there were no differences regarding G2677 (A/T) genotype in CSF concentration of PB [40]. It was also showed that there was no correlation with seizure frequency [27].

The literature data did not indicate an important role of *ABCB1/MDR1* gene polymorphisms in epilepsy treatment. There is still not clear influence on P-gp expression and function in response to AED therapy. It seems that more precise knowledge of the frequency of *ABCB1/MDR1* polymorphisms may contribute to a better understanding of disease pathomechanism and its implications for the effective treatment.

4. Genes important for homocysteine and ADMA metabolism and antiepileptic drug therapy in epilepsy

The polymorphisms in genes *MTHFR, MTR, MTHFD1,* and *CBS* involved in Hcy metabolism, as shown in **Figure 1**, are not unique to epilepsy and are also involved in heart diseases, neural tube defects, migraine, stroke, Parkinson's and Alzheimer's diseases, schizophrenia, and a few other disorders [43–45].

Hcy

Gene	Locus
MTHFR	1p36.3
MTR	1q43
MTRR	5p15.31
MTHFD1	14q24
CBS	21q22.3

ADMA

Gene	Locus
DDAH1	1p22
eNOS	7q36

Figure 1. Genes associated with homocysteine (Hcy) and asymmetric dimethylarginine (ADMA) metabolism.

MTHFR gene encodes methylenetetrahydrofolate reductase, MTHFR enzyme. The most common polymorphisms of this gene, C677T and A1298C, are associated with this enzyme deficiency. The *MTHFR* C677T polymorphism leads to the substitution of alanine for valine within the N-terminal catalytic domain of the enzyme. The mean activity of MTHFR enzyme in individuals carrying the CT genotype is 65%, while in TT variant carriers it reaches only 30%, both in comparison to the CC genotype. The *MTHFR* C677T TT is a cause of HHcy [46, 47]. Recent meta-analysis has shown that *MTHFR* C677T polymorphism is a risk factor for epilepsy [45]. The relation between C677T variants and HHcy in patients with epilepsy treated with AEDs was widely studied, but the results are ambiguous. The elevated Hcy level was observed among adult patients with CT and TT genotype [16, 48]. Moreover, it has been shown that children and young adults with TT genotype treated with AEDs have higher Hcy level and lower IQ score compared to those with CC genotype [49]. No contribution in HHcy was found in children treated with CBZ or VPA [50].

The *MTHFR* A1298C polymorphism leads to the substitution of glutamate for alanine within the C-terminal regulatory domain of the MTHFR enzyme. The mean activity of MTHFR protein in subjects with AC genotype is 70%. Furthermore, double heterozygotes of mentioned polymorphism in MTHFR (CT and AC) have an additional loss of activity [43]. Also the frequency of diplotype CT677/AC1298 was higher in epileptic patients than in controls and could be a risk factor for HHcy [51]. The effect of only A1298C polymorphism on Hcy level is minimal [43, 52]. According to meta-analysis the influence of *MTHFR* A1298C polymorphism on epilepsy remains inconsistent [45].

MTR gene encodes methionine synthase, MTR enzyme, while *MTRR* encodes methionine synthase reductase, MTRR enzyme. MTRR protein catalyzes the conversion of inactive form of MTR into active. Both enzymes, MTR and MTRR, are essential for Hcy remethylation to methionine. *MTR* A2756G polymorphism converts aspartic acid to glycine and in *MTRR* A66G methionine replaces isoleucine. It was observed that *MTR* A2756G and *MTRR* A66G polymorphisms are associated with increased Hcy level due to reduction in enzyme activity and may be risk factors for HHcy [53, 54]. On the other hand, other studies deny the influence of G allele of *MTR* A2756G on Hcy level, also in epileptic patients [16, 55]. The G allele of this polymorphism occurred more frequent in epileptics than in controls [16].

MTHFD1 gene encodes three-functional enzyme methylenetetrahydrofolate dehydrogenase/ methyltetrahydrofolate cyclohydrolase/formyltetrahydrofolate synthetase, MTHFD1 that regulates the Hcy circulation. *MTHFD1* G1958A polymorphism results in the substitution of an arginine by a glutamine. According to Sniezawska et al. [16], the AA genotype was more frequent in epileptic patients than in controls, but only wild-type genotype was associated with increased Hcy level in AED-treated patients.

CBS gene encodes cystathionine beta-synthase, CBS, an enzyme responsible for Hcy degradation to cystathionine. Missense mutation in *CBS* gene leads to its deficiency and homocystinuria. Reversible cerebral white matter lesions were found in MRI among patients with CBS deficiency [56]. *CBS* T833C polymorphism results in substitution of threonine for isoleucine. Another widely studied polymorphism is 844ins68. The T833C/844ins68 polymorphism is associated with mild HHcy [57]. However, *CBS* T833C polymorphism increases the risk of HHcy in patients treated with AEDs. Moreover, among 20% of patients with TC genotype and increased level of Hcy, the seizures were observed [13].

What is interesting, polymorphisms in Hcy metabolism genes also influence the ADMA level. It was demonstrated that epileptic patients treated with AEDs with gene polymorphisms *MTHFR* (C677T), *MTR* (A2756G), and *MTHFD1* (G1958A) had increased level of ADMA [16].

DDAH1 gene encodes dimethylarginine dimethylaminohydrolase, DDAH enzyme that degrades ADMA, as shown in **Figure 1**. Isoform 1 of DDAH is highly expressed in brain. Lind et al. [58] showed that several polymorphisms in *DDAH1* gene are related to ADMA level, but not to endothelium-dependent vasodilatation. Another group identified 4-nucleotide deletion/ insertion variant in the promoter region that leads to reduction of *DDAH1* transcription activity and mRNA level, which increase the ADMA concentration and is a risk factor for thrombosis stroke and coronary heart disease [59]. Polymorphisms in *DDAH1* gene have not been studied in epilepsy yet.

eNOS gene encodes endothelial isoform of nitric oxide synthase, an enzyme that can be inhibited by ADMA. It was observed that polymorphisms in *eNOS* can influence the ADMA level. Studies performed on rats with pilocarpine-induced status epileptics indicated that increased eNOS are related with DDAH1 overexpression via augmented ADMA inhibition [60]. Overexpression of DDAH1 protects against HHcy-induced cerebral vascular dysfunction [61]. The possible role for ADMA-DDAH pathway in neuronal activity modulation was

http://dx.doi.org/10.5772/64445

proposed due to increased ADMA concentration and DDAH1 expression in brain and spinal cord [62].

5. Antiepileptic drugs and other risk factors of vascular diseases

In the literature, there have been many publications indicating an increase in the plasma Hcy level in patients with epilepsy treated with AEDs [16, 63]. It has been showed that elevated level of Hcy above 15 μM (HHcy) in epileptic patients treated with AEDs may be associated with a number of clinical complications. Older publications indicate that HHcy may lead to three times increase the risk of myocardial infarction and twice increase the risk of stenosis of the coronary artery [64] and development of vascular disease [65, 66], neuropsychiatric [13] and considered a risk factor in seizure resistance and resistance to AEDs treatment [15].

Currently, it is believed that the impact of the AED risk of vascular disease depends on the type of drug used in patients with epilepsy. AEDs can be divided into two groups: hepatic enzyme-inducing AEDs (CBZ, PB, PHT) leading to an increase in cholesterol, low-density lipoprotein (LDL), total cholesterol, triglycerides, C-reactive protein (CRP), and Hcy level and hepatic enzyme-inhibiting AEDs (VPA) whose impact on the level of Hcy is not clear [16, 24, 67]. It is believed that the action of liver cytochrome P450-inducing AEDs leads to metabolic changes of macromolecular compounds, in particular lipids [68]. On the other hand, the liver cytochrome P450 inhibition of AEDs is not associated with metabolic changes but exhibits a proatherogenic effect by the impact on insulin resistance, body weight gain, and elevated oxidative stress [69]. At the same time, the share of inducing- and inhibiting AEDs in the pathogenesis of ischemic stroke and myocardial infarction is diverse.

Although, the study on a cohort of 252,407 patients aged above 18 years of age using inducing and inhibiting liver enzyme AEDs has shown that inducing AEDs do not lead to an increased risk of ischemic stroke and cause a small increase in myocardial infarction. While inhibiting AEDs also do not lead to an increased risk of ischemic stroke and lead to a reduction in the risk of myocardial infarction [24]. Moreover, according to Renoux et al. [24], only prolonged use of inducing AEDs led to an increase in the risk of myocardial infarction.

So far there is no effective therapy leading to a reduction in the level of Hcy and/or ADMA and other risk factors for vascular lesions, e.g., lipids and proteins following the AEDs used in epilepsy treatment. These issues require further study.

6. Summary

AEDs especially the older generation, including CBZ, PB, and PHT may lead to increased plasma Hcy concentrations and changes in the level of plasma ADMA in patients with epilepsy, as shown in **Figure 2**. It is believed that CBZ, PB, and PHT lead to elevated levels of plasma Hcy and/or ADMA by inducing liver enzyme. On the other hand, VPA does not lead to activation of liver enzymes, and its effect on plasma levels of Hcy and/or ADMA is varied.

Longer duration of the use of AEDs associated with impaired intestinal absorption of FA (CBZ, PB, and PHT) leads to an increase in incidents of myocardial infarction involving elevated levels of Hcy and/or ADMA or by other mechanisms of vascular lesions. However, VPA does not lead to an increase in incidents of ischemic stroke and leads to a decrease of myocardial infarction. It seems that the toxic effect of AEDs not only involves production of neurotoxic Hcy but also involves induction of apoptosis.

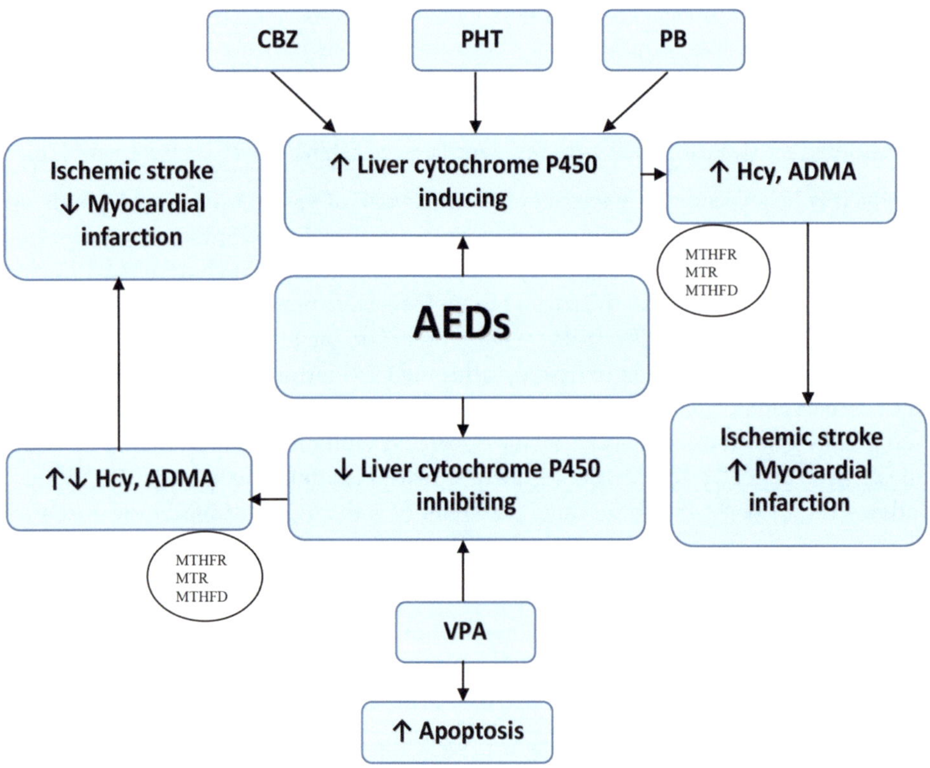

Figure 2. Antiepileptic drugs (AEDs) and risk factors of vascular diseases in epilepsy. Enzymes associated with Hcy-homocysteine metabolism, MTHFR, MTR, MTHFD1. ADMA, asymmetric dimethylarginine; CBZ, carbamazepine; VPA, valproic acid; PHT, phenytoin; PB, phenobarbital; ↑, increase; ↓, decrease level.

Supplementation with B-group vitamins and FA, and arginine may improve the effectiveness of AED therapy in patients with epilepsy.

Acknowledgements

This study was supported by the Poznan University of Medical Sciences grant, no. 502-01-11111-45-07-467.

Author details

Jolanta Dorszewska[1*], Urszula Lagan-Jedrzejczyk[1,2], Marta Kowalska[1], Katarzyna Wize[1] and Wojciech Kozubski[2]

*Address all correspondence to: dorszewskaj@yahoo.com

1 Laboratory of Neurobiology, Department of Neurology, Poznan University of Medical Sciences, Poznan, Poland

2 Department of Neurology, Poznan University of Medical Sciences, Poznan, Poland

References

[1] Lagan-Jedrzejczyk U, Lianeri M, Kozubski W, Dorszewska J. Homocysteine and apoptotic factors in epileptic patients treated with antiepileptic drugs. In: Kilmer McCully, editor. Homocysteine: structure, biosynthesis and health implications. NOVA Sciences Publishers, Inc., NY, USA; 2014, p. 83–111.

[2] Karabiber H, Sonmezgoz E, Ozerol E, Yakinci C, Otlu B, Yologlu S. Effects of valproate and carbamazepine on serum levels of homocysteine, vitamin B12, and folic acid. Brain and Development; 2003, 25:113–115. DOI: 10.1016/S0387-7604(02)00163-8.

[3] Attilakos A, Papakonstantinou E, Schulpis K, Voudris K, Katsarou E, Mastroyianni S, Garoufi A. Early effect of sodium valproate and carbamazepine monotherapy on homocysteine metabolism in children with epilepsy. Epilepsy Research; 2006, 71:229–232. DOI: 10.1016/j.eplepsyres.2006.06.015.

[4] Hamed SA, Hamed EA, Hamdy R, Nabeshima T. Vascular risk factors and oxidative stress as independent predictors of asymptomatic atherosclerosis in adult patients with epilepsy. Epilepsy Research; 2007, 74:183–192. DOI: 10.1016/j.eplepsyres.2007.03.010.

[5] Badiou S, Breton H, Peyriere H, Charasson V, Crespel A, Gelisse P, Cristol JP, Hillaire-Buys D. Comparison of carbamazepine and oxcarbazepine effects on aminothiol levels. European Journal of Clinical Pharmacology; 2008, 64:83–87. DOI: 10.1007/s00228-007-0388-z.

[6] Gidal B, Tamura T, Hammer A, Vuong A. Blood homocysteine, folate and vitamin B-12 concentrations in patients with epilepsy receiving lamotrigine or sodium valproate for initial monotherapy. Epilepsy Research; 2005, 64:161–166. DOI: 10.1016/j.eplepsyres.2005.03.005.

[7] Boger RH, Bode-Boger SM, Sydow K, Heistad DD, Lentz SR. Plasma concentration of asymmetric dimethylarginine, an endogenous inhibitor of nitric oxide synthase is elevated in monkey with hyperhomocysteinemia or hypercholesterolemia. Arterio-

sclerosis, Thrombosis, and Vascular Biology; 2000, 20:1557–1564. DOI: 10.1161/01.ATV. 20.6.1557.

[8] Verrotti A, Pascarella R, Trotta D, Giuva T, Morgese G, Chiarelli F. Hyperhomocysteinemia in children treated with sodium valproate and carbamazepine. Epilepsy Research; 2000, 41:253–257. DOI: 10.1016/S0920-1211(00)00150-9.

[9] Yoo JH, Hong SB. A common mutation in the methylenetetrahydrofolate reductase gene is a determinant of hyperhomocysteinemia in epileptic patients receiving anticonvulsants. Metabolism; 1999, 48:1047–1051. DOI: 10.1016/S0026-0495(99)90204-4.

[10] Apeland T, Mansoor MA, Strandjord RE. Antiepileptic drugs as independent predictors of plasma total homocysteine levels. Epilepsy Research; 2001, 47:27–35. DOI: 10.1016/S0920-1211(01)00288-1.

[11] Unal O, Deda G, Teber S, Ertem M, Akar N. Thrombophilic risk factors in epileptic children treated with valproic acid. Pediatric Neurology; 2009, 40:102–106. DOI: 10.1016/j.pediatrneurol.2008.10.005.

[12] Sener U, Zorlu Y, Karaguzel O, Ozdamar O, Coker I, Topbas M. Effects of common antiepileptic drug monotherapy on serum levels of homocysteine, vitamin B12, folic acid and vitamin B6. Seizure; 2006, 15:79–85. DOI: 10.1016/j.seizure.2005.11.002.

[13] Siniscalchi A, Mancuso F, Gallelli L, Ibbadu G, Mercuri NB, De Sarro G. Increase in plasma homocysteine levels induced by drug treatments in neurologic patients. Pharmacological Research; 2005, 52: 367–375. DOI: 10.1016/j.phrs.2005.05.013.

[14] Yoo JH, Lee SC. Elevated levels of plasma homocyst(e)ine and symmetric dimethylarginine in elderly patients with stroke. Atherosclerosis; 2001, 158:425–430. DOI: 10.1016/S0021-9150(01)00444-0.

[15] Kubova H, Folbergrova J, Mares P. Seizures induced by homocysteine in rats during ontogenesis. Epilepsia; 1995, 36:750–756. DOI: 10.1111/j.1528-1157.1995.tb01611.x.

[16] Sniezawska A, Dorszewska J, Rozycka A, Przedpelska-Ober E, Lianeri M, Jagodzinski PP, Kozubski W. MTHFR, MTR, and MTHFD1 gene polymorphisms compared to homocysteine and asymmetric dimethylarginine concentrations and their metabolites in epileptic patients treated with antiepileptic drugs. Seizure; 2011, 20:533–540. DOI: 10.1016/j.seizure.2011.04.001.

[17] Ozdemir O, Yakut A, Dinleyici EC, Aydogdu SD, Yarar C, Colak O. Serum asymmetric dimethylarginine (ADMA), homocysteine, vitamin B(12), folate levels, and lipid profiles in epileptic children treated with valproic acid. European Journal of Pediatrics; 2011, 170:873–877. DOI: 10.1007/s00431-010-1366-5.

[18] Kielstein JT, Bode-Boger SM, Frolich JC, Ritz E, Haller H, Fliser D. Asymmetric dimethylarginine, blood pressure, and renal perfusion in elderly subjects. Circulation; 2003, 107:1891–1895. DOI: 10.1161/01.CIR.0000060496.23144.A7.

[19] Chan JR, Boger RH, Bode-Boger SM, Tangphao O, Tsao PS, Blaschke TF, Cooke JP. Asymmetric dimethylarginine increases mononuclear cell adhesiveness in hypercholesterolemic humans. Arteriosclerosis, Thrombosis, and Vascular Biology; 2000, 20:1040–1046. DOI: 10.1161/01.CIR.0000060496.23144.A7.

[20] Cooke JP, Oka RK. Atherogenesis and the arginine hypothesis. Current Atherosclerosis Reports; 2001, 3:252–259.

[21] Kielstein JT, Bode-Boger SM, Frolich JC, Haller H, Boger RH. Relationship of asymmetric dimethylarginine to dialysis treatment and atherosclerosis disease. Kidney International; 2001, 78:9–13. DOI: 10.1046/j.1523-1755.2001.59780009.x.

[22] Miyazaki H, Matsuoka H, Cooke JP, Usui M, Ueda S, Okuda S, Imaizumi T. Endogenous nitric oxide synthase inhibitor: a novel marker of atherosclerosis. Circulation; 1999, 99:1141–1146. DOI: 10.1161/01.CIR.99.9.1141.

[23] Olesen JB, Abildstrøm SZ, Erdal J, Gislason GH, Weeke P, Andersson C, Torp-Pedersen C, Hansen PR. Effects of epilepsy and selected antiepileptic drugs on risk of myocardial infarction, stroke, and death in patients with or without previous stroke: a nationwide cohort study. Pharmacoepidemiology and Drug Safety; 2011, 20:964–971. DOI: 10.1002/pds.2186.

[24] Renoux C, Dell'Aniello S, Saarela O, Filion KB, Boivin JF. Antiepileptic drugs and the risk of ischaemic stroke and myocardial infarction: a population-based cohort study. BMJ Open; 2015, 5:e008365. DOI: 10.1136/bmjopen-2015-008365.

[25] Vyas MV, Davidson BA, Escalaya L, Costella J, Saposnik G, Burneo JG. Antiepileptic drug use for treatment of epilepsy and dyslipidemia: systematic review. Epilepsy Research; 2015, 113:44–67. DOI: 10.1016/j.eplepsyres.2015.03.002.

[26] Fisher RS, Acevedo C, Arzimanoglou A, Bogacz A, Cross JH, Elger CE, Engel J Jr, Forsgren L, French JA, Glynn M, Hesdorffer DC, Lee BI, Mathern GW, Moshé SL, Perucca E, Scheffer IE, Tomson T, Watanabe M, Wiebe S. ILAE official report: a practical clinical definition of epilepsy. Epilepsia; 2014, 55:475–482. DOI: 10.1111/epi.12550.

[27] Lagan-Jedrzejczyk U, Oczkowska A, Florczak A, Florczak-Wyspianska J, Karczewski J, Swiejkowska A, Wiktorowicz K, Przedpelska-Ober E, Kozubski W, Dorszewska J. ABCB1/MDR1 gene polymorphisms and the level of apoptotic factors in epilepsy patients treated with antiepileptic drugs. European Journal of Neurology. 2015, 22:Suppl 1, 341.

[28] Striano P, Vari MS, Mazzocchetti C, Verrotti A, Zara F. Management of genetic epilepsies: from empirical treatment to precision medicine. Pharmacological Research; 2016, 11:426–429. DOI: 10.1016/j.phrs.2016.04.006.

[29] Florczak A, Florczak J, Dorszewska J. Antiepileptic drugs and apoptosis. Farmakoterapia w Psychiatrii Neurologii; 2010, 26:145–152 (in Polish).

[30] Santulli L, Coppola A, Balestrini S, Striano S. The challenges of treating epilepsy with 25 antiepileptic drugs. Pharmacological Research; 2016, 107:211–219. DOI: 10.1016/j.phrs.2016.03.016.

[31] Foldvary-Schaefer N, Fong JS, Morrison S, Wang L, Bena J. Lacosamide tolerability in adult patients with partial-onset seizures: impact of planned reduction and mechanism of action of concomitant antiepileptic drugs. Epilepsy Behavior; 2016, 57:155–160. DOI: 10.1016/j.yebeh.2016.02.007.

[32] Pack AM. Perampanel: another choice for patients with idiopathic generalized epilepsy who have tonic-clonic seizures. Epilepsy Currents; 2016, 16:27–28. DOI: 10.5698/1535-7597-16.1.27.

[33] Lynch BA, Lambeng N, Nocka K, Kensel-Hammes P, Bajjalieh SM, Matagne A, Fuks B. The synaptic vesicle protein SV2A is the binding site for the antiepileptic drug levetiracetam. Proceedings of the National Academy of Science of United States of America. 2004, 101:9861–9866. DOI: 10.1073/pnas.0308208101.

[34] Strickler SM, Dansky LV, Miller MA, Seni MH, Andermann E, Spielberg SP. Genetic predisposition to phenytoin-induced birth defects. Lancet; 1985, 2:746–749. DOI: 10.1016/S0140-6736(85)90629-4.

[35] Holmes LB, Harvey EA, Coull BA, Huntington KB, Khoshbin S, Hayes AM, Ryan LM. The teratogenicity of anticonvulsant drugs. New England Journal of Medicine; 2001, 344:1132–1138. DOI: 10.1056/NEJM200104123441504.

[36] Gidal BE. P-glycoprotein expression and pharmacoresistant epilepsy: cause or consequence? Epilepsy Currents; 2014, 14:136–138. DOI: 10.5698/1535-7597-14.3.136.

[37] Siddiqui A, Kerb R, Weale ME, Brinkmann U, Smith A, Goldstein DB, Wood NW, Sisodiya SM. Association of multidrug resistance in epilepsy with a polymorphism in the drug-transporter gene ABCB1. New England Journal of Medicine; 2003, 348:1442–1448. DOI: 10.1056/NEJMoa021986.

[38] Vahab SA, Sen S, Ravindran N, Mony S, Mathew A, Vijayan N, Nayak G, Bhaskaranand N, Banerjee M, Satyamoorthy K. Analysis of genotype and haplotype effects of ABCB1 (MDR1) polymorphisms in the risk of medically refractory epilepsy in an Indian population. Drug Metabolism and Pharmacokinetics; 2009, 24: 255–260. DOI: 10.2133/dmpk.24.255.

[39] Sterjev Z, Trencevska GK, Cvetkovska E, Petrov I, Kuzmanovski I, Ribarska JT, Nestorovska AK, Matevska N, Naumovska Z, Jolevska-Trajkovic S, Dimovski A, Suturkova L. Mint. The association of C3435T single-nucleotide polymorphism, Pgp-glycoprotein gene expression levels and carbamazepine maintenance dose in patients with epilepsy. Neuropsychiatr Disease and Treatment; 2012, 8:191–196. DOI: 10.2147/NDT.S28285.

[40] Basic S, Hajnsek S, Bozina N, Filipcic I, Sporis D, Mislov D, Posavec A. The influence of C3435T polymorphism of ABCB1 gene on penetration of phenobarbital across the

blood–brain barrier in patients with generalized epilepsy. Seizure; 2008, 17:524–530. DOI: 10.1016/j.seizure.2008.01.003.

[41] Qiang LU, Liwen WU, Liri JIN, Qi XU, Yan SHEN. Association analysis of a polymorphism of MDR1 Gene and refractory temporal lobe epilepsy in a Chinese population. Neurology Asia; 2007, 12:94–95.

[42] Haerian BS, Lim KS, Tan HJ, Mohamed EH, Tan CT, Raymond AA, Wong CP, Wong SW, Omar H, Roslan H, Mohamed Z. Association between ABCB1 polymorphism and response to sodium valproate treatment in Malaysian epilepsy patients. Epileptic Disorder; 2011, 13:65–75. DOI: 10.1684/epd.2011.0419.

[43] Weisberg I, Tran P, Christensen B, Sibani S, Rozen R. A second genetic polymorphism in methylenetetrahydrofolate reductase (MTHFR) associated with decreased enzyme activity. Molecular Genetics and Metabolism; 1998, 64:169–172.

[44] Casas JP, Bautista LE, Smeeth L, Sharma P, Hingorani AD. Homocysteine and stroke: evidence on a causal link from Mendelian randomisation. Lancet; 2005, 365:224–232. DOI: 10.1016/S0140-6736(05)17742-3.

[45] Wu YL, Yang HY, Ding XX, Zhao X, Chen J, Bi P, Sun YH. Association between methylenetetrahydrofolate reductase C677T polymorphism and epilepsy susceptibility: a meta-analysis. Seizure; 2014, 23:411–416. DOI: 10.1016/j.seizure.2014.01.018.

[46] Liu A, Menon S, Colson NJ, Quinlan S, Cox H, Peterson M, Tiang T, Haupt LM, Lea RA, Griffiths LR. Analysis of the MHTFR C677T variant with migraine phenotypes. BMC Research Notes; 2010, 3:213–218. DOI: 10.1186/1756-0500-3-213.

[47] Schürks MM, Rist PM, Kurth T. MTHFR 677C>T and ACE D/I polymorphisms in migraine: a systematic review and meta-analysis. Headache; 2010, 50:588–599. DOI: 10.1111/j.1526-4610.2009.01570.x.

[48] Belcastro V, Striano P, Gorgone G, Costa C, Ciampa C, Caccamo D, Pisani LR, Oteri G, Marciani MG, Aguglia U, Striano S, Ientile R, Calabresi P, Pisani F. Hyperhomocysteinemia in epileptic patients on new antiepileptic drugs. Epilepsia 2010;51:274–279. DOI: 10.1111/j.1528-1167.2009.02303.x.

[49] Di Rosa G, Lenzo P, Parisi E, Neri M, Guerrera S, Nicotera A, Alibrandi A, Germanò E, Caccamo D, Spanò M, Tortorella G. Role of plasma homocysteine levels and MTHFR polymorphisms on IQ scores in children and young adults with epilepsy treated with antiepileptic drugs. Epilepsy Behavior; 2013, 29:548–551. DOI: 10.1016/j.yebeh.2013.09.034.

[50] Vurucu S, Demirkaya E, Kul M, Unay B, Gul D, Akin R, Gokçay E. Evaluation of the relationship between C677T variants of methylenetetrahydrofolate reductase gene and hyperhomocysteinemia in children receiving antiepileptic drug therapy. Progress in Neuro-Psychopharmacology & Biological Psychiatry; 2008, 32:844–848. DOI: 10.1016/j.pnpbp.2007.12.018.

[51] Caccamo D, Condello S, Gorgone G, Crisafulli G, Belcastro V, Gennaro S, Striano P, Pisani F, Ientile R. Screening for C677T and A1298C MTHFR polymorphisms in patients with epilepsy and risk of hyperhomocysteinemia. Neuromolecular Medicine; 2004, 6: 117–126.

[52] Meisel C, Cascorbi I, Gerloff T, Stangl V, Laule M, Müller JM, Wernecke KD, Baumann G, Roots I, Stangl K. Identification of six methylenetetrahydrofolate reductase (MTHFR) genotypes resulting from common polymorphisms: impact on plasma homocysteine levels and development of coronary artery disease. Atherosclerosis; 2001, 154:651–658. DOI: 10.1016/S0021-9150(00)00679-1.

[53] Laraqui A, Allami A, Carrié A, Coiffard AS, Benkouka F, Benjouad A, Bendriss A, Kadiri N, Bennouar N, Benomar A, Guedira A, Raisonnier A, Fellati S, Srairi JE, Benomar M. Influence of methionine synthase (A2756G) and methionine synthase reductase (A66G) polymorphisms on plasma homocysteine levels and relation to risk of coronary artery disease. Acta Cardiologica; 2006, 61:51–61. DOI: 10.2143/AC.61.1.2005140.

[54] Kluijtmans LA, Young IS, Boreham CA, Murray L, McMaster D, McNulty H, Strain JJ, McPartlin J, Scott JM, Whitehead AS. Genetic and nutritional factors contributing to hyperhomocysteinemia in young adults. Blood; 2003, 101:2483–2488.

[55] Klerk M, Lievers KJ, Kluijtmans LA, Blom HJ, den Heijer M, Schouten EG, Kok FJ, Verhoef P. The 2756A>G variant in the gene encoding methionine synthase: its relation with plasma homocysteine levels and risk of coronary heart disease in a Dutch case–control study. Thrombosis Research; 2003, 110:87–91. DOI: 10.1016/S0049-3848(03)00341-4.

[56] Sasai H, Shimozawa N, Asano T, Kawamoto N, Yamamoto T, Kimura T, Kawamoto M, Matsui E, Fukao T. Successive MRI findings of reversible cerebral white matter lesions in a patient with cystathionine β-synthase deficiency. Tohoku Journal of Experimental Medicine; 2015, 237:323–327. DOI: 10.1620/tjem.237.323.

[57] Gaustadnes M, Ingerslev J, Rütiger N. Prevalence of congenital homocystinuria in Denmark. New England Journal of Medicine; 1999, 340:1513. DOI: 10.1056/NEJM199905133401915.

[58] Lind L, Ingelsson E, Kumar J, Syvänen AC, Axelsson T, Teerlink T. Genetic variation in the dimethylarginine dimethylaminohydrolase 1 gene (DDAH1) is related to asymmetric dimethylarginine (ADMA) levels, but not to endothelium-dependent vasodilation. Vascular Medicine; 2013, 18:192–199. DOI: 10.1177/1358863X13496488.

[59] Ding H, Wu B, Wang H, Lu Z, Yan J, Wang X, Shaffer JR, Hui R, Wang DW. A novel loss-of-function DDAH1 promoter polymorphism is associated with increased susceptibility to thrombosis stroke and coronary heart disease. Circulation Research; 2010, 106:1145–1152. DOI: 10.1161/CIRCRESAHA.109.215616.

[60] Hirotsu C, Matos G, Tufik S, Andersen ML. Changes in gene expression in the frontal cortex of rats with pilocarpine-induced status epilepticus after sleep deprivation. Epilepsy Behavior; 2013, 27:378–384. DOI: 10.1016/j.yebeh.2013.02.024.

[61] Rodionov RN, Dayoub H, Lynch CM, Wilson KM, Stevens JW, Murry DJ, Kimoto M, Arning E, Bottiglieri T, Cooke JP, Baumbach GL, Faraci FM, Lentz SR. Overexpression of dimethylarginine dimethylaminohydrolase protects against cerebral vascular effects of hyperhomocysteinemia. Circulation Research; 2010, 106:551–558. DOI: 10.1161/CIRCRESAHA.109.200360.

[62] Greco R, Ferrigno A, Demartini C, Zanaboni A, Mangione AS, Blandini F, Nappi G, Vairetti M, Tassorelli C. Evaluation of ADMA-DDAH-NOS axis in specific brain areas following nitroglycerin administration: study in an animal model of migraine. Journal of Headache Pain; 2015, 16:560. DOI: 10.1186/s10194-015-0560-2.

[63] Bochyńska A, Lipczyńska-Łojkowska W, Gugała-Iwaniuk M, Lechowicz W, Restel M, Graban A, Lipska B, Ryglewicz D. The effect of vitamin B supplementation on homocysteine metabolism and clinical state of patients with chronic epilepsy treated with carbamazepine and valproic acid. Seizure; 2012, 21:276–281. DOI: 10.1016/j.seizure.2012.01.013.

[64] Selhub J, Jacques PF, Bostom AG, D'Agostino RB, Wilson PW, Belanger AJ, O'Leary DH, Wolf PA, Schaefer EJ, Rosenberg IH. Association between plasma homocysteine concentrations and extracranial carotid-artery stenosis. New England Journal of Medicine; 1995, 332:286–291. DOI: 10.1056/NEJM199502023320502.

[65] Verrotti A, Domizio S, Angelozzi B, Sabatino G, Morgese G, Chiarelli F. Changes in serum lipids and lipoproteins in epileptic children treated with anticonvulsants. Journal of Paediatrics and Child Health; 1997, 33:242–245. DOI: 10.1111/j.1440-1754.1997.tb01588.x.

[66] Tan TY, Lu CH, Chuang HY, Lin TK, Liou CW, Chang WN, Chuang YC. Long-term antiepileptic drug therapy contributes to the acceleration of atherosclerosis. Epilepsia; 2009, 50:1579–1586. DOI: 10.1111/j.1528-1167.2009.02024.x.

[67] Katsiki N, Mikhailidis DP, Nair DR. The effects of antiepileptic drugs on vascular risk factors: a narrative review. Seizure; 2014, 23:677–684. DOI: 10.1016/j.seizure.2014.05.011.

[68] Mintzer S. Metabolic consequences of antiepileptic drugs. Current Opinion in Neurology; 2010, 23:164–169. DOI: 10.1097/WCO.0b013e32833735e7.

[69] Verrotti A, Scardapane A, Franzoni E, Manco R, Chiarelli F. Increased oxidative stress in epileptic children treated with valproic acid. Epilepsy Research; 2008, 78:171–177. DOI: 10.1016/j.eplepsyres.2007.11.005.

Chapter 10

Epidemiological Study of Acute Poisoning for Antiepileptic Drugs: A 2-Year Retrospective Study in Cracow, Poland

Anna Staniszewska, Marta Dąbrowska-Bender,
Aleksandra Czerw, Dominik Olejniczak,
Grzegorz Juszczyk and
Magdalena Bujalska-Zadrożny

Additional information is available at the end of the chapter

http://dx.doi.org/10.5772/64455

Abstract

The aim of this study was designed to examine the rate of occurrence of antiepileptic drug overdose in 2002 and 2012 in Cracow, Poland, and analyze the demographics and clinical features of the patients Antiepileptic drugs (AEDs) intoxication. A retrospective study included all the patients admitted in to the Toxicology Units in Cracow for AED intoxications in 2002 and in 2012. Patients were identified of discharge diagnoses (ICD-10). AED intoxication were 5.40% of the total admissions. Mean age of the patients was 35.88 ± 12.54 years. The female-to-male ratio was 1:1.7. The most frequent AED was carbamazepine (n = 140), followed by valproate (n = 31). The most frequent motivation was intentional intoxication (n = 166, 94.86%). Ethanol was coingested by 51 patients (29.14%). Most of the patients ingested other drugs (32%). Antiepileptic drugs intoxication accounted for only of 7.13% of all cases admitted to the abovementioned toxicology units in 2002 and 2012 in Cracow. Our studies show that most of the AED poisoning cases in those years were caused by drugs belonging to the old generation antiepileptic drugs, including carbamazepine and valproic acid. The majority of the intoxication cases was related to suicidal poisoning and commonest identified reason of self-intoxication were issues with self including attention-seeking behavior.

Keywords: antiepileptic drugs, acute intoxication, clinical manifestations, drug serum level, suicide attempts

INTECH
open science | open minds

1. Introduction

Antiepileptic drugs (AEDs) are mainly used in the treatment of epilepsy and treatment of some mental disorders. Patients suffering from it are at increased risk of suicidal ideation, suicide attempts, and completed suicides. The widespread use of AEDs resulted also in the fact that this group of drugs is frequently encountered as the cause of acute toxicity among patients treated at the toxicology unit around the world. Few data are available regarding the rate of AED overdose in individual countries. For example, AEDs are approximately 3% of the intoxication cases in the USA [1]. Other studies shows a 25% increase in the rate of occurrence of antiepileptic drug overdose between 2000 and 2006 [2, 3] in the USA. Annual Report of the American Association of Poison Control Centers Toxic Exposure Surveillance System states that AEDs comprise 3.2% of all causes of poisoning in adults (>19 years old) [4]. The Brazilian study by Bonilha et al. show that in Saõ Paulo and its outskirts in 2001, AED poisoning accounted for 16% of all the poisonings [5]. In Edinburgh (the UK, Scotland) for the period from 2000 to 2007, AED poisonings accounted for 3.4% of all poisonings [6]. In Marmara region (Uludag) in west Turkey for the period 1996–1999, 6.7% of medicinal intoxications was due to AEDs [7]. In France (Paris emergency departments), the prevalence of poisoning with AEDs for the period 1992–1993 was 2.9% and for 2001–2002 was 0.9% [8]. In Iran (studies conducted in the referral center for all cases of poisoning occurring in Tehran), AED poisoning accounted for 4.8% of all the pharmaceutical intoxications [9].

2. Aim

This study was designed to examine the rate of occurrence of antiepileptic drug overdose in 2002 and 2012 in Cracow, Poland, and to analyze the demographics and clinical features of the patients AED intoxication.

3. Material and methods

A retrospective study included all patients admitted for AED intoxications to Specialist Hospital Louis Rydgier's Co. o.o. in Cracow, in 2002 (in 2002, Cracow was the only toxicological unit), and all the persons were admitted for the same reason in to University Hospital in Cracow as well as Specialist Hospital Louis Rydgier's Co. o.o in Cracow in 2012. Patients were identified on the basis of discharge diagnoses (using International Classification of Diseases, ICD-10) with the code for poisoning by antiepileptic, sedative-hypnotic, and antiparkinsonism drugs (T42, excluded T42.0, T42.1, T42.3, T42.4, T42.8).

The data gathered included age, gender, mode of poisoning, reasons for attempt, and history of attempting suicide. The clinical spectrum of data analyzed consisted of serum level of AEDs, severity of poisoning, and effects of treatment.

The project was approved by the Ethics Committee, Medical University of Warsaw (No. AKBE/32/13).

3.1. Area of the survey

In Poland, there lives about 38 million people. Today's Poland consists of 16 provinces (voivodships), according to the last changes implemented in 1999. In Poland, toxicological units are located in nine large cities, which hospitalized patients with individual provinces. The University Hospital in Cracow and Specialist Hospital Louis Rydgier's Co. o.o in Cracow are responsible for all inhabitants of the Malopolskie (comprises 3.4 million of the country's population) and Swietokrzyskie provinces (comprises 1.26 million of the country's population) in Poland.

3.2. Statistical analysis

The data were collected in a Microsoft Excel database. Data are presented as mean and standard deviation (SD). Statistical analysis was performed using Statistical Programme for Social Sciences (SPSS). We used Pearson's χ^2 test to evaluate the association (and its strength) of the frequencies of data distribution among the different drug groups. A value of $p<0.05$ was considered to be statistically significant.

4. Results

Of all the poisoning cases ($n = 2455$ patients), 175 (7.13%) patients with AED intoxications were admitted to the Toxicology Unit in Cracow, Poland, in 2002 and 2012. Females accounted for 37.14% of the cases and males accounted for 62.86% with a female-to-male ratio of 1:1.7. The mean age of patients in the sample was 35.88 years (SD ± 12.54). **Table 1** describes the demographic characteristics of the patients.

	2002	2012	Total N (%)
Gender			
Female	37	28	65 (37.14%)
Male	73	37	110 (62.86%)
Total	110	65	175 (100%)
Age			
Range	14–58 years	18–82 years	14–82 years
Mean ± SD	34.93 ± 11.,80	37 ± 13.64	35.88 ± 12.54

Table 1. Demographic characteristics of study population.

Out of 175 patients with AED intoxications, 170 took one of the antiepileptic drugs, while 5 patients received more than one AED (carbamazepine [CBZ] + valproid acid [VPA]). The majority of patients receiving AED took carbamazepine only ($n = 140$). Valproate ($n = 31$) was the second most common (but 5 out of 31 have taken VPA in combination with CBZ). Smaller numbers were found for the remaining AEDs (<1% each): lamotrigine ($n = 1$), phenytoin ($n = 1$), and topiramate ($n = 2$)—see **Table 2**. Men were more likely to ingest carbamazepine than women (Person $\chi^2 = 11.7$, $p < 0.0001$).

Drug	2002	2012	Total N (%)
Carbamazepine	96	44	140 (80%)
Valproic acid	8	18	26 (14.86%)
Carbamazepine + Valproic acid	4	1	5 (2.86%)
Topiramate	0	2	2 (1.14%)
Lamotrigine	1	0	1 (0.57%)
Phenytoin	1	0	1 (0.57%)

Table 2. Characteristics of antiepileptic drugs associated with analyzed poisoning cases ($n = 175$).

The distribution of serum levels of AEDs was found as follows: 11 patients had therapeutic serum levels, 4 patients had subtherapeutic level of drugs, while in 141 cases, the drug concentrations were at the toxic level. AED concentrations in serum could not be measured in 23 patients (13.14%). **Table 3** shows the serum-level distributions for individual antiepileptic drugs.

Carbamazepine level	**N (%)**
Subtherapeutic level (<4 μg/ml)	1
Therapeutic level (4–12 μg/ml)	10
Toxic level (>12 μg/ml)	113
Toxicological analysis confirmed presence of CBZ in blood.	21
Range: 3.88–56.2 μg/ml. Mean: 26.94 ± SD 11.59	
Valproic acid level	N (%)
Subtherapeutic level (<50 μg/ml)	3
Therapeutic level (50–100 μg/ml)	1
Toxic level (>100 μg/ml)	27
Range: 5–660 μg/ml. Mean: 263 ± SD 174.17	
Topiramate level	**N (%)**
Toxicological analysis confirmed presence of TPM in blood.	1
Lamotrigine level	**N (%)**
Toxicological analysis confirmed presence of LTG in blood	1
Phenytoin level	**N (%)**
Subtherapeutic level (<10 μg/ml)	0
Therapeutic level (10–20 μg/ml)	0
Toxic level (>20 μg/ml)	1
Mean: 53 μg/ml	

Table 3. Serum levels of valproic acid ($n = 31$), carbamazepine ($n = 145$), topiramate ($n = 2$), lamotrigine ($n = 1$), phenytoin ($n = 1$) stratified by toxicological status of drug concentrations.

http://dx.doi.org/10.5772/64455

	2002	2012	Total N (%)
Mode of poisoning			
Suicidal	106	60	166 (94.86%)
Accidental	3	3	6 (3.43%)
Not available	1	2	3 (1.71%)
Poisoning Severity Score (PSS)			
Minor	60	33	93 (53.14%)
Moderate	45	26	71 (40.57%)
Severe	4	6	10 (5.71%)
Fatal	1	0	1 (0.57%)
No. of suicide attempts			
Not available	65	43	108 (61.71%)
Another	41	18	59 (33.71%)
Not applicable	4	4	8 (4.57%)
Treatment effect			
Cured	62	57	119 (68%)
Psychiatric ward	32	1	33 (18.9%)
Death	1	0	1 (0.57%)
Discharged from hospital at his own request	15	7	22 (12.57%)
Ethanol			
N	36	15	51 (29.14%)
Range	0–3, 59‰	0–2, 92‰	
Mean ± SD	0.43 ± 0081	0.42 ± 0.85	
Reason for attempting suicide			
Person to person conflicts	0	22	22 (12.57%)
Reason not identified or not recorded	82	25	107 (61.14%)
Issues with school/work	1	4	5 (2.86%)
Issues with self-including attention-seeking behavior	22	6	28 (16%)
Mentally challenged	5	8	13 (7.43%)
Comorbidity			
Depression	29	14	43 (24.57%)
Alcohol dependence syndrome	42	24	66 (37.71%)
Personality disorder	14	13	27 (15.43%)
Bipolar disorder	1	3	4 (2.28%)
Schizophrenia	1	6	7 (4%)
Other mental disorder	23	15	38 (21.71%)
Somatic disease	3	12	15 (8,57%)
Epilepsy	41	23	64 (36.57%)
Other drugs			
Antipsychotics	12	9	21 (12%)
Antidepressants	6	5	11 (6.28%)
Barbiturates	4	1	5 (2.86%)
Benzodiazepines	17	3	20 (11.43%)
Nonsteroidal anti-inflammatory drugs	1	2	3 (1.71%)
Opioids	0	2	2 (1.14%)

Table 4. Characteristics of suicide attempts.

Severity of intoxication was classified according to Poisoning Severity Score (PSS). The PSS grades severity as (0) none—no symptoms or signs related to poisoning: (1) minor—mild, transient, and spontaneously resolving symptoms, (2) moderate—pronounced or prolonged symptoms, (3) severe—severe or life-threatening symptoms, and (4) fatal poisoning—death [10].

The PSS was minor in 93 patients, moderate in 71 patients, severe in 10 patients, and fatal in 1 patient. Alcohol was involved in 29.14% of cases. An alcohol consumption did not differ significantly depending on the gender (Pearson's $\chi^2 = 0.1$, $p = 0.745$).

It is noteworthy that of the 56 ($n = 36$ in 2002, $n = 20$ in 2012) patients (32%), one patient took 1 or >1 antiepileptic drug and more than one (i.e., antiepileptic only) drug, including antipsychotics (12%), benzodiazepines (11.43%), antidepressants (6.28%), barbiturates (2.86%), nonsteroidal anti-inflammatory drugs (1.71%), and opioids (1.14%).

One-third of the patients (33.71%) had at least one suicide attempt before hospitalization; however, no information was available regarding the severity of these suicide attempts. Two patients (1.14%) had attempted suicide during hospitalization.

Suicidal and accidental poisoning, respectively, represented 94.86% and 3.43% of acute intoxications cases. The cause of poisoning in three cases (1.71%) could not be found. The most frequent reason of intoxication was issues with self—including attention-seeking behavior (16%), followed by person to person conflicts (12.57%). The frequency of poisoning cases between different circumstances did not differ significantly depending on the gender (Pearson's $\chi^2 = 0.5$, $p = 0.920$). There was no association between previous history of parasuicide, gender, and AED intoxication ($p > 0.05$).

Nearly half of the poisoned patients (44.57%) described in this report were treated with AEDs because of epilepsy or psychotic disorders prior to the poisoning.

More than half of the patients had a diagnostic history of psychiatric disorders, and 66 (37.71%) a diagnostic history of alcoholism.

Most patients (68%, $n = 119$) were discharged to homes in good condition, 33 (18.9%) were transferred to a psychiatric ward. As many as 22 patients (12.57%) did not complete hospitalization because they left the hospital at their own request.

The characteristics of the suicide attempts are shown in **Table 4**.

5. Discussion

Our results show a lower probability of AED intoxication in women than in men (37.1% vs. 62.9%). However, most studies observe that women were more likely than men to undergo drugs intoxications, including antiepileptic drugs [7, 11–14]. In Poland, women more often than men attempted suicide; however, men tend to be more successful than women in actual lethality. Other studies have confirmed this result [15–17]. In Poland, according to the data by the Police Headquarters the most common way to commit suicide is hanging (72%), other popular methods often include: jumping from a height (6.9%) and poisoning (4.6%) [18]. The Polish study by Bolechała et al. show that in Cracow, in 1991–2000, suicidal poisoning was in the male-to-female ratio of 1.8:1 [19].

In 2002, 5100 people died by suicide in Poland. According to the data, the vast majority of the suicides were committed by males (n = 4215). Whereas, in 2012, in Poland 4177 people committed suicide, including 3569 men [18]. In our study, twofold more men in 2002 committed suicide than in 2012.

In our study, the most commonly encountered drug was carbamazepine which generally corresponded with community prescribing patterns. It is also compatible with reports from Edinburgh [6], Iran (Tehran) [9], and São Paulo [5]. Another frequently used drug in our study was valproic acid. It is known from the literature that the number of overdose cases of sodium valproate is steadily increasing in civilized countries [20, 21]. Carbamazepine and sodium valproate were the most frequently used AEDs. In the present study, men were more likely to use carbamazepine than women ($p < 0.0001$). However, in a study by Nixon et al. (data from Edinburgh, the UK), women were more likely to ingest lamotrigine than men ($p < 0.0001$) and less likely to ingest sodium valproate ($p = 0.0234$) [6].

In our study, a higher than expected proportion of patients had coingested other (taken for reasons other than epilepsy) drugs (32%), which was in concordance with a previous report from Turkey [22]. However, this proportion was higher in the study by Nixon et al. in Edinburgh (65.4%) [6]. In our study, the most frequently taken drug types were antipsychotics (12%) as in the study by Çelenk et al. (12.5%) [22] concerning 1987 patients admitted to the Mayıs University Faculty of Medicine Emergency Department (Samsun, central Black Sea Region, Turkey). In Poland, in 2002, 211 people died by an overdose of hypnotics drugs, in 2012—193 people [18].

The suicide risk in patients with epilepsy is significantly higher than in the general population. Standardized mortality ratio for suicides among epileptic patients is estimated at 3.5–5.8 in comparison with the general population [23, 24]. In a review of 21 studies, a mean of 11.5% (range: 0–67%) of the deaths of patients with epilepsy were attributed to suicide [25]. The proportion of deliberate self-poisoning was 94.86% in our study. Suicide attempt was the most frequent circumstance observed in Brazil (Saõ Paulo) [5] and Iran (Tehran, 98.9%) [9], too.

In a study by Harris et al., suicide attempt among patients with epilepsy increases future suicide risk to 38.4% compared with the general population [26]. Similar results were obtained in the Swedish study (data from Stockholm county area), where that percentage was 46.2% [17]. Our study show that every third patient had a history of previous parasuicide. Our findings are consistent with those of Hassanian-Moghaddam et al. [9]. Previous suicide attempt is a risk factor for suicide attempts in future.

The most important reasons for suicide attempts in epileptic patients are common to general population and other chronic disease. Some authors suggest that concomitant depression and other psychiatric disorders are the main risk factors of suicidal thoughts [27]. Danish study confirmed that 2.32% (n = 492) individuals who committed suicide had epilepsy compared with 0.74% (n = 3140) controls. In case of comorbid psychiatric disease, overall risk of suicide in epileptic patients appears to be nearly 14-fold higher, including 32-fold for affective disorders and 12-fold for anxiety disorders [28], and it is almost twice higher in the case of those with previous mental disorders and 12.5-fold for schizophrenia [29]. Similarly, Swedish study showed that epilepsy concomitant with psychiatric disorders is associated with ninefold higher risk of suicide [23]. Logistic regression analysis in a study by Hassanian-Moghaddam et al. revealed that the presence of medical disorders and history of psychiatric events is associated with AED intoxication [9]. In the present study, most patients had a history of psychiatric disorders (i.e., depression, personality disorders, bipolar disorder, and schizophrenia) or somatic disorders.

The mental illness (including depression, bipolar disorder, schizophrenia, and others) was the cause for the vast majority of suicides in Poland, in both 2002 and 2012 (respectively, n = 1017 and n = 808) [18].

On the other hand, Buljan et Santić demonstrated that among hospital-treated epilepsy patients, beside psychiatric comorbidity, difficult family situation is a significant factor of higher suicide risk. Study results showed that 14.6% of the epileptic patients treated at one hospital in Zagreb (Croatia) have attempted suicide [30]. This study revealed that person-to-person conflicts were reasons for attempting suicide for 12.57% of the patients. In our study, in 107 if the cases, the cause of suicide is unknown because some patients discharged from hospital at their own request refused to answer the question on the reason for attempting suicide.

Alcoholism is associated with a high risk for suicidality, suicide attempts, and completed suicides [31, 32]. Up to 40% of the persons with alcoholism attempt suicide at some time or other, and 7% end their lives by committing suicide [33]. Alcohol dependence syndrome was diagnosed in 37.71% of our patients. Ethanol was coingested by 51 patients (29.14%) in this study and by 94 patients (15.3%) in a study by Nixon et al. [16]. Alcohol use is associated with risk behaviors [34, 35]. People who are under the influence of alcohol are more likely to attempt suicide. Alcohol intoxication increases suicide risk up to 90 times in comparison with abstinence [34].

In Poland, in 2002 and in 2012 among the suicides, the vast majority was under the influence of alcohol (respectively, n = 1069 and n = 1438) [18].

In 2008, the FDA issued an alert contained a warning against an increased risk of suicidality (suicidal ideation or behavior) for antiepileptic drugs [36]. The FDA analyzed the reports of suicidality from placebo-controlled clinical studies of 11 antiepileptic drugs. In this analysis, patients receiving antiepileptic drugs had approximately twice the risk of suicidal behavior or ideation (0.43%) compared with patients receiving placebo (0.22%). In the present study, 44.57% of the patients described in this report were treated with AED because of the epilepsy or psychotic disorders prior to the poisoning. The number of cases of AED overdose is less in 2012 than in 2002, almost half. Some explanation for this may be that currently, there is a widespread use of drugs in the new generation. These newer drugs are more efficacious and have a better safety as compared with conventional (older) AED.

http://dx.doi.org/10.5772/64455

The patients' clinical condition was evaluated according to PSS and measuring serum level of AEDs. It was found that 93 persons (53.14%) had minor, 71 (40.57%) moderate, and 10 patients (5.71%) had severe clinical findings and symptoms. Only one patient (0.57%) died due to CBZ poisoning. A 56-year-old man reportedly poisoned intentionally was admitted to Toxicology Department. History from family members revealed that patient had ingested together 320 tablets of carbamazepine and clomipramine. His carbamazepine serum concentration was 56.2 microg/mL. Urine analysis revealed clomipramine presence. Serum levels of other drugs and ethanol were all negative. He had a history of psychiatric illness, including depression. During whole hospitalization the patient was unconscious, unresponsive to the pain (Glasgow Coma Scale, GCS = 3). His pupils were broad in size with no reaction to light. His vital signs were as follows: pulse rate 70 beats/min, blood pressure 90/40 mmHg, temperature 36.4 C, and respiratory insufficiency. He was immediately intubated, and gastric lavage was performed to give a small amount of tablet. Patient was shifted to intensive care unit. Despite intense treatment and decrease of carbamazepine level to therapeutic values, there were no signs of patient recovery. Despite intensive resuscitation, in the third day of treatment the patient died. The corpse was transferred for investigation to the Forensic Medicine Department, the section was performed. In literature, CBZ serum level of 37 mcg/ml has been potentially lethal [37], but death due to CBZ overdose has been observed at lower concentrations [38–40].

Celenk et al. reported that 38 of the cases (59.4%) had no clinical symptoms, 18 cases (28%) had minor, 5 cases (7.8%) had moderate.

In our study, most of the patients had toxic serum drug levels ($n = 141$, 80.57%). In the abovementioned study from north Turkey, 28 patients (43.8%) had toxic serum AED level [22]. The knowledge of concentration range is significantly useful in clinical practice.

After treatment in the Toxicology Unit, a higher proportion of overdose patients discharged to go home (68%), whereas 18.9% of the patients required transfer to a psychiatric facilities. One death occurred in this study. Like our observation, Nixon et al. reported in the UK study that 14% of antiepileptic drug-overdose patients required transfer to a psychiatric facility, and 78.3% were discharged home [6].

6. Conclusion

Antiepileptic drugs intoxication accounted for only of 7.13% of all the cases admitted to the abovementioned toxicology units in 2002 and 2012 in Cracow, Poland, and AED poisoning is more common among males. Our studies show that most of AED poisoning cases in those years were caused by drugs belonging to the old generation antiepileptic drugs, including carbamazepine and valproic acid. The majority of intoxication cases were related to suicidal poisoning (94.86%), and commonest identified reason of self-intoxication were issues with self-including attention-seeking behavior (16%). Second leading established cause of suicide attempts were person-to-person conflicts (12.57%). Drugs combinations (AED + other drugs) were recorded in 32% of the cases and in 29.14% there occurred combinations between AEDs and alcohol.

Our study was a university hospital-based study, so these results may not be representative of the general population. However, these data still provide important information on the characteristics of the poisoning in this part of Poland. Further work is required to determine the rate of occurrence of antiepileptic drug overdose.

Acknowledgements

We thank the staff of University Hospital and Specialist Hospital Louis Rydgier's Co. o.o. in Cracow, Poland, for available of medical histories.

Author details

Anna Staniszewska[1*], Marta Dąbrowska-Bender[2], Aleksandra Czerw[2], Dominik Olejniczak[2], Grzegorz Juszczyk[2] and Magdalena Bujalska-Zadrożny[3]

*Address all correspondence to: anna.staniszewska@wum.edu.pl

1 Department of Experimental and Clinical Pharmacology, Medical University of Warsaw, Warsaw, Poland

2 Department of Public Health, Medical University of Warsaw, Warsaw, Poland

3 Department of Pharmacodynamics, Medical University of Warsaw, Warsaw, Poland

References

[1] Litovitz TL, Klein-Schwartz W, Rodgers Jr GC, et al. 2002 Annual Report of the American association of poison control centers toxic exposure surveillance system. Am J Emerg Med 2002;20(5):391–452. DOI: 10.1016/S0735-6757(03)00088-3.

[2] Litovitz TL, Klein-Schwartz W, White S, et al. 2000 Annual Report of the American Association of Poison Control Centers Toxic Exposure Surveillance System. Am J Emerg Med 2001;19:337–395. DOI: 10.1053/ajem.2001.25272.

[3] Bronstein AC, Spyker DA, Cantilena LR, et al. 2006 Annual Report of the American Association of Poison Control Centers National Poison Data System (NPDS). Clin Toxicol 2007;45:815–917. DOI: 10.1080/15563650701754763.

[4] Watson WA, Litovitz TL, Klein-Schwartz W, et al. 2003 Annual Report of the American Association of Poison Control Centers Toxic Exposure Surveillance System. Am J Emerg Med. 2004;22:335–404. DOI:10.1016/j.ajem.2004.06.001.

[5] Bonilha L, Collares CF, Alves do Amaral D, et al. Antiepileptic drugs: a study of 1028 cases registered by São Paulo Intoxication Control Center. Seizure 2005;14:170–174. DOI:10.1016/j.seizure.2005.01.003.

[6] Nixon AC, Doak MW, Crozier H, et al. Patterns of antiepileptic drug overdose differ between men and women: admissions to the Edinburgh Poisons Unit, 2000–2007.Q J Med 2009;102:51–56. DOI:10.1093/qjmed/hcn148.

[7] Akkose S, Bulut M, Armagan E, et al. Acute poisoning in adults in the years 1996–2001 treated in the Uludag University Hospital, Marmara Region, Turkey. Clin Toxicol (Phila) 2005;43:105–109. DOI: 10.1081/CLT-50429.

[8] Staikowsky F, Theil F, Mercadier P, et al. Change in profile of acute self drug-poisonings over a 10-year period. Hum Exp Toxicol 2004;23:507–511. DOI: 10.1191/0960327104ht487oa.

[9] Hassanian-Moghaddam H, Zarei MR, Kargar M, et al. Factors associated with non-benzodiazepine antiepileptic drug intoxication: Analysis of 9,809 registered cases of drug poisoning. Epilepsia 2010;51(6):979–983. DOI:10.1111/j.1528-1167.2010.02553.x.

[10] Persson H, Sjöberg G, Haines J, et al. Poisoning Severity Score: Grading of acute poisoning. J Toxicol—Clin Toxicol 1998;36:205–213.

[11] Townsend E, Hawton K, Harriss L, et al. Substances used in deliberate self-poisoning 1985–1997: trends and associations with age, gender, repetition and suicide intent. Soc Psychiatry Psychiatr Epidemiol 2001;36:228–234. DOI:10.1007/s001270170053.

[12] Waring WS, Laing WJ, Good AM, et al. Pattern of lithium exposure predicts poisoning severity: evaluation of referrals to a regional poisons unit. Q J Med 2007;100:271–276. DOI:10.1093/qjmed/hcm017.

[13] Wilson AD, Howell C, Waring WS. Venlafaxine ingestion is associated with rhabdomyolysis in adults: a case series. J Toxicol Sci 2007;32:97–101. DOI:10.2131/jts.32.97.

[14] Waring WS, Good AM, Bateman DN. Lack of significant toxicity after mirtazapine overdose: a five-year review of cases admitted to a regional toxicology unit. Clin Toxicol 2007;45:45–50. DOI: 10.1080/15563650601005837.

[15] Hołyst B. Ocena tendencji rozwojowych samobójstw w Polsce i niektórych innych państwach. Lęk Depr. 1997;3:157–172.

[16] Jarosz M. Samobójstwa. Wydawnictwo Naukowe PWN, Warszawa 1997, 44–73 p.

[17] Lester D. Samobójstwa w Polsce na tle trendów światowych. Psychiatr. Pol. 2000;34(5): 773–781.

[18] Liczba zamachów samobójczych zakończonych zgonem. [Internet]. Available from: http://http://statystyka.policja.pl/st/wybrane-statystyki/samobojstwa [Accessed: 2015-10-04]

[19] Bolechała F., Polewka A., Trela F., Zięba A., Kołodziej J.: Samobójstwa kobiet i mężczyzn w materiale krakowskiego Zakładu Medycyny Sądowej—analiza porównawcza. Arch. Med. Sądowej Krym. 2003;53(3):301–311.

[20] Spiller HA, Krenzelok EP, Klein-Schwartz W, et al. Multicenter case series of valproic acid ingestion: serum concentrations and toxicity. J Toxicol Clin Toxicol 2000;38:755–760. DOI: 10.1081/CLT-100102388.

[21] Isbister GK, Balit CR, Whyte IM, et al. Valproate overdose: a comparative cohort study of self-poisonings. Br J Clin Pharmacol 2003;55:398–404. DOI:10.1046/j.1365-2125.2003.01772.x.

[22] Çelenk Y, Katı C, Duran L, et al. The Evaluation of Patients Admitted to the Emergency Department with Non-Benzodiazepine Antiepileptic Drug Poisoning. JAEM. 2013;12:199–204. DOI: 10.5152/jaem.2013.41646.

[23] Nilsson L, Tomson T, Farahmand BY, et al. Cause-specific mortality in epilepsy: a cohort study of more than 9,000 patients once hospitalized for epilepsy. Epilepsia. 1997;38:1062–1068. DOI:10.1111/j.1528-1157.1997.tb01194.x.

[24] Rafnsson V, Olafsson E, Hauser WA, et al. Cause-specific mortality in adults with unprovoked seizures. A population-based incidence cohort study. Neuroepidemiol. 2001;20:232–236. DOI:10.1159/000054795.

[25] Jones JE, Hermann BP, Barry JJ, et al. Rates and risk factors for suicide, suicidal ideation, and suicidal attempts in chronic epilepsy. Epilepsy & Behav 2003;4(3):31–38. DOI: 10.1016/j.yebeh.2003.08.019.

[26] Harris EC, Barraclough B. Suicide as an outcome for mental disorders. A meta-analysis. Br J Psychiatry. 1997;170(3):205–228. DOI:10.1192/bjp.170.3.205.

[27] Lim HW, Song HS, Hwang YH, et al. Predictors of suicidal ideation in people with epilepsy living in Korea. J Clin Neurol 2010; 6:81–88. DOI: 10.3988/jcn.2010.6.2.81.

[28] Kanner AM. Suicidality and Epilepsy: A complex relationship that remains misunderstood and underestimated. Epilepsy Curr. May 2009;9(3):63–66. DOI: 10.1111/j.1535-7511.2009.01294.x.

[29] Christensen J, Vestergaard M, Mortensen PB, et al. Epilepsy and risk of suicide: a population-based case–control study. Lancet Neurol 2007;6:693–698. DOI: 10.1016/S1474-4422(07)70175-8.

[30] Buljan RAM, Santić AM. Suicide attempts in hospital-treated epilepsy patients. Acta Clin Croat. 2011;50(4):485–490.

[31] Murphy G, Wetzel R, Robins E, et al. Multiple risk factors predict suicide in alcoholism. Arch. Gen. Psychiatry 1992;49:459–466. DOI:10.1001/archpsyc.1992.01820060039006.

[32] Inskip H, Harris, E., Barraclough, B. Lifetime risk of suicide for affective disorder, alcoholism and schizophrenia. Br. J. Psychiatry 1998;172:35–37. DOI:10.1192/bjp.172.1.35.

[33] Sher L. Risk and Protective Factors for Suicide in Patients with Alcoholism. The Scientific World JOURNAL, 2006;6:1405–1411. DOI:10.1100/tsw.2006.254.

[34] Hufford MR. Alcohol and suicidal behavior. Clin Psychol Rev 2001;21:797–811. DOI: 10.1016/S0272-7358(00)00070-2.

[35] Cherpitel CJ, Borges GL, Wilcox HC. Acute alcohol use and suicidal behavior: a review of the literature. Alcohol Clin Exp Res. 2004;28(Suppl.):18–28S. DOI: 10.1097/01.ALC.0000127411.61634.14.

[36] Information for Healthcare Professionals. Suicidality and Antiepileptic Drugs. [Internet] 2008. Available from: http://www.fda.gov/Drugs/DrugSafety/PostmarketDrugSafetyInformationfor PatientsandProviders/ucm100192.htm [Accessed date: 2015-08-30].

[37] Schmidt S, Smitz-Buhl M. Signs and symptoms of carbamazepine overdose. J. Neurol. 1995;242:169–173.

[38] Kłys M, Bystrowska B, Bujak-Giżycka B. Postmortem toxicology of carbamazepine. J. Anal. Toxicol. 2003;27:243. DOI: 10.1093/jat/27.4.243.

[39] Montgomery VL, Richman BJ, Goldsmith LJ, et al. Severity and carbamazepine level at time of initial poison center contact correlate with outcome in carbamazepine poisonong, J. Toxicol. Clin. Toxicol. 1995;33;311–323. DOI: 10.3109/15563659509028916.

[40] Spiller HA, Carlisle RD. Timely ante mortem and postmortem concentrations in a fatal carbamazepine overdose. J. Forensic Sci. 2001;46:1510–1512.

Chapter 11

Acute Valproic Acid Intoxication: An Attempt at Estimating the Correlation Between Serum Level and Clinical Manifestations

Anna Staniszewska and
Magdalena Bujalska-Zadrożny

Additional information is available at the end of the chapter

http://dx.doi.org/10.5772/64453

Abstract

We investigated the association between serum valproic acid (VPA) levels and clinical conditions in patients after acute intoxication with this drug. We performed a retrospective study of cases of VPA intoxications hospitalized in Toxicology Unit in Cracow in 2 years of observation. The study included 26 patients (age: 35.69 ± 12.93 years). In all patients, the VPA plasma level was higher than the therapeutic range, mean ± SD: 275.32 ± 135.97 μg/ml. About half of poisoned patients described in this report were treated with VPA prior to the poisoning. We noted four cases of mixed VPA intoxications with ethanol. Acute pulmonary failure was observed in two persons. The mean hospital stay for all patients was 4.69 days. This analysis demonstrates that increased serum VPA levels, in acute intoxication with this drug, were associated with the severity of poisoning — in PSS ($P = 0.019$) and in Matthews coma scale ($P = 0.022$), diastolic pressure ($P = 0.022$) and length of stay in hospital ($P = 0.001$). No correlation was detected between the serum VPA concentration and the heart rate and systolic blood pressure. In persons treated with VPA earlier, the course of poisoning was less severe, although these results were not statistically significant.

Keywords: valproic acid, acute intoxication, clinical manifestations, drug serum level, toxicity

1. Introduction

Valproic acid (VPA) (and its derivatives) is a commonly used conventional antiepileptic drugs (AED) for pharmacotherapy in epileptic patients. VPA was introduced in 1978 as AED [1]. Valproic acid is characterized by multidirectional action that involves increased gamma-aminobutyric acid (GABA)-ergic transmission, reduced release and/or effects of excitatory amino acids, blockage of voltage gated sodium channels and modulation of dopaminergic and serotonergic transmission [2]. This drug is effective in patients with all types of seizures, and especially in those with idiopathic generalized epilepsy [3, 4]. It is also prescribed to treat bipolar and schizoaffective disorders, social phobias and neuropathic pain, as well as for prophylaxis and treatment of migraine headache [5–9]. Valproic acid is a fatty acid which is about 90% bound to plasma proteins and the main metabolic transformations of valproic acid take place in liver, including that of the cytochrome P-450. Valproic acid follows a non-linear pharmacokinetic profile in terms of protein-binding saturation [10]. Acute VPA intoxication also occurs as a consequence of suicidal or accidental overdose. VPA intoxication incidence is increasing [11–14], probably because of its use in psychiatric disorders. It usually results in mild and self-limited central nervous system depression. However, serious toxicity and even deaths have been reported [15, 16]. The therapeutic serum concentrations for VPA are 50–100 μg/ml [17, 18]. Monitoring VPA serum levels helps to evaluate therapeutic response, compliance and possible toxicity.

2. Aim

The aim of study was to evaluate plasma concentrations of VPA and the clinical symptoms of acute intoxication.

3. Materials and methods

We performed a retrospective study of all cases of VPA intoxications ($n = 31$) hospitalized in Toxicology Unit in Cracow in 2 years of observation. A total of 26 patients who fulfilled inclusion and exclusion criteria were included in this study. The inclusion criteria were patients should be at least 18 years of age and documented serum VPA concentration should be ≥100 μg/ml. Patients taking VPA with other drugs which have an effect on VPA pharmacokinetic (i.e. carbamazepine, benzodiazepine, barbiturate) and patients with abnormal renal or liver function tests were excluded. From the medical records, relevant demographic data were taken, i.e. age and gender. The clinical spectrum consisted of consciousness disturbances, breath, heart rate, blood pressure, serum level of VPA, severity of poisoning, length of stay in hospital and treatment effect (survival/death). The project was reviewed and approved by the Ethics Committee, Medical University of Warsaw (no. AKBE/32/13).

The level of consciousness was graded on a scale of 0–IV according to Matthew and Lawson coma scale. Matthew-Lawson coma scale of determining severity of coma: grade 0—fully conscious, alert; grade I—drowsy but responds to verbal command; grade II—unconscious patient but responds to minimal painful stimuli, reflexes intact; grade III—unconscious patient but responds to maximal painful stimuli, absence of superficial reflexes and sluggish deep reflexes; grade IV—unconscious patient with no response to painful stimuli, loss of all reflexes including corneal, laryngeal, pharyngeal. Grades III and IV are considered as severe grades of poisoning [19].

Severity of intoxication was classified according to Poisoning Severity Score (PSS). The PSS is a classification scheme for cases of poisoning in adults and children. The PSS grades severity as (0) none—no symptoms or signs related to poisoning, (1) minor—mild, transient and spontaneously resolving symptoms, (2) moderate—pronounced or prolonged symptoms, (3) severe—severe or life-threatening symptoms, and (4) fatal poisoning—death [20].

3.1. Statistical analysis

The data were collected in a Microsoft Excel database. Data are presented as mean and standard deviations. Statistical analysis of all data was performed by Statistica version 12 using the Pearson's r, Spearman's rho, Mann-Whitney U test. Differences were considered statistically significant at $P < 0.05$.

4. Results

We studied episodes of hospitalization for VPA intoxication in 26 patients, of whom 9 were men (34.61%). The mean age was 35.69 ± 12.93 years (range: 18–73 years) (**Table 1**).

Characteristics	***N* (%)**
Gender	
Female	17 (65.39%)
Male	9 (34.61%)
Total	26 (100%)
Age, years	
Range: 18–73	
Mean ± SD: 35.69 ± 12.93	

Table 1. Demographics characteristics of study population.

Half of the poisoned patients (50%) described in this report were treated with valproic acid due to epilepsy or psychotic disorders prior to the poisoning. These patients had a less severe clinical course of poison, although these results were not statistically significant ($P = 0.09$).

The following intensity of quantitative consciousness disturbances according to Matthew's scale was observed: grade 0—26.92%, I—26.92%, II—30.77%, and III—15.39%.

Parameters	
Systolic blood pressure (SBP), mmHg	
Range	100–160
Mean ± SD	127.15 ± 16.55
Diastolic blood pressure (DBP), mmHg	
Range	50–100
Mean ± SD	79.23 ± 12.25
Heart rate (HR), beats/min	
Range	58–122
Mean ± SD	88.46 ± 17.58
Breath	
Competence of a respiration	24 (92.31%)
Intubation	2 (7.69%)
Matthew coma scale (MCS)	
Grade 0	7 (26.92%)
Grade 1	7 (26.92%)
Grade 2	8 (30.77%)
Grade 3	4 (15.39%)
Grade 4	0 (0%)
Poisoning severity score (PSS)	
Minor	14 (53.85%)
Moderate	7 (26.92%)
Severe	5 (19.23%)
Ethanol, ‰	
Range	0–2.92
Mean ± SD	0.305 ± 0.77
Yes	4 (15.38%)
No	22 (84.62%)
Co-morbidity	
Depression	7 (26.92%)
Alcohol dependence syndrome	4 (15.38%)
Personality disorder	5 (19.23%)
Somatic disease	3 (11.54%)
Bipolar disorder	2 (7.69%)
Schizophrenia	4 (15.38%)
Other mental disorder	5 (19.23%)
Epilepsy	9 (34.62%)
Length of stay in hospital, days	
Range	2–13
Mean ± SD	4.69 ± 2.57
Treatment effect	
Discharged from hospital in good condition	17 (65.39%)
Discharged from hospital on a voluntary distractions	7 (26.92%)
Referral to mental hospital/ward	2 (7.69%)
Toxic valproic acid level, μg/ml	
Range	110–660
Mean ± SD	275.32 ± 135.97

Table 2. Clinical parameters distribution in examined population.

http://dx.doi.org/10.5772/64453

The serum VPA concentration showed moderate positive correlations with Matthew's scale (*Spearman's rho* = 0.45, $P = 0.022$).

The minimal and maximal values of blood pressure were: 100–160 and 50–100 mmHg, respectively, for systolic and diastolic blood pressure; heart rate: 58–122 beats/min; breathing rate in non-intubated patients: 13–20 breaths/min.

Correlational analysis (Pearson's *r*) revealed a moderate negative correlation between the VPA concentration and diastolic blood pressure ($r = -0.45$, $P = 0.022$). This negative correlation means that when the VPA level is higher, the diastolic blood pressure is lower.

In the study population, no statistical correlation was found between the serum VPA concentration and the heart rate ($r = -0.01$, $P = 0.944$), and systolic blood pressure ($r = -0.09$, $P = 0.655$).

Severity of intoxication was classified according to poisoning severity score (PSS). The PSS was minor in 14 patients, moderate in 7 patients and severe in 5 patients.

A positive relationship between the decrease in number of PSS and the increasing VPA serum level was demonstrated (*Spearman's rho* = 0.46, $P = 0.019$).

A significant proportion of patients had comorbid mental health disorders (e.g. depression, personality disorders, schizophrenia, and bipolar disorder).

Only two patients were inefficient to breathe and they required intubation. No patients had arrhythmias and seizures.

Alcohol was co-ingested by four patients. The mean ethanol concentration was 0.305‰.

The mean length of hospital stay was 4.69 days. We observed strong correlation between the serum level of VPA and the number of days of stay in hospital ($r = 0.96$; $P = 0.001$).

Seventeen of these 26 patients were discharged to home in good condition and two to a psychiatric ward. There were no reported mortalities among the cases of VPA intoxications.

The mean of serum level of valproic acid was 275.32 ± 135.97 μg/ml.

The characteristics of clinical parameters are shown in **Table 2**.

5. Discussion

Despite the fact that valproic acid is an old generation antiepileptic drug, in the literature, there is little information about the case series of VPA overdose. However, there is a description of case reports of VPA intoxication [21–24].

In our study, a positive relationship between the decrease in number of PSS and the increasing VPA serum level was demonstrated (*Spearman's rho* = 0.46, $P = 0.019$). It has been observed that the higher the concentration of VPA, the more severe the poisoning. In the literature, a serum level of >450 μg/ml was more likely to be associated with a moderate or major adverse outcome ($P < 0.005$) [11].

Symptoms of VPA intoxication are diverse. The most common manifestation of overdose is central nervous system (CNS) depression [25, 26]. Other studies show that some patients have mild to moderate lethargy [13, 27]. It was noted that patients who ingest more than 200 mg/kg VPA and/or have plasma concentrations greater than 180 μg/ml usually develop severe CNS depression [28]. Taking VPA at higher doses (>400 mg/kg) is associated with serious consequences such as coma, cerebral oedema [29], metabolic acidosis, hyperammonemia, thrombocytopenia and leukopenia, and circulatory collapse [11, 30, 31]. The study by Spiller et al. [11] show that the concentration of VPA > 850 μg/ml was more likely to be associated with coma ($P < 0.005$). In a large multicentre review of 134 patients (80 with VPA levels in the toxic range), 71% of patients presented with lethargy, and 15% were in coma [8]. In our study, 15.39% of patients were in stage III coma (Matthew's scale). This study shows that the serum VPA concentration showed moderate positive correlations with Matthew's coma scale (*Spearman's rho* = 0.45, $P = 0.022$). This means that the higher the VPA concentration, the higher its score on Matthew's coma scale.

Other possible adverse effects of valproic acid on the nervous system include agitation, hallucinations, tremors, myoclonus and seizures [28].

In addition to generally known symptoms, valproic acid intoxication may also be associated with hypotension [32]. In this study, correlational analysis (*Pearson's r*) revealed a moderate negative correlation between VPA concentration and diastolic blood pressure ($r = -0.45$, $P = 0.022$). This negative correlation means that when the VPA level is higher, the diastolic blood pressure is lower.

Other clinical findings include respiratory depression and acute respiratory distress syndrome [33, 34]. In the study by Tank et al. [35], all patients with serum levels higher than 850 μg/ml were comatose, and 63% of these patients needed intubation.

In our study, out of 26 patients, only two experienced respiratory depression and required intubations. The first patient was a 49-year-old man, reportedly poisoned intentionally, admitted to Toxicology Department. His valproate sodium serum concentration was 224.8 μg/ml. The serum level of other drugs and ethanol were all negative. He had a history of psychiatric illness, including personality disorder and alcohol dependence syndrome. His vital signs were as follows: pulse rate 115 beats/min, blood pressure 155/100 mmHg, temperature 36.6°C and respiratory insufficiency. On the day of admission, the patient was unconscious, in the third stage coma by Matthew's scale, with features of overt respiratory failure. The patient was immediately intubated and connected to a respirator. After the first day the patient was extubated, had efficient breathing, but with persistent disturbances of consciousness, periodically extremely agitated and psychotic. Gradually, the patient's condition experienced an improvement. From the fifth day there was a logical, calm. When the serum levels returned to normal, the patient made a complete recovery. On the seventh day of treatment, after psychiatric review, the patient was discharged home in good condition. The second patient was a 24-year-old woman admitted to the Toxicology Department after attempting suicide by ingesting tablets of valproic acid. Her valproate sodium serum concentration was high and peaked at 315 μg/ml. The serum level of other drugs and ethanol were all negative. She had a history of psychiatric illness, including paranoid schizophrenia. The patient was confused, hallucinated

http://dx.doi.org/10.5772/64453

and developed deep coma. In addition, the physical examination revealed tachycardia 120 beats/min and normal blood pressure (110/70 mmHg). Her core body temperature was 36.8°C. In the early hours of observation, there were repeated spasms and respiratory insufficiency—the patient was intubated and connected to a respirator. Gradually, the patient's condition improved, and after 4 days of mechanical ventilation, the patient was extubated. In the fourth day the patient was in contact and began to walk in the fifth. Because of the high risk of recurrence of attempted suicide, the patient was urgently addressed without consent to the psychiatric ward for further treatment. At the time of discharge, the patient did not require hospitalization for toxicological reasons.

Haematological disturbances are rare, but there are potentially serious complication of chronic valproate therapy and overdose [11, 13]. Spiller et al. [11] demonstrated that thrombocytopaenia (<150 tys/μl), occurred with valproate concentrations >450 μg/ml, but did not correlate it with dose ingested, whereas fatal leukopenia (WBC < 1200 tys/μl) was observed in patients with VPA concentrations >1200 μg/ml. Hypernatremia (Na+ > 145 mmol/l) and hypocalcaemia were observed in patients with peak VPA concentrations >450 μg/ml [13].

In our study, there were no reported haematological disturbances among the cases of VPA intoxications.

In our study, mean length of hospital stay for all patients was 4.69 days; in the study by Spiller et al. [11], it was 42 ± 33.1 hours. In this study, statistical analysis found the relationship between the serum concentration of VPA and the duration of stay in hospital ($P = 0.001$) and that the higher the drug concentration, the longer the length of stay in hospital for the patients.

In the case series by Spiller et al. [11], patients with peak valproic acid concentrations above 450 μg/ml were more likely to develop significant clinical effects and have longer hospital stays ($P < 0.05$). Also, acute toxicity seems to be less severe in patients who are regularly taking valproate [36].

Few fatalities of valproic acid overdose are reported in the literature [11, 27, 35–41]. Deaths were associated with plasma concentrations ranging from 305.4 μg/ml [37] to 1970 μg/ml [27]. In our study, the highest related VPA level was 660 μg/ml; however, the intoxication in this case was non-lethal.

6. Conclusions

1. Positive correlation of the serum VPA concentrations with diastolic blood pressure, poisoning severity score, Matthew's coma scale and length of stay in hospital has been found.

2. We failed to find any significant correlation between the VPA plasma level and the remaining parameters.

Acknowledgements

We thank staff of University Hospital and Specialist Hospital Louis Rydgier's in Cracow, Poland, for the availability of medical histories.

Author details

Anna Staniszewska[1*] and Magdalena Bujalska-Zadrożny[2]

*Address all correspondence to: anna.staniszewska@wum.edu.pl

1 Department of Experimental and Clinical Pharmacology, Medical University of Warsaw, Warsaw, Poland

2 Department of Pharmacodynamics, Medical University of Warsaw, Warsaw, Poland

References

[1] Lisa KH, Philip AM. Valproic acid overdose and hemodialysis. Nephrol Transplant. 2001;16:1483–1486. DOI: 10.1093/ndt/16.7.1483

[2] Perruca E. Pharmacological and therapeutic properties of valproate: a summary after 35 years of clinical experience. CNS Drugs. 2002;16(10):695–714.

[3] Kyngas H. Compliance with health regimens of adolescents with epilepsy. Seizure. 2000;9:598–604. DOI: 10.1053/seiz.2000.0470

[4] Kubotsu K, Goto S, Fujita M, et al. Automated homogeneous liposome immunoassay systems for anticonvulsant drugs. Clin Chem. 1992;38(6):808–812.

[5] Davis LL, Ryan W, Adinoff B, et al. Comprehensive review of the psychiatric use of valproate. J Clin Psychopharmacol. 2000;20(suppl. 1):1S–17S.

[6] Goldberg JF. Treatment guidelines: current and future management of bipolar disorder. J Clin Psychiatry. 2000;61(suppl. 13):12–18. DOI: 10.1017/S1461145708009231

[7] Norton J. Use of intravenous valproate sodium in status migraine. Headache. 2000;40:755–757. DOI: 10.1046/j.1526-4610.2000.00133.x

[8] Hardy JR, Rees EAJ, Gwillian B, et al. A phase II study to establish the efficacy and toxicity of sodium valproate in patients with cancer-related neuropathic pain. J Pain Symptom Manage. 2001;21(3):204–209. DOI: 10.1016/S0885-3924(00)00266-9

[9] Johannessen CU, Johannessen SI. Valproate: past, present, and future. CNS Drug Rev. 2003;9:199–216. DOI: 10.1111/j.1527-3458.2003.tb00249.x

[10] Hoofnagle JH. Drug-induced liver injury network (DILIN). Hepatology. 2004;40:773. DOI: 10.1002/hep.1840400403

[11] Spiller HA, Krenzelok EP, Klein-Schwartz W, et al. Multicenter case series of valproic acid ingestion: serum concentrations and toxicity. J Toxicol Clin Toxicol. 2000;38:755–760. DOI: 10.1081/CLT-100102388

[12] Watson WA, Litovitz TL, Klein-Schwartz W, et al. 2003 annual report of the American Association of Poison Control Centers Toxic Exposure Surveillance System. Am J Emerg Med.2004;22:335–404. DOI: 10.1016/j.ajem.2004.06.001

[13] Sztajnkrycer MD. Valproic acid toxicity: overview and management. J Toxicol Clin Toxicol. 2002;40:789–801. DOI: 10.1081/CLT-120014645

[14] Bedry R, Parrot F. Severe valproate poisoning [in French]. Réanimation. 2004;13:324–333. DOI: 10.1016/j.reaurg.2004.03.014

[15] Ellenhorn M. Diagnosis and treatment of human poisoning. In: Ellenhorn M, editor. Medical Toxicology. Baltimore: Williams and Wilkins; 1997:pp. 609–610.

[16] Leikin JPF. Poisoning and Toxicology Handbook. 3rd ed. Hudson: Lexi-Comp; 2002.

[17] Chadwick DW. Concentration-effect relationship of valproic acid. Clin Pharmacokinet. 1985;10:155–165.

[18] Shakya G, Malla S, Shakya KN, et al. Therapeutic drug monitoring of antiepileptic drugs. J Nepal Med Assoc. 2008;47(171):94–97.

[19] Matthew H, Lawson AAH. Treatment of Common Acute Poisonings. Edinburgh, London, New York: Churchill Livingstone; 1975.

[20] Persson H, Sjöberg G, Haines J, Pronczuk de Garbino J. Poisoning Severity Score: Grading of acute poisoning. J Toxicol Clinical Toxicol. 1998;36:205–213. DOI: 10.3109/15563659809028940

[21] Berthelot-Moritz F, Chadda K, Chanavaz I, et al. Fatal sodium valproate poisoning. Intensive Care Med. 1997;23:599.

[22] Brubacher JR, Dahghani P, McKnight D. Delayed toxicity following ingestion of enteric-coated divalproex sodium (Epival). J Emerg Med. 1999;17:463–467. DOI: 10.1016/S0736-4679(99)00008-6

[23] Van Keulen JG, Van der Deure J, Gemke RJBJ, et al. Treatment of valproic acid overdose with continuous arteriovenous hemofiltration. J Toxicol Clin Toxicol. 2000;38:219.

[24] Ishikura H, Matsuo N, Matsubara M, et al. Valproic acid overdose and L-carnitine therapy. J Anal Toxicol. 1996;20:55–58. DOI: 10.1093/jat/20.1.55

[25] Khoo SH, Leyland MJ. Cerebral edema following acute sodium valproate overdose. J Toxicol Clin Toxicol. 1992;30:209–214. DOI: 10.3109/15563659209038632

[26] Andersen GO, Ritland S. Life threatening intoxication with sodium valproate. J Toxicol Clin Toxicol. 1995;33:279–284. DOI: 10.3109/15563659509018000

[27] Garnier R, Boudignat O, Fournier PE. Valproate poisoning. Lancet. 1982;2:97. DOI: 10.1016/S0140-6736(82)91713-5

[28] Lheureux PER, Penaloza A, Zahir S, et al. Science review: carnitine in the treatment of valproic acid-induced toxicity—what is the evidence? Crit Care. 2005;9(5):431–440. DOI: 10.1186/cc3742

[29] Dupuis RE, Lichtman SN, Pollack GM. Acute valproic acid overdose. Clinical course and pharmacokinetic disposition of valproic acid and metabolites. Drug Saf. 1990;5:65-71.

[30] Garnier R, Fournier E. Intoxication associated with sodium valproate. Nouv Presse Med., 1982:11: 678.

[31] Jones AL, Proudfoot AT. Features and management of poisoning with modern drugs used to treat epilepsy. Q J Med. 1998;91:325–332. DOI: 10.1093/qjmed/91.5.325

[32] Ota KS. Probable valproate sodium-associated hypotension, Am J Geriatr Pharmacol. 2010;8(3):281–284. DOI: 10.1016/j.amjopharm.2010.04.005

[33] Graudins A, Aaron CK. Delayed peak serum valproic acid in massive divalproex overdose—treatment with charcoal hemoperfusion. J Toxicol Clin Toxicol. 1996;34:335–341. DOI: 10.1046/j.1365-2125.2003.01772.x

[34] Snodgrass WR. Critical Care Toxicology. In: Brent J, Phillips SD, Wallace KL, Donovan JW, Burkhart KK, editors. Diagnosis and Management of the Critically Poisoned Patient. Philadelphia: Elsevier Mosby; 2005. pp. 565–570.

[35] Tank JE, Palmer BF. Simultaneous "in series" hemodialysis and hemoperfusion in the management of valproic acid overdose. Am J Kidney Dis. 1993;22(2):341–344. DOI: 10.1016/S0272-6386(12)70329-3

[36] Chadwick DW, Cumming WJK, Livingstone I, et al. Acute intoxication with sodium valproate. Ann Neurol. 1978;6:552–553. DOI: 10.1002/ana.410060616

[37] Oamilleri C, Albertson T, Offerman S. Fatal cerebral edema after moderate valproic acid overdose. Ann Emerg Med. 2005;45(3):337–338.

[38] Schnabel R, Rambeck B, Janssen F. Fatal intoxication with sodium valproate. Lancet. 1984;1:221–222. DOI: 10.1016/S0140-6736(84)92140-8.

[39] Connacher AA, Macnab MS, Moody JP, et al. Fatality due to massive overdose of sodium valproate. Scott Med. J. 1987;32:85–86. DOI: 10.1177/003693308703200312

[40] Lokan RJ, Dinan AC. An apparent fatal valproic acid poisoning. J. Anal. Toxicol. 1988;12:35–37. DOI: 10.1093/jat/12.1.35

[41] Ryall JE. Fatal overdose sodium valproate. Bull. Int. Assoc. Forensic Toxicol. 1992;22:23–26.

Chapter 12

Therapeutic Monitoring of Anticonvulsants: Use of Saliva as Biological Fluid

Marta Vázquez and Pietro Fagiolino

Additional information is available at the end of the chapter

http://dx.doi.org/10.5772/64108

Abstract

Plasma drug concentration is not homogeneous within the intravascular space, being the arterial (P_A) concentrations higher or lower than that in veins (P_V) depending on whether the samples are taken during the drug absorption or the elimination phases, respectively. However, blood samples are currently withdrawn from peripheral veins and total (bound plus unbound) plasma drug concentration is assayed. Despite the fact that free plasma drug levels (P_{fV}) are not determined in routine therapeutic drug monitoring (TDM), they could be assayed for research purposes. Salivary drug concentrations (S) approximate to their free plasma levels in the arteries of the great circulation. Saliva is recommended to be collected with stimulation to minimize the difference between the pHs of both fluids (saliva and blood), and thus, artery/vein-free drug concentration ratios (P_{fA}/P_{fV}) could be surrogated by the stimulated saliva/free-plasma in vein drug concentration ratios (S_S/P_{fV}). It is possible in this way not only to assess this S/P ratio but also to infer the brain (B)/P_{fV} ratio, which is actually the most relevant for antiepileptic drugs (AEDs). Different cases of AEDs are considered in this review, taking into account their physiochemical properties and their ability to be transported by membrane carriers.

Keywords: drug concentration in saliva, saliva-to-plasma concentration ratio, brain-to-saliva concentration ratio

1. Introduction

The concept of therapeutic drug monitoring (TDM) in plasma or serum of antiepileptic drugs (AEDs) is led by the assumption that the pharmacodynamic effects of drugs correlate better with circulating concentrations than with administered doses. TDM encompasses both drug quantification in a sample and pharmacological interpretation for dosage adjustment. Although TDM has been used as a tool to optimize treatment of epilepsy for almost 50 years, evidence for its usefulness in improving clinical outcome is scarce and controversial. The main potential pitfall regarding TDM interpretation is that we are still measuring drug levels in a fluid far away from the site of action. Plasma drug concentration is not homogeneous within the intravascular space, while all arteries have the same drug level value, each vein coming from different organs may have different drug concentrations, among them and in relation with their respective arteries. Arterial drug concentration is higher than the respective venous concentration during input of the active substance either after intravenous or oral administration. The opposite is observed when drug elimination predominates. This circulatory issue has been well referenced in the literature both in animals [1] and in humans [2], and gives evidence to understand the discrepancy between plasma venous drug concentrations, which are commonly measured, and drug effects [2, 3]. Blood samples are currently withdrawn from peripheral veins and total (bound plus unbound) plasma drug concentration is assayed although only the free drug is responsible for the pharmacological effect.

Measurement of AED concentrations in brain interstitial fluid (BIF) could be the solution as such concentrations are considered to reflect those occurring in the brain, which result in the pharmacological effect of the drug. Furthermore, BIF concentrations would reflect the free serum concentration. However, the impossibility of obtaining this fluid turns it in an inappropriate biological matrix for AEDs TDM purpose.

Saliva has been investigated by our group as an alternative biological fluid for TDM of AEDs. Saliva is produced in the salivary glands by ultrafiltration of arterial plasma. For this reason, of particular advantage, apart from the easiness to collect and the fact that saliva can be sampled repetitively, is that the concentration in saliva approximates to its free plasma levels in the arteries of the great circulation.

Saliva is recommended to be collected with stimulation to minimize the difference between the pHs of both fluids, and thus, artery/vein free drug concentration ratios could be surrogated by the stimulated-saliva/free-plasma-in-vein drug concentration ratios. It is possible in this way not only to assess this saliva/plasma (S/P) ratio but also to infer the brain/free plasma drug ratio, which is actually the most relevant for AEDs.

Different chemical structures and mechanism actions identify AEDs. Acting on ion movements (voltage-gated sodium and calcium channels) or postsynaptic receptors (gamma-aminobutyric acid and glutamate receptors) characterized first-generation AEDs. Second- and third-generation AEDS focused on ion movements but through different channels such as the neuronal KCNQ potassium channels [ritagabine (RTG)], or targeting the voltage-gated sodium channels but enhancing the slow inactivation of the channel [lacosamide (LCM)]. Some drugs were synthesized as GABA analogs [(gabapentin (GBP) and pregabalin (PGB)] but they do not act directly on GABA receptors. They bind to a subunit of presynaptic voltage-gated N-type Ca^{2+} channels, decreasing calcium entry and avoiding therefore glutamate release. Regarding their chemical structure, AEDs are carboxamide derivatives [phenobarbital (PHB), phenytoin (PHT), ethosuximide (ESM), carbamazepine (CBZ), oxcarbamazepine (OXC), levetiracetam (LEV), RTG, LCM], sulfonamides and sulfamates [felbamate (FBM), zonisamide (ZNS), topiramate (TPM)], amino acid compounds [vigabatrin (VGT), GBP, PGB], carboxylic acids [valproic acid (VPA), tiagabine (TGB)], and heterocycle amines [lamotrigine (LTG)].

In accordance with their chemical structures most of them are not ionized in body fluids, except for PHB, amino acid and carboxylic acid drugs, and LTG. Despite some extent of ionization, non-ionized moieties of AEDs have enough lipophilicity to cross the blood-brain barrier (BBB) rapidly. Plasma (P) and saliva (S) are the main biological fluids used for drug monitoring. Because of the lower pH found in saliva (6.4) than in plasma (7.4) [4] and the acidic characteristic of PHB, VGT, GBP, PGB, VPA, and TGB, a lower S/P concentration ratio than their respective free/total plasma concentration ratio is obtained [5]. Conversely, LTG has a preference for saliva due to its basic properties, and then a higher S/P than free/total plasma ratio can be foreseen. All the other antiepileptic compounds are expected to have similar S/P and free/total concentration ratios. However, not only pH-partition considerations have to be taken into account to forecast S/P concentration ratios.

The aim of this review is to discuss the potential use of saliva as a biological matrix to perform AED TDM.

2. Arteriovenous (A-V) difference in plasma drug concentration

During drug input, arteries have higher drug concentrations than all the veins of the large circulation, except for the vein through which the substance enters the body. So, while the drug is entering the body arteries are transporting an amount of substance that exceeds the one previously eliminated. This is repeated after each circulatory cycle until the steady state is reached. At this point, the amount of drug entering the body is the same as the one that is being eliminated, and the concentrations in veins and arteries become equal.

Once the administration is interrupted, drug decay proceeds from all branches of the circulatory apparatus. After drug input ceases, the veins exhibit higher concentrations than the arteries, except for those veins coming from eliminating organs. This inversion during the elimination phase is because the blood entering the arteries of the large circulation suffered a dilution caused by the lesser content of solute that veins coming from the eliminatory organs had.

It is important to bear in mind that not only the absorption or elimination of a drug rules the A-V difference in drug concentration but also changes in the migration of substances outside the vessels. These changes take place during physical activity of individuals and they could modify the A/V drug concentration ratio. A sudden increase in the distribution of cardiac output [6] to the muscles might force the drug to disappear from the intravascular space, rendering a decrease in the A/V drug concentration ratio at those organs not involved in the migration of solute. This situation reverts once subjects stop doing muscular activity, and the A/V ratio increases up to the previous value as if a process of drug absorption is operating from the muscles.

3. Saliva production

Saliva is the fluid produced by the salivary glands, and is made up mainly of water, electrolytes, mucus and enzymes. Humans have three major pairs of salivary glands that differ in the type of secretion they produce: 1—parotid glands, which produce a serous watery secretion; 2—submaxillary (mandibular) glands, which produce a mixed serous and mucous secretion; and 3—sublingual glands, which secrete saliva that is predominantly mucous in character.

The basic secretory units of salivary glands are clusters of cells called acini. These cells secrete a fluid that contains water, electrolytes, mucus and enzymes, all of which flow out of the acinus into collecting ducts. Within the ducts, the composition of the secretion is altered. Much of the sodium is actively reabsorbed, potassium and protons secreted, and large quantities of bicarbonate ion reabsorbed [7]. Small collecting ducts within salivary glands lead into larger ducts, eventually forming a single large duct that empties into the oral cavity.

Secretion of saliva is under control of the autonomic nervous system. Traditionally, acetylcholine is the parasympathetic postganglionic transmitter and noradrenaline the sympathetic postganglionic transmitter that act on the secretory elements of the glands. Noradrenaline acts on α1-adrenoceptors and β1-adrenoceptors, whereas acetylcholine acts on muscarinic M1 and M3 receptors. Parasympathetically induced vasodilatation may generate a 20-fold increase in gland blood flow, which ensures the secretory cells produce large volumes of saliva over a long period of time. The parasympathetic transmitter vasoactive intestinal peptide, besides acetylcholine, plays a major role in the vasodilator response, which also involves the action of NO. Stimulation of the sympathetic innervation initially causes vasoconstriction by α1-adrenergic receptors and then a vasodilatation mediated by β1-adrenoceptors increasing the gland blood flow.

4. Saliva drug concentration and saliva-to-plasma level ratio

Saliva has been used as an alternative biological fluid for TDM for more than three decades. Nowadays it is emerging again as a valuable matrix for AED TDM because it is associated with several advantages over the conventional sampling fluids: plasma, serum, or blood [5]. Nevertheless, few articles deal with the most relevant advantage that drug monitoring in saliva has [8, 9], that is, a measure of the drug directly available (free in the arterial plasma) for all body tissues, including the brain.

As other organs, salivary glands receive substances from the arterial part of capillaries and thereafter solutes are transferred through the basal and apical membranes of acinar cells into the upper zone of salivary ducts. The fluid recently formed in acini has a similar pH and a similar composition in free substances to the plasma in the artery [8]. This is true for substances which have no restriction in their passage through lipophilic membranes, such as AEDs. During its transit through the luminal space of ducts the fluid interchanges protons, other ions and solutes with the interior of ductal cells through the apical membrane, and thereafter with

http://dx.doi.org/10.5772/64108

the interstitial space through the basal membrane [7]. So, drug molecules located in the arterial space of the circulatory system pass through the acini into the salivary conducts, returning back to the circulatory system through the veins from ductal cells.

When saliva is secreted into the oral cavity, drug concentration and pH differ sensitively from the value they have at the upper zone of ducts. Saliva becomes more acidic and more or less concentrated in AEDs depending on their physicochemical characteristics. The volume withdrawn determines whether the drug concentration in this fluid would be closer to the free plasma venous value or to the arterial one. For non-ionized AEDs, the smaller the volume of saliva is (usually obtained without stimulation, or the first fraction obtained after stimulation), the closer to free plasma venous concentration becomes. In the case of weak acid molecules, lower values than the corresponding free ones in venous plasma are obtained since the pH at the lower part of the ducts is more acidic than in blood (and in the acinus). Conversely, in the case of basic AEDs, a higher value than the free plasma venous concentration should be expected.

When saliva volumes are large, or when saliva is obtained with stimulation (chewing parafilm®, or putting small amounts of citric acid crystals on the tongue), saliva AED concentrations become closer to the upper part of the ducts (acini). As it was reported in the literature [10, 11], the variability in saliva drug concentration could be diminished by using stimulated saliva sampling.

Figures 1 and **2** show saliva collection without or with stimulation, respectively.

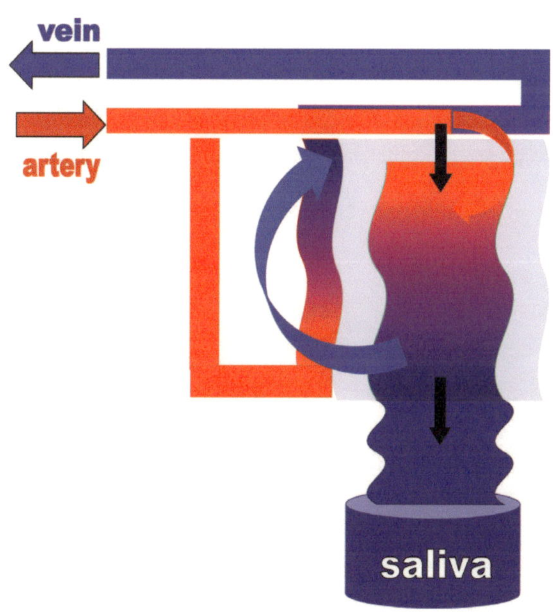

Figure 1. Schematic representation of saliva collection without stimulation.

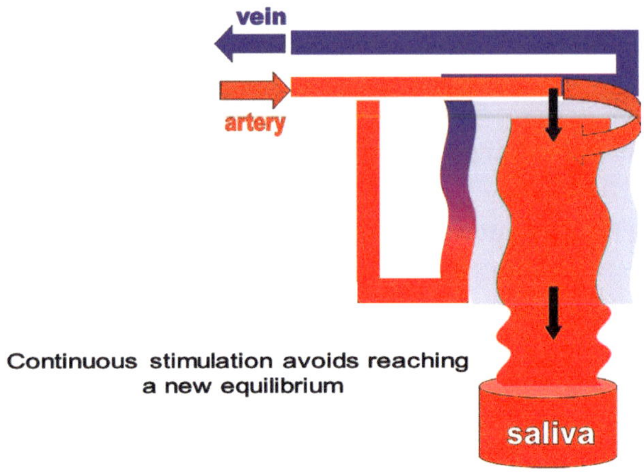

Figure 2. Schematic representation of saliva collection with stimulation.

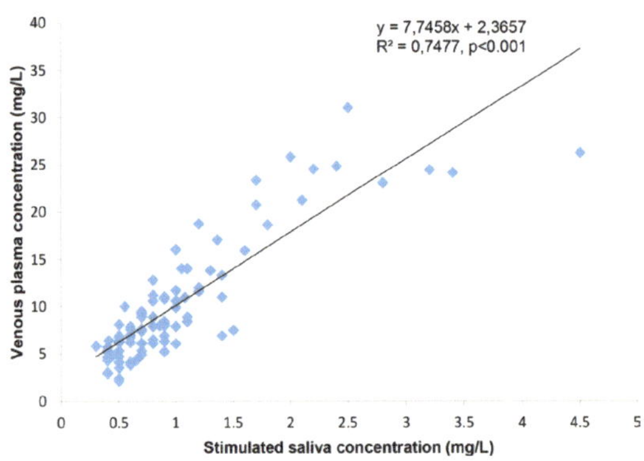

Figure 3. Predose venous plasma concentration versus predose stimulated saliva concentration in patients receiving PHT.

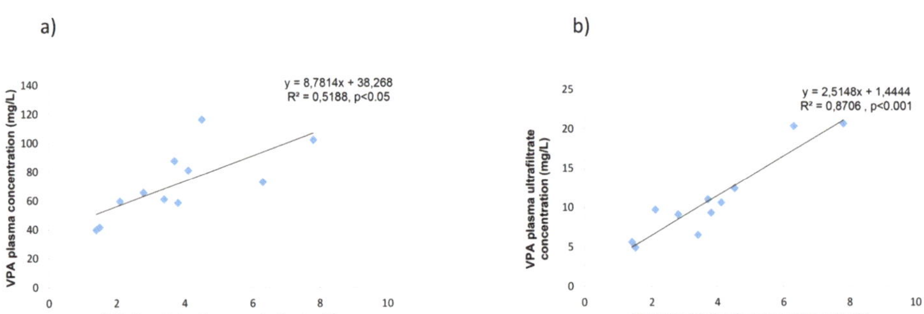

Figure 4. VPA plasma concentration versus VPA stimulated saliva concentration (a) and VPA plasma ultrafiltrate concentration versus VPA stimulated saliva concentration (b) in 11 pediatric patients.

http://dx.doi.org/10.5772/64108

For a number of AEDS drugs, mainly those which are lipophilic and non-ionized at salivary pH range (i.e. PHT), stimulated or non-stimulated saliva concentrations highly correlated with plasma concentrations. **Figure 3** shows pre-dose venous plasma and citric acid-stimulated saliva samples obtained in 94 patients taking PHT for seizure control. For VPA, which is more ionized in plasma than in saliva, citric acid stimulation seemed to be adequate to diminish pH variability. A great volume of saliva was drained from salivary ducts and thereafter its pH became closer to blood pH. Stimulated saliva and blood samples (prior to the morning dose) were withdrawn from eleven children diagnosed with epilepsy receiving VPA as monotherapy. Interestingly, as it is shown in **Figure 4**, saliva concentrations correlated with plasma concentrations (**Figure 4a**, $p < 0.05$) but a higher correlation was found between saliva levels and VPA ultrafiltrate plasma concentrations (**Figure 4b**, $p < 0.001$).

It is also noteworthy that no matter the time after dose the samples were taken, during the absorption or the elimination phase, the stimulated saliva (S_S) drug level would always be linked with the free serum level at the arterial plasma.

Under this mode of sampling, the S_S/P concentration ratio should be understood as an approach for measuring the A/V drug concentration ratio since P levels usually come from venous blood specimens. Performed as such, saliva drug concentration would be closer to the free plasma drug concentration in all arteries (P_{fA}) of the great circulation and above (during the absorption), or below (during the elimination), free plasma level in the vein (P_{fV}) of almost all the organs that do not participate either in drug entry or exit from the body.

It is currently known that efflux pumps belonging to the ABC (ATP binding cassette) family of transporters, such as P-glycoprotein (Pgp) and multidrug resistance protein 2 (MRP2), are located at the apical membrane of both acinar and ductal cells [12]. Some AEDs are substrate of these transporters, and then, the S/P ratio could be effectively affected by changes in the activity or the expression of efflux carriers. Because of this, salivary levels were used for assessing the systemic modification in efflux transporters [13]. Pre-dose sampling is preferred to minimize the contribution of drug absorption in the S/P ratio. Significant increases in the pre-dose S/P concentration ratio for CBZ and PHT, throughout the time-course of their chronic administrations [14, 15] revealed their inductive effect over their own membrane transporters [16, 17].

On the basis of current literature data [2, 18] it is possible to retrieve the same conclusion issued by our group, since the S_S/P_{fV} ratios assessed for PHT and PHB, two recognized efflux transporter inducers, were above 1 (average value: 1.10 and 1.06, respectively). This ratio should be approximately 1 or below 1 if there is no drug entrance. Due to the higher clearance that CBZ has after chronic administration, pre-dose S_S/P_{fV} should be theoretically much lower than 1 [19], but because of its inductive effect [14] the obtained value resulted practically 1 [18]. It is important to remark that to reach a reliable conclusion about overexpression of efflux carriers, S_S/P_{fV} must be determined when drug absorption is not operating. If this is not considered, misleading results could be obtained. For instance, CBZ yielded higher S_S/P_{fV} ratios (1.39–1.44) when samples were taken from 1 to 5 h after dose intake [20]. These higher ratios are related more to the effect of drug absorption than to its inductive effect on efflux transporters.

On the other hand, drugs that are not recognized as inducers of membrane carriers, such as LTG or LEV, rendered S_S/P_{fV} values of 0.82 [21] and 0.36–0.41 [22] respectively.

Interestingly, LCM given to healthy subjects [23] or to controlled epileptic patients after a single dose [24] rendered S_S/P_{fV} lower than 1 during the elimination phase of the drug, with a consistent plasma protein binding of 15%. However, when LCM was given as adjunctive therapy to patients with intractable epilepsy [25], not only its protein binding increased to around 90% but also the S_S/P_{fV} rose to 1.44. In most of the patients, co-medications were efflux transporter inducers. This last fact could have resulted in a preferential transfer of LCM to saliva due to its affinity for Pgp [26]. It is known that seizures are associated with an increased inflammatory response [27], which in turn enhances alpha-1-acid glycoprotein (AAG) plasma levels [28] and overexpresses efflux transporters at the BBB and tissues far away from the central nervous system (CNS) [29]. This overexpression could reinforce the transport of LCM from blood to saliva. On the other hand, the increased protein binding rate of LCM in refractory epilepsy patients could be related to its eventual binding to AAG, but up to date this issue has not been studied.

5. Saliva-to-brain drug concentration ratio

The main objective in TDM is to follow-up patient's pharmacotherapy by means of drug levels to predict the evolution of the treatment, or to interpret both the occurrence of adverse reactions and therapeutic failures; in other words, to infer drug concentration at its action site (in the case of AEDs, for effectiveness, at the brain). Which drug concentration, plasma or saliva, can be the appropriate as a surrogate for assessing CNS exposure? The answer to this question is not an easy issue, since no decision has been made for the best matrix to pursuit AED TDM so far. Past and current approaches were carried out just to correlate saliva with plasma AED concentrations. Maybe, this objective is substantially more affordable and suitable than the main issue, or perhaps because either with plasma or with saliva the main problem of refractoriness to AEDs still remains as a great challenge.

Strong evidence [29–33] supports the hypothesis of an overexpression of efflux transporter, not only in the brain but also in the rest of the body, caused by uncontrolled seizures.

As previously discussed, two scenarios can be possible: (1) the AED used in the treatment is not a substrate of efflux transporter or (2) it is a substrate. In the first case, pre-dose stimulated saliva is a valuable tool to follow-up the treatment of non-ionized AEDs that are not so highly bound to plasma protein. Advantages of saliva TDM of AEDs as an alternative to plasma TDM include: (a) sample collection is painless and non-invasive, (b) it is more economical and with reasonable sensitivity, specificity, accuracy, precision of the analytical methods. In the case of acidic ionized compounds the use of stimulated saliva increases its concentration up to the corresponding free serum value since saliva pH value rises and becomes comparable to that of plasma. A decreased salivary level for basic drugs would be attained. To sum up, AEDs that are not transported by efflux carriers would have in the brain the same levels as their stimulated salivary concentrations.

Some considerations should be taken into account for AEDs substrate of efflux transporters to infer their concentrations in the brain. If the AED is an efflux transporter inducer, if the clinical response of the patient is worsening throughout the time course of the treatment, and if the response is not appropriately related with plasma or saliva drug concentration, a decreased brain concentration should be suspected. To corroborate this fact, pre-dose stimulated saliva and venous plasma samples should be taken and the S_S/P_{fV} evaluated. If this ratio is above 1, there is a great chance of developing refractoriness to the treatment. Discontinuation of the drug, or a change in its dosage regime [34] could be assayed.

When the AED is a substrate of efflux transporters but it does not induce them, such as LCM [26] and LTG [35], apart from following-up the anticonvulsant treatment through measurements of AED in saliva, the evolution of silent antiepileptic responses could be monitored by assessing the S_S/P_{fV} throughout the time course of the treatment. If the ratio lowers, the observed control of seizures might be additionally supported with a favorable prognostic. If the ratio tends to increase, dose reinforcement of the AED or some other therapeutic alternative should be considered.

In conclusion, in all the cases dealing with an efflux transporter substrate, an inverse relationship between brain-to-plasma and saliva-to-plasma would be inferred.

6. Conclusions

Salivary drug concentration measurement is an efficient clinical practice for monitoring epileptic patients. This cost-saving and easy-to-obtain fluid gives valuable information not only of the AED treatment but also of the clinical evolution of the epilepsy.

Author details

Marta Vázquez* and Pietro Fagiolino

*Address all correspondence to: mvázquez@fq.edu.uy

Pharmaceutical Sciences Department, University of the Republic, Montevideo, Uruguay

References

[1] Lam G, Chiou WL. Determination of the steady-state volume of distribution using arterial and venous plasma data from constant infusion studies with procainamide. J Pharm Pharmacol 1982;34:132–134.

[2] Gourlay SG, Benowitz NL. Arteriovenous differences in plasma concentration of nicotine and catecholamines and related cardiovascular effects after smoking, nicotine nasal spray, and intravenous nicotine. Clin Pharmacol Ther 1997;62:453–463.

[3] Galeazzi RL, Benet LZ, Sheiner LB. Relationship between the pharmacokinetics and pharmacodynamics of procainamide. Clin Pharmacol Ther 1976;20:278–289.

[4] Haeckel R, Hänecke P. Application of saliva for drug monitoring. An in vivo model for transmembrane transport. Eur J Clin Chem Clin Biochem 1996;34:171–191.

[5] Patsalos PN, Berry DJ. Therapeutic drug monitoring of antiepileptic drugs by use of saliva. Ther Drug Monit 2013;35:4–29.

[6] Fagiolino P, Eiraldi R, Vázquez M. The influence of cardiovascular physiology on dose-pharmacokinetic and pharmacokinetic-pharmacodynamic relationships. Clin Pharmacokinet 2006;45:433–448.

[7] Thaysen JH, Thor NA, Schwartz IL. Excretion of Na, K, Cl, CO_2 in human parotid saliva. Am J Physiol 1954;178:155–159

[8] Posti J. Saliva-plasma drug concentration ratios during absorption: theoretical considerations and pharmacokinetic implications. Pharm Acta Helv 1982;57:83–92

[9] Fagiolino P. Drug monitoring in saliva: biopharmaceutical, pharmacokinetic and therapeutic applications. (Monitorización de fármacos en saliva: aplicaciones biofarmacéuticas, farmacocinéticas y terapéuticas [in Spanish]). Sectorial Commission of Scientific Research , Comisión Sectorial de Investigación Científica (CSIC)—Universidad de la República Montevideo [ISBN 9974-39-187-3], 1999:3–122

[10] Haeckel R, Mühlenfeld HM. Reasons for intraindividual inconstancy of the digoxin saliva to serum concentration ratio. J Clin Chem Clin Biochem 1989;27:653–658.

[11] Siegel IA, Ben-Aryeh H, Gozal D, Colin AA, Szargel R, Laufer D. Comparison of unbound and total serum theophylline concentrations with those of stimulated and unstimulated saliva in asthmatic children. Ther Drug Monit 1990;12:460–464.

[12] Uematsu T, Yamaoka M, Doto R, Tanaka H, Matsuura T, Furusawa K. Expression of ATP-binding cassette transporter in human salivary ducts. Arch Oral Biol 2003;48:87–90.

[13] Fagiolino P, Vázquez M, Maldonado C et al. Usefulness of salivary drug monitoring for detecting efflux transporter overexpression. Curr Pharm Des 2013;19:6767–6774.

[14] Maldonado C, Fagiolino P, Vázquez M, et al. Time-dependent and concentration-dependent upregulation of carbamazepine efflux transporter. A preliminary assessment from salivary drug monitoring. Lat Am J Pharm 2011;30:908–912.

[15] Alvariza S, Ibarra M, Vázquez M, Fagiolino P. Different oral phenytoin administration regimens could modify its chronic exposure and its saliva/plasma concentration ratio. J Med Pharm Innov 2014;1(6S):35–43.

[16] Fagiolino P, Vázquez M, Eiraldi R, Maldonado C, Scaramelli A. Efflux transporter influence on drug metabolism: Theoretical approach for bioavailability and clearance prediction. Clin Pharmacokinet 2011;50:75–80.

[17] Loscher W, Potschka H. Drug resistance in brain diseases and the role of drug efflux transporters. Nat Rev Neurosci 2005;6: 591–602.

[18] McAuliffe JJ, Sherwin AL, Leppik IE, Fayle SA, Pippenger CE. Salivary levels of anticonvulsants: a practical approach to drug monitoring. Neurology 1977;27:409–413.

[19] Fagiolino P, Vázquez M, Eiraldi R. Clearance and bioavailability study through arterio-venous drug concentrations relationship. Eur J Pharm Sci 2013;48:825–829.

[20] MacKichan, Duffner PK, Cohen ME. Salivary concentrations and plasma protein binding of carbamazepine and carbamazepine-10,11-epoxide in epileptic patients. Br J Clin Pharmac 1981;12:31–37.

[21] Tsiropoulos I, Kristensen O, Klitgaard NA. Saliva and serum concentration of lamotrigine in patients with epilepsy. Ther Drug Monit 2000;22:517–521.

[22] Grim SA, Ryan M, Miles MV, et al. Correlation of levetiracetam concentrations between serum and saliva. Ther Drug Monit 2003;25:61–66.

[23] Cawello W, Bökens H, Nickel B, Andreas JO, Halabi A. Tolerability, pharmacokinetics, and bioequivalence of the tablet and syrup formulations of lacosamide in plasma, saliva and urine: Saliva as a surrogate of pharmacokinetics in the central compartment. Epilepsia 2013;54:81–88.

[24] Fountain N, Staelens L, Tytgat D, Rudd GD, Jacques P, Cawello W. Low lacosamide plasma protein binding in lacosamide-naïve patients. Neurology 2012;78(Meeting Abstracts 1):P01.077.

[25] Greenaway C, Ratnaraj N, Sander JW, Patsalos PN. Saliva and serum lacosamide concentrations in patients with epilepsy. Epilepsia 2011;52:258–263.

[26] Zhang C, Chanteux H, Zhong Z, Kwan P, Baum L. Potential role for human P-glycoprotein in the transport of lacosamide. Saliva and serum lacosamide concentrations in patients with epilepsy. Epilepsia 2013;54:1154–1160.

[27] Lorigados Pedre L, Morales Chacón LM, Orozco Suárez S., Rocha L. Pharmacoresitant epilepsy and immune system. In: Rocha L, Cavalheiro EA, eds. Pharmacoresistance in Epilepsy: From Genes and Molecules to Promising Therapies. Springer, New York Heidelberg Dordrecht London 2013: 149–168.

[28] Morita K, Yamaji A. Changes in the concentration of serum alpha 1-acid glycoprotein in epileptic patients. Eur J Clin Pharmacol 1994;46:137–142.

[29] Lazarowski A, Czornyj L, Lubienieki F, Girardi E, Vazquez S, D'Giano C. ABC-transporters during epilepsy and mechanisms underlying multidrug resistance in refractory epilepsy. Epilepsia 2007;48:140–149.

[30] Potschka H, Fedrewitz M, Löscher W. Multidrug resistance protein MRP2 contributes to blood-brain-barrier function and restricts antiepileptic drug activity. J Pharmacol Exp Ther 2003;306:124–31.

[31] Luna-Munguia H, Orozco-Suarez S, Rocha L. Effects of high frequency electrical stimulation and R-verapamil on seizure susceptibility and glutamate and GABA release in a model of phenytoin-resistant seizures. Neuropharmacology 2011;61:807–814.

[32] Lazarowski A, Seviever G, Taratuto A, Massaro M, Rabinowicz A. Tuberous sclerosis associated with MDR1 gene expression and drug-resistant epilepsy. Pediatr Neurol 1999;21:731–734.

[33] Remy S, Beck H. Molecular and cellular mechanism of pharmacoresistance in epilepsy. Brain 2006;129:18–35.

[34] Fagiolino P, Vázquez M, Orozco Suárez S, et al. Contribution of the antiepileptic drug administration regime in the development and/or establishment of pharmacoresistant epilepsy. In: Rocha L, Cavalheiro EA, eds. Pharmacoresistance in Epilepsy: From Genes and Molecules to Promising Therapies. Springer, New York Heidelberg Dordrecht London 2013: 169–184.

[35] Römermann K, Helmer R, Löscher W. The antiepileptic drug lamotrigine is a substrate of mouse and human breast cancer resistance protein (ABCG2). Neuropharmacology 2015;93:7–14.

Chapter 13

Role of ABC-Transporters in Epileptogenesis and Pharmacoresistant Epilepsy

Lazarowski Alberto and Czornyj Liliana

Additional information is available at the end of the chapter

http://dx.doi.org/10.5772/64349

Abstract

According to a recently published article by our group [*The complexity of roles of P-glycoprotein in refractory epilepsy: pharmacoresistance, epileptogenesis, SUDEP and relapsing marker after surgical treatment ADMET & DMPK 3(2) (2015) 110-121*], we have written a chapter related to these concepts.

The manuscript reviews the structure and function of several ABC-transporters, their roles in the transport of different natural compounds, as well as a wide spectrum of drugs. In this regard, it is important to remember that their expression is also related to the highly specialized functions of specific types of cells. In each of these the expression can be transient, permanent or "*de-novo*" induced, also secondary to a wide spectrum of factors. As described initially in cancer, overexpression of ATP-binding cassette (ABC) transporters such as P-glycoprotein (ABCB1, P-gp), multidrug resistance-associated protein (ABCC1, MRP), and breast cancer–resistance protein (ABCG2, BCRP) confers a multidrug-resistant phenotype, by transporting a diverse range of compounds out of the cell against a concentration gradient. This characteristic was also later demonstrated in epilepsy, particularly in cases receiving simultaneously more than 3 antiepileptic drugs (AEDs).

Additional information related to genetic variants such as the Single Nucleotide Polymorphism (SNP) of these transporters, whether alone or associated with a Cytochrome (CYP) system, can modify their functional expression level inducing changes in their pharmacokinetics, their bio-distribution and their brain access to more common AEDs, producing an imbalance in their dose–response equilibrium. Furthermore, the increased production and design of new AEDs, as observed during the last 30 years, has not decreased the high percentage (30–40%) of drug-resistant epileptic cases.

The AEDs design is based on experimental models of seizures induced in "normal/non-epileptic" animals (mice or rats). For this reason, a discussion on the current experimental models of epilepsy will be included, as well as a suggestion that the next generation of AEDs should be developed and assayed via new experimental models where the current AEDs have failed.

One important aspect regarding pharmacoresistant phenotype is that it can be present at the onset of diseases, or it can be acquired progressively. Differences in both conditions can be related with therapeutic error, loss of compliance, or with the specific epileptic syndrome. Of particular interest results is the fact that ABC transporters "P-gp and BCRP" are also the biomarkers of stem cells. In this regard, some epileptic syndromes, secondary to malformations of cortical development or brain tumors, may also serve as a biomarker of risk for seizure relapse after epilepsy surgery.

Finally, we assume that the pathophysiological condition of "hypoxic stress" is produced during each seizure, and this mechanism induces a wide spectrum of biological responses at cellular levels (neurons, astrocytes) in the brain, and on peripheral organs such as the heart. This complex regulatory system can also induce ABC-transporter overexpression in the cells of these different organs. Because P-gp is not expressed in both normal neurons and cardyomiocytes, and P-gp expression can produce membrane depolarization, we can speculate that P-gp could play a role in changing the electric properties of each of these cells. Furthermore, our previous studies suggest that P-gp overexpression in neurons plays a role in epileptogenesis and its expression in cardyomiocytes could be related with Sudden Unexpected Death in Epilepsy (SUDEP).

Keywords: ABC-transporters, Epileptogenesis, Pharmacoresistant Epilepsy, SUDEP, Stem-cell markers

---

1. Introduction

Epilepsy was described as a clinical entity by Hippocrates in the 5th century BC, however, the oldest inscriptions date from 4000 years BC. Epilepsy, one of the world's oldest recognized disorders, affects currently around 50 million people worldwide. Furthermore, it is the second most common neurological disorder after stroke, with approximately 1-2% of the population being affected by some form of epilepsy. Two features are characteristic of this disease, around 30-40% of epileptic patients are drug refractory and nearly 90% of epilepsy cases are in low-income countries, where both social consequences and different stratagem of treatments affects seriously their gross national product. Several of, if not all, the described properties of ABC-transporters, particularly P-gp, could be involved in the development of AEDs resistance phenotype as well as playing a part in the intimate mechanisms of epileptogenesis. Hence, not only is the control of pharmacoresistnace important, but the prevention of epileptogenesis too, represents challenges to arresting the development of this disease or reach their clinical manifestation full control.

2. ABC transporters and multidrug resistance (MDR) phenotype

P-glycoprotein (P-gp) is member of the ABC (ATP-binding cassette) superfamily of transporters, discovered in pharmacoresistant cancer cells as a 170 kDa plasma membrane protein (**Figure 1**). The ABCB-1 gene, which is also named MDR-1 gene, encodes P-gp, which was the first transporter related to the MDR phenotype [1]. P-gp also named as MDR protein 1 (MDR1); in spite that it is commonly reported as the gene product of the ABCB1 gene, can be also encoded by the ABCB4 gene, and this P-gp sister is named MDR-3 protein – mainly expressed in hepatocytes [2].

Biochemical, molecular, and structural analysis have definitively established that the involvement of P-gp in pharmacoresistance results from its primary function as an ATP- and Ca^{2+}-dependent detoxifying pump, that extrudes potentially toxic compounds out of the cells and can confer resistance levels of 1,000-fold or more to the expressing cells [3]. In spite of the fact that P-gp pumps aqueous soluble drugs, it can also function as a "hydrophobic vacuum cleaner", because many P-gp substrates (largely hydrophobic) bind to P-gp from the lipid bilayer rather than from the aqueous phase.

Currently, 49 different members have been identified in the human genome - these are classified into seven families by the Human Genome Organization (ABC-A to ABC-G). They are encoded in almost all chromosomes [except 5, 8, 15, 18, 20, and Y] [4], and 22 of them have been associated with physiologic or pathological functions. Additional to P-gp, are the

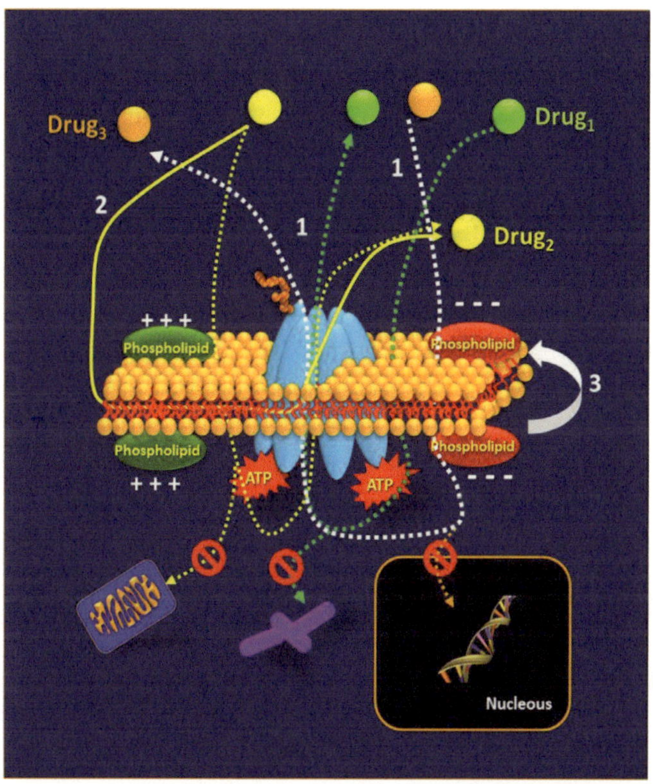

Figure 1. Schematic structure of P-glycoprotein and its typical functional properties. 1. Efflux system as a pore model. **2.** hydrophobic vacuum cleaner. Both these mechanisms are related to substrate exporting and the pharmacoresistance phenotype in different diseases, including epilepsy. **3.** Phospholipid flippase, related with membrane polarity and suggested as an epileptogenic mechanism.

MDR-associated proteins (MRPs) and breast cancer resistant protein (BCRP) which have also been related to the MDR phenotype. P-gp, MRPs, and BCRP are normally expressed in the luminal surface of most excretory tissues including the capillary endothelial cells in the blood–brain barrier (BBB) or the blood–cerebrospinal fluid (BCSF) barrier (BCSFB), playing together a combined role, i.e., to reduce the brain penetration of many drugs [5].

These three transporters are key in the MDR phenotype of cancer cells and mediate the ATP-dependent unidirectional efflux of different drugs as well as being natural to both endogenous and exogenous compounds.

P-gp and BCRP can export unmodified drugs as well as conjugates, while MRPs can export mainly glutathione and other drug conjugates. Both P-gp and BCRP can transport neutral or cationic compounds, whereas MRPs can transport anionic compounds [6].

A wide spectrum of differentiating agents, hormones, oncogenes, and transcription factors, known to be evolved in apoptosis, stress, inflammation, and hypoxia (e.g., p53, NFkB, NF-IL6, AP-1, HIF-1α, E2F1, and EAPP) can up-regulate the expression of these transporters [7–10], including previously non-expressive cells such as neurons or cardiomyocytes [11, 12]. This property suggests that P-gp and other MDR-like proteins may be also involved in cell survival death–related biological processes [13, 14].

Furthermore, overexpression of microRNAs miR-27a and miR-451 are directly involved in overexpression and activity of P-gp, and treatment of P-gp positive cells with the antagomirs of miR-27a or miR-451 decreased the expression of P-gp and MDR1 mRNA [15].

In the classical pump model, the P-gp alternates between an inward-facing and an outward-facing conformation, and these changes in the transporter induced by either substrate binding or ATP hydrolysis leads to the formation of a hydrophilic channel that permits the release of the substrate from the cytosol to the extracellular space.

On the other hand, some evidence indicates that P-gp can also decrease the plasma membrane potential of several cell types from normal values (−60 mV) to −10 or 0 mV [16, 17], and under this condition, it can also reduce the convulsive thresholds, and additionally modulates the swelling activated Cl^- currents – both physiologic disturbances observed during brain hypoxia and convulsive stress [18–20].

3. Epilepsy and Refractory Epilepsy

Seizures are defined as "the abnormal excessive or synchronous neuronal activity in the brain" that can be produced secondary to a wide spectrum of injuries. However, "epileptic seizures" are produced spontaneously, so, a seizure is an event and epilepsy is a disorder involving recurrent unprovoked seizures.

So, what is epilepsy? Throughout the last five decades, the definition of epilepsy has been subjected to extensive controversy and debate by different neurological schools. After several years of deliberations on this issue results have been published by the International League

Against Epilepsy (ILAE) commissioned second task force, to develop a practical (operational) definition of epilepsy, designed for use by doctors and patients and adopted as a position of the ILAE.

The Epilepsy Dictionary, recently published by the ILAE and the World Health Organization (WHO), indicate that epilepsy is defined as a chronic affliction of diverse etiology, characterized by recurring seizures due to excessive neuronal discharge (epileptic seizures), associated with diverse clinical and paraclinical manifestations. However, many variables such as age, risk factors, or genetic mutations, were not included within this definition.

The seizures themselves are the clinical manifestation of an underlying transient abnormality of cortical neuronal activity and the phenotypic expression of each seizure is determined by the point of origin of the hyperexcitability and its degree of spread throughout the brain. From such a minimal expression as loss of awareness to more complex manifestations as tonic–clonic seizures, crisis can last between a few seconds and a few minutes, can be isolated, or can occur in series. All these variations, contribute to the design of the current epilepsy classification. Several causes of sporadic or recurrent seizures include different etiologies such as acquired structural brain damage, altered metabolic states, or inborn brain malformations, and all of them present genetic differences as compared with nonconvulsive individuals. Furthermore, despite the observation that several different illnesses can develop secondary epilepsy, it is clear that only a fraction and not all of the affected patients will develop an epileptic syndrome from the same primary disease. According with this observation, we need to say that epilepsy secondary to other disease cannot be explained only by the primary disease "per se". Perhaps, this difference in susceptibility, could be also based on genetic variants between them, or perhaps all of them share a particular epileptogenic mechanism that is not present in other patients with the same disease but without epilepsy.

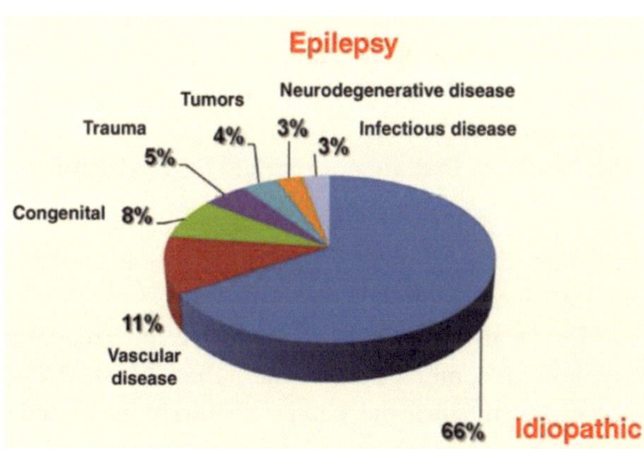

Figure 2. Different causes of epilepsy. In spite the majority of epilepsies are characterized as idiopathic (66%), near 30–40% of epileptic syndromes are secondary to different process that also can induce overexpression of P–gp.

A wide spectrum of syndromes – as diverse as neurodegenerative disorders, mental retardation syndromes, as well as neuronal migration disorders and mitochondrial encephalomyopathies – have been described as capable of developing severe epileptic phenotypes, and to date, more than 200 single-gene disorders are known in which the presence of recurrent seizures are an important part of the phenotype. In 1975, the majority of epilepsies were characterized as 'idiopathic', but today, several of these idiopathic epilepsies comprise autoimmune epilepsies, epilepsies with lesions previously undetected, and the newly defined epilepsies secondary to genetic cause [21]. However, a large group of idiopathic epilepsies have unknown etiologies or epileptogenic intrinsic mechanisms (**Figure 2**).

The treatment of choice for control of epileptic seizures is pharmacologic therapeutics with antiepileptic drugs (AEDs), and the success of this treatment depends on the right selection of AEDs for the specific epileptic syndrome [22].

It is clear the wrong choice of AEDs or lack of therapeutic compliance by the patients may be the cause of treatment failure. However, if a drug resistant phenotype is observed under correct therapeutic stratagem, then patients, who were considered drug resistant, may not remain so because newer AEDs are being developed, targeting newly discovered pathophysiological mechanisms. Furthermore, individuals defined as being drug resistant with their epilepsy considered "drug resistant", perhaps have not yet been prescribed appropriate drugs.

4. Definition of Drug Resistance in Epilepsy

Resistance to drug treatment is a critical problem in the therapy of many brain disorders including epilepsy. When a patient has failed trials of two appropriate AEDs, the probability of achieving seizure freedom with subsequent AED treatments is modest. A useful functional criterion of refractory epilepsy (RE) is the failure to control seizures despite the use of two or more appropriate AEDs, even when maximum tolerated doses are administered (**Figure 3**). Interestingly, it was suggested that patients who were considered drug resistant under a given definition may not remain so as newer AEDs are developed, or designed, to target previously unappreciated underlying pathophysiological mechanisms. Additionally, individuals who we could define as being drug resistant, perhaps his epilepsy is considered "drug resistant" simply because we do not yet have drugs that are appropriate for the treatment of that individual's epilepsy [23].

During the last decade, more than 15 new AEDs have become available, however, the percentage of patients with RE remains near 30–40%, as observed during the early era of treatment with common, older AEDs. In all these cases, the failure of pharmacological therapeutics is observed after altering different combinations of more than 2 or 3 AEDs [24]. This particular phenotype, suggests a common intrinsic mechanism should be evaluated to better design new AEDs able to avoid the pharmacoresistance, and the subsequent development of a new crisis. These observations strongly suggest that all AEDs were wrongly developed using experimental models of seizures induced in healthy animals (without epilepsy), when they should have been developed via models of epilepsy in which all current AEDs have failed. In this regard, developing therapeutics to block P-gp activity, the main factor related with MDR-phenotype, should be addressed [25].

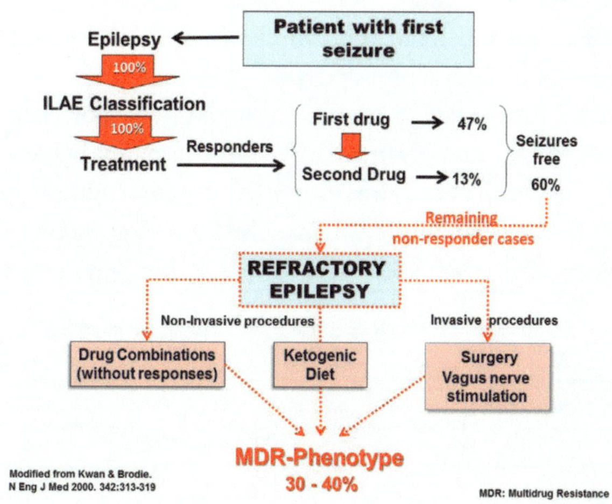

Figure 3. Schematic flow of therapeutic decision: Despite the administration of different therapeutic strategies that include more than two AEDs, almost 30–40% of patients will develop a phenotype of multidrug-resistant (MDR) epilepsy.

5. ABC-transporters and RE

The most important factor regulating the balance between dose and response with a direct impact in the plasmatic levels of drugs is related to the higher expression of the ABC transporters in the transporting epithelia, including the intestine, liver, or kidney, and playing a key role in the absorption, distribution, and removal of AEDs. Consequently, increased functional expression of multidrug transporter proteins, particularly P-gp, which are able to prevent access of AEDs to the brain, and decrease concentration in the sites of action, is an emerging concept of pharmacoresistance in epilepsy, based on extensive clinical and experimental evidence [26–29]. The particular location of these transporters in different excretory organs will induce a unidirectional route for the drugs from the inner to the external body.

The confirmation that P-gp can transport major AEDs (**Table 1**) is in concordance with the potential increased washout of AEDs which could be present in patients with RE [30–32]. The first evidence showing the upregulation of the *mdr1* gene, after experimentally induced seizures, was reported by several different authors showing a highly increased P-gp expression in reactive astrocytes after intracerebroventricular administration of kainite; in BBB and unidentified brain cells after kainate-induced epilepsy [33, 34]; and progressively in neurons after repetitive seizures induced by 3-mercaptopropionic acid [35].

Refractory epilepsy is described in patients receiving recommended AED doses and having adequate therapeutic levels of AEDs in plasma, but who remain without control of seizures. Additionally, it was also demonstrated that therapeutic levels of phenytoin (PHT) in the blood and Cerebrospinal fluid (CSF) can be achieved after 2 hours - enough to reach steady state concentrations within therapeutic range [36]. Sometimes, persistently low levels in the plasma of at least one of the AEDs administered at recommended doses has been observed during the daily follow-up of patients with different epileptic syndromes' who underwent polytherapy. Interestingly, these cases are currently assumed as non-detectable laboratory errors in the procedures or methods of AED measurement, or a non-complains behavior of the patient with the physicians′ therapeutic indication. However, this particular situation can also be observed in patients with pharmacoresistant epilepsy, for who high expression of P-glycoprotein was also observed in their biopsy specimens from epileptogenic brain areas after surgical treatment [37, 38].

AEDs as ABC-transporters (ABC-t) substrates	
Antiepileptic drug	**ABC-t substrate**
Phenobarbital	P-gp
Phenytoin	P-gp/MRP
Carbamazepine	P-gp/MRP
Valproate	P-gp/MRP
Benzodiazepines	P-gp
Ethosuximide	?
Vigabatrin	P-gp
Lamotrigine	P-gp
Gabapentin	P-gp
Felbamate	P-gp
Topiramate	P-gp
Tiagabine	?
Oxcarbazepine	?
Levetiracetam	MRP
Pregabalin	?

P-gp: P-glycoprotein; *MRP:* multidrug resistant-associated proteins

Table 1. Several AEDs share their status as substrates of P-gp, and some of them are also substrates of MRP (multidrug resistant related protein).

All these data, suggests that several, if not all AEDs, could be substrates of P-gp - brain overexpression being related to RE phenotype and a simultaneous systemic P-gp overexpression, something which can induces persistent subtherapeutic levels in plasma, of at least one AED administered.

Over the last 20 years, subsequent to the firsts three clinical reports [37, 39, 40], more than 300 clinical and experimental publications, related to P-gp and/or MDR-1 gene and refractory epilepsy, were registered (**Figure 4**). One of the hypotheses of RE proposes that P-gp as well as others ABCt, could play a significant role in pharmacoresistance in epilepsy by extruding AEDs from their intended site of action to brain outside. Both *in-vitro* and *in-vivo* experiments have demonstrated that several AEDs such as phenytoin, phenobarbital, lamotrigine, and levetiracetam, are substrates of human P-gp and MRPs [41–43].

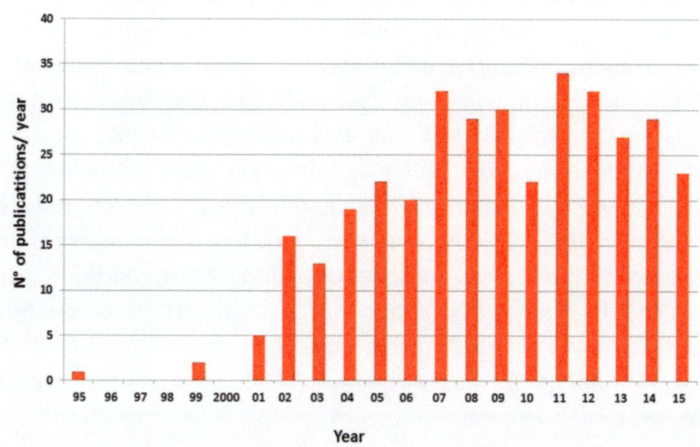

Figure 4. Number of publications each year focusing on ABC-transporters and epilepsy.

The initial interpretation of these investigations was that ABC-transporters such as P-gp, MRPs, and BCRP, whether individually or combined, could be responsible for the phasmacoresistant phenotype, RE. These transporters can induce the efflux of AEDs from the brain as well as increasing bodily excretion and/or inhibiting absorption, via the alteration of the pharmacokinetics of these agents [30–32].

Additionally, experimental evidence has demonstrated that seizures can induce the overexpression of these transporters, particularly P-gp, not only at the BBB level, but also in neurons and astroglial cells. Furthermore, these seizure-induced expressions can be progressively increased, according to the number and/or severity of the crisis. Consequently, we can assume that seizures without control can increase the risk of developing pharmacoresistant epilepsy because seizures can also induce a progressively increased brain expression of P-gp [33–35].

Interestingly, epilepsy is the second most common neurological disorder after cerebrovascular accident (CVA) (stroke). This very important position in the international statistics of brain diseases is concordant with the wide spectrum of very different factors causing epilepsy [44]. Furthermore, these particular and multifactorial processes can advance in clinically silent ways, and later can lead to a first spontaneous crisis, something which is recognized as latency phase or "epileptogenesis". Under this context, persistent neuronal excitability, secondary to an also wide spectrum of chronic mechanisms, in response to complex and progressive processes, leads to a prolonged and increased depolarization and reduces the convulsive thresholds which precede seizures.

In this regards, as previously mentioned, an alternative mechanism to the classic pumping function of P-gp was described in cells expressing the MDR-1 gene, exhibiting significantly low membrane potential ($\Delta\Psi0= -10$ to -20 mV) compared to physiological potential ($\Delta\psi0$ of -60 mV) [16, 17].

The main function of neurons is electrical conductivity which depends on the action potential of the membrane and its polarity. Neurones, therefore, are key to communication, with interneuronal connections being dependent on both chemical and electrical synaptic transmission [45]. Near the rest potential, low glutamic acid concentration induces a "weak" stimulus and only activates the AMPA/Kainate receptors with the NMDA receptor remaining closed. Interestingly, neurons from epileptogenic brain areas overexpressing P-gp could exhibit a pre-depolarized membrane potential, and lead to a persistent reduced threshold to stimulate these cells. So, they could become more sensitive to new seizures under normal or lightly elevated concentrations of glutamic acid. So, under these conditions, the same normal "weak" stimulus could open KA/AMPA and NMDA channels producing total activation of neurons and inducing a new seizure. Furthermore, recently it was demonstrated that chronically elevated extracellular glutamate is a common pathological feature among epilepsies with different etiology [46].

All these observations suggest that P-gp dependent membrane potential alterations ($\Delta\psi0$), not only could contribute to the development of the refractory phenotype, but also to the intrinsic mechanisms of the epileptogenicity. In agreement with these concepts, a preliminary collaborative study showed the first evidence that repetitive seizures induce high neuronal P-gp overexpression associated with refractoriness and a concomitant progressive enrollment of hippocampal cells with a depolarized membrane. Both refractoriness and depolarization were reversed after administration of nimodipine, a calcium channel blocker that also inhibits P-gp activity [47].

P-gp overexpression in neurons can be induced by many silent non-convulsive processes such as inflammation, hypoxia, and toxic agents, and can also constitutively be expressed in immature brain cells. All these conditions can contribute to a progressive lowering of membrane potential, particularly in neurons.

Consequently, how much time P-gp can be expressed in brain cells after an initial inducer insult, waiting a new stimulus producing a persistent chronically P-gp expression, and ending in spontaneous seizures commonly named EPILEPSY?.

So, irrespective of the well-known drug transport property, there could be an additional mechanism that increases the risk that new seizures play a role in epileptogenesis. Because seizures also induce a greater expression of P-gp, all these mechanisms could explain popular comments like: "seizures induce seizures" and "seizures without control induce refractoriness".

Patients with RE carry an increased mortality risk than patients with well-controlled seizures. This clinical phenomenon named Sudden Unexpected Death in Epilepsy (SUDEP), needs a

http://dx.doi.org/10.5772/64349

mechanistic or molecular explanation because post-mortem examination does not reveal a toxicological or anatomical cause of death [48]. Several clinical behaviors of these particular RE cases are in concordance with the MDR phenotype, and different studies have suggested seizure activity as an inducer of cardiovascular alterations. Again, potential membrane alterations, secondary to a high expression of P-gp, but now in cardiomyocytes, could also explain sudden death in these patients. Interestingly, P-gp overexpression in this type of cell, was demonstrated in both chronic and acute heart hypoxic models, as well as in induced fatal status epilepticus after repetitive, induced seizures in rats [49–51].

It was reported that the potential pathomechanisms of SUDEP comprise cardiac arrhyth-mia, due to electrolyte disturbances, arrhythmogenic drugs, or transmission of epileptic activity via the autonomic nervous system to the heart, central or obstructive apnea, and myocardial ischemia [52].

A variety of seizure-related cardiac dysrhythmias such as lengthening of the QT interval, ST depression and T-wave inversion, ventricular fibrillation and asystole, bradyarrhythmias, as well as atrial fibrillation and sinus and supraventricular tachycardias were documented. Interestingly, atrial and ventricular premature depolarizations were also documented under the same conditions [53–54]. So, we could suggest that a similar mechanism of progressive P-gp overexpression, inducing an also progressive depolarization in the brain, is related with epileptogenesis, and that a progressive P-gp overexpression in cardiomycoites may induce an also progressive heart depolarization increasing heart dysfunction.

It was mentioned above that RE is observed in approximately one-third of patients with epilepsy. In the same way, it was described that refractory status epilepticus (RSE), defined as status epilepticus (SE) that fails to respond to acute administration of two antiepileptic medications, also occurs in approximately one- third of patients with SE, and is associated with an increase in the length of time patience stay in hospital, functional disability, as well as mortality [55].

Taking these data together, we can speculate that after a long period of RE, an accumulated high brain and heart P-gp expression, increases the risk of SE development and, under severe stress, can also increase the risk of sudden and fatal heart failure.

6. ABC-t genetic polymorphisms, Refractory Epilepsy and Epileptogenesis

One intriguing and unresolved question is whether the ABC-transporter's polymorphisms could play a role in pharmacoresistance to AED treatment, as well as in epileptogenesis. Remembering that epilepsy constitutes a heterogeneous group of disorders that is characterized by recurrent unprovoked seizures due to widely different etiologies, discrepant observation in genetic studies related with refractoriness could be attributed to variety of factors such as variable definitions of AED-resistance, variable epilepsy phenotypes, and ethnicities among studies. In this regard, a significant number of studies have been developed to establish whether different haplotypes, resulting from the combination of polymorphisms of ABC-t and enzyme systems of drug metabolism, are associated with the development of drug-resistant phenotype in epilepsy.

To date, all scientific literature indicates controversial results, where several studies suggest a positive relationship and several others indicate the opposite. A trend showing a negative correlation appears to be observed in caucasian cases [60–62], and a positive correlation in Mexican or Asiatic patients [56–59].

According to these contradictory observations, a more recent study of 738 ethnically matched Malayalam speaking subjects were enrolled into a genetic study of the ABC-transporter. All of them were residents of Kerala, south India, for more than three generations, of which 259 were RE (AED resistant), 201 were AED responsive, and the remaining 275 were non-epilepsy control subjects. Interestingly, this study concluded that variants in the ABCB1 and ABCG2 do not confer a significant risk to AED-resistance in the south Indian population of Kerala, but instead demonstrate an increased vulnerability to epilepsy and associated phenotypes [63].

Perhaps, irrespective of genetic polymorphisms, the final result of a high histological brain expression of these transporters could be the prognostic hallmark for the clinical evolution of the disease. Neuropathological alterations secondary to repetitive seizures may be adaptive and reversible, while other alterations may be permanent. Furthermore, in others cases, similar brain alterations can be present as constitutive lesions, playing a role in the epileptogenesis, as proposed in epilepsies secondary to mesial temporal sclerosis [64], brain malformations [65], or tumors [66].

Epilepsy surgery has been established as an effective treatment option in pharmacoresistant epilepsies [67]. However, in one study of long-term outcomes in 325 people having anterior temporal resection, the rate of seizure freedom was 41% after 10 years [68]. More recently, the long-term outcome of surgery for epilepsy in 615 adults, indicated that although most patients showed a substantial reduction in seizures, only 40% entered long-term remission by virtue of having no seizures from the time of surgery, and only 28% of those who were seizure-free at last follow-up had discontinued antiepileptic drugs and could therefore be regarded as being cured [69]. Furthermore, ABC-transporters, such as P-gp and BCRP, could be interpreted as stem-cell markers present in several brain cortical malformations, as previously described in epileptogenic subependimal giant astrocytoma (SEGA) [70], being constitutive components of immature not fully differentiated cells, as observed in dysplastic neurons and ballooned cells or brain tumor cells. Interestingly, all these abnormal cells play a role in epileptogenesis, have high expression of ABC-transporters, and are also refractory to AEDs.

Malformations of cortical development as well as brain tumors arise from abnormal progenitor cells where ABC-transporters, together with others stem cell markers, could help to improve the identification of these abnormal progenitor cells and serve as biomarkers for seizure relapse risk after epilepsy surgery [71].

In this regard, the functional activity of P-gp measured at the BBB level was evaluated in patients with temporal lobe epilepsy by a positron emission tomography (PET) study using [^{11}C]-verapamil, before and after temporal lobe surgery, to assess whether postoperative changes in seizure frequency and antiepileptic drug load are associated with changes in P-gp function. In this study, only 7 cases were enrolled and followed up for a median of 6 years after surgery. P-gp immunoreactivity in surgically resected hippocampal specimens was also determined. Patients with optimal surgery outcomes, defined as seizure freedom and withdrawal of AEDs, had global PET scan parameter increases as compared with presurgery PET scans, suggesting a reduced P-gp function at the BBB of different evaluated brain areas. Consequently, an optimal surgical outcome, defined as seizure freedom and withdrawal of AEDs, was associated with higher temporal lobe P-gp function before surgery, higher P-gp-positive staining in surgically resected hippocampal specimens, and reduction in global P-gp function postoperatively, compared with nonoptimal surgery outcomes. This pilot study suggests that Pgp overactivity in epilepsy is dynamic, and complete seizure control and elimination of antiepileptic medication is associated with reversal of overactivity [72].

These particular observations indicate that presurgery overexpression and overactivity of P-gp can be a reactive process secondary to chronic stimulation that can disappear when convulsive stress is also eliminated by surgical treatment, with a minimal risk of seizure relapse. In contrast, abnormal stem cells with aberrant location have a constitutive P-gp (or BCRP) overexpression which can induce a persistent membrane depolarization associated refractoriness and epileptogenesis. So, ABC-transporters and other stem cell markers, if they are presents in those mentioned abnormal cells, could contribute to build a risk score or prognostic profile for long-time seizure relapse [71].

In spite of the high success rate of many surgical procedures for pharmacoresistant epilepsy, a substantial number of patients do not become seizure-free. Alternative strategies using brain electrical modulation by deep brain/vagal nerve/transcraneal magnetic stimulations, have gained considerable interest in the last decade as potential therapies in medically refractory epilepsy. Under these conditions, it was suggested that electrical modulation of the brain may reduce the overexpression of P-gp, and combined with pharmacotherapy, may represent an innovative approach to avoid epileptogenesis, reduce seizure activity, induce beneficial effects during the postictal state, diminish the amount of antiepileptic drugs, and improve alertness, memory, and mood in pharmacoresistant epilepsy [73].

The transporter theory of pharmacoresistance in epilepsy could also be completed with additional properties of P-gp such as:

1. P-gp expression inducible by a wide spectrum of factors such as hypoxia, convulsions, inflammation, trauma, cancer, toxics, metabolic imbalance, infection, etc.

2. P-gp inducing membrane depolarization and possibly being related with epileptogenesis when P-gp is expressed in neurons.

3. Seizures also inducing P-gp overexpression at the BBB, neurons, and in the heart.

4. Further expression of P-gp related with further pharmacoresistance, more severity of seizures, and increased risk of develop of SE and/or SUDEP.

Perhaps, pharmacological modulation of expression and function of P-gp could avoid invasive surgical treatment of refractory epilepsy, the relapse of seizures after surgery, and SE and/or the SUDEP.

7. Conclusion and remarks

The drug transporter properties of P-gp producing pharmacokinetic changes and pharmacoresistance phenotype should be distinguished from those related to plasmatic membrane depolarization directly related with epileptogenesis. ABC-transporters, such as P-gp and BCRP, could also be markers of the presence of stem cells or immature, not fully differentiated, brain cells, as observed in dysplastic neurons and ballooned cells in several brain cortical malformations, or brain tumor cells. In all these cases, high expression of ABC-transporters, were documented and they are also refractory to AEDs. The condition of ABC-transporters as stem cell markers, if they are present in those mentioned abnormal cells, could contribute to the creation of a risk score or predictive profile for long-time seizure relapse after surgical treatment.

Finally, repetitive seizures and/or apneas can induce simultaneous P-gp overexpression in both the brain and heart, and it could represent a high-risk factor for developing an acute heart failure under severe stress triggered by SE resulting in death (SUDEP) (**Figure 5**).

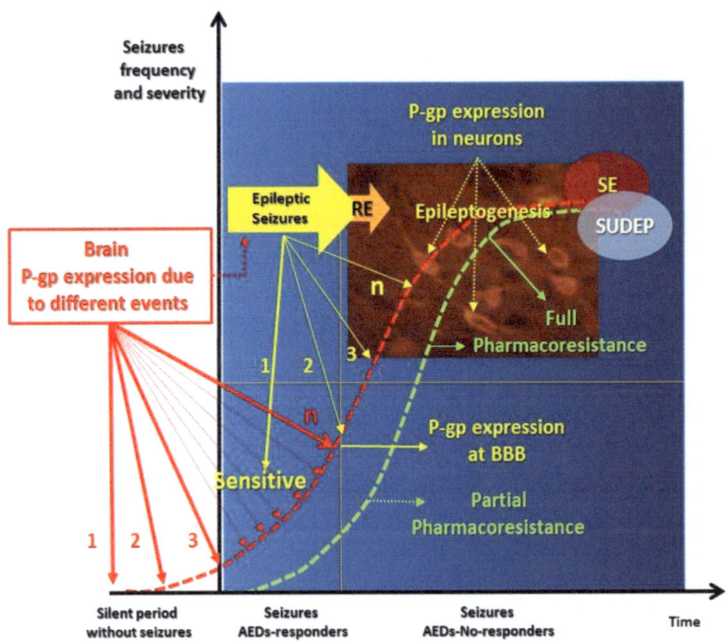

Figure 5. Progressive brain overexpression of P-gp. Initially, a wide spectrum of different stimuli can affect the brain without seizures, however, with a light induction of P-gp expression, it is most noticeable at the BBB level. This upregulation can be reversible, except if new stimuli are added and spontaneous epileptic seizures are also started. The early pharmacological control of seizures is the key to avoiding the installation of a secondary epileptic syndrome. If not, the progressive increased expression of P-gp will develop epilepsy with drug resistant phenotype, and later expression of P-gp, at neurons, will have a direct participation in epileptogenesis. Under these conditions, SE and/or SUDEP can be the final scenario.

http://dx.doi.org/10.5772/64349

Author details

Lazarowski Alberto[1,2*] and Czornyj Liliana[2,3]

*Address all correspondence to: nadiatom@ffyb.uba.ar

1 INFIBIOC-School of Pharmacy and Biochemistry, University of Buenos Aires, Buenos Aires, Argentina

2 Fundación INVESTIGAR, Buenos Aires, Argentina

3 Children´s Hospital "Juan P Garrahan", Buenos Aires, Argentina

References

[1] Ling V. Does P-Glycoprotein predict response to chemotherapy? J Natl Cancer Inst. 1989 Jan 18;81(2):84-5.

[2] van der Bliek AM, Kooiman PM, Schneider C, P PB Sequence of mdr3 cDNA encoding a human P-glycoprotein. Gene 1988;71: 401-411.

[3] Gottesman MM, Pastan I. (1993) Biochemistry of multidrug resistance mediated by the multidrug transporter. Annual Review of Biochemistry 62:385–427.

[4] Dean M, Rzhetsky A, Allikmets R. The human ATP-binding cassette (ABC) transporter superfamily. Genome Res. 2001;11(7):1156-66.

[5] Cordon-Cardo. Immunological analysis of P-glycoprotein expression in normal and tumor tissues in human, in Roninson IB (ed): Molecular and cellular biology of multidrug resistance in tumor cells. NY, Premium Press, 1991, pp303-318.5.

[6] Combates NJ, Rzepka RW, Pan Chen Y-N, Cohen D. NF-IL6, a member of the C/EBP family of transcription factors, binds and transactivates the human MDR1 gene promoter. J Biol Chem 1994;269:29715–29719.

[7] Sharom FJ. ABC multidrug transporters: structure, function and role in chemoresistance. Pharmacogenomics 2008;9,1:105-127.

[8] Goldsmith ME, Gudas JM, Schneider E, Cowan KH. Wild type p53 stimulates expression from the human multidrug resistance promoter in a p53-negative cell line. J Biol Chem 1995;270:1894–1898.

[9] Comerford K, Wallace T, Karhausen J, Louis N, Montalto M, Coglan S. Hypoxia-inducible factor-1-dependent regulation of the multidrug resistance (MDR1) gene. Cancer Res 2002;62:3387–3394.

[10] Andorfer P, Rotheneder H. Regulation of the MDR1 promoter by E2F1 and EAPP. FEBS Letters 587 (2013) 1504–1509

[11] Lazarowski A, Caltana L, Merelli A, Rubio MD, Ramos AJ, Brusco A. Neuronal mdr-1 gene expression after experimental focal hypoxia: A new obstacle for neuroprotection. J Neurol Sciences 2007;258:84–92.

[12] Laguens RP, Lazarowski AJ, Cuniberti LA, Vera Janavel GL, Cabeza Meckert PM, Yannarelli GG, del Valle HF, Lascano EC, Negroni JA, Crottogini AJ. Expression of the MDR-1 gene-encoded P-glycoprotein in cardiomyocytes of conscious sheep undergoing acute myocardial ischemia followed by reperfusion. J Histochem Cytochem 2007;55(2):191–197.

[13] Friesen C, Fulda S, Debatin KM. Deficient activation of the CD95 (APO-1/Fas) system in drug-resistant cells. Leukemia 1997;11:1833–1841.

[14] Abolhoa A, Wilson AE, Ross H, Danenberg P, Burt M, Scotto KW. Rapid activation of MDR1 gene expression in human metastatic sarcoma following in vivo exposure to doxorubicin. Clin Cancer Res 1999; 5:3352–3356

[15] Zhua H, Wua H, Liub X,. Evansa BR, Medinaa DJ, Liub Ch-G, Yang J-M. Role of MicroRNA miR-27a and miR-451 in the regulation of MDR1/P-glycoprotein expression in human cancer cells. Biochem Pharmacol 2008;76,5:582–588.

[16] Wadkins RM, Roepe PD. Biophysical aspect of P-glycoprotein mediated multidrug resistance. Int Rev Cytol 1997; 171: 121-65.

[17] Roepe PD. What is the precise role of human MDR 1 protein in chemotherapeutic drug resistance? Curr Pharm Des 2000; 6: 241-60.

[18] Vanoye C, Castro A, Pourcher T, Reuss L, Altenberg G. Phosphorylation of P-glycoprotein by PKA and PKC modulates swelling-activated Cl- currents. Am J Physiol 1999; 276: C370-C378.

[19] Müller M. Effects of chloride transport inhibition and chloride substitution on neuron function and on hypoxic-spreading depression-like depolarization in rat hippocampal slices. Neuroscience 2000;97:33-45.

[20] Le Duigou C, Bouilleret V, Miles R. Epileptiform activities in slices of hippocampus from mice after intra-hippocampal injection of kainic acid. J Physiol 2008; 586: (Pt 20): 4891-904

[21] Rhys H. Thomas & Samuel F. Berkovic The hidden genetics of epilepsy —a clinically important new paradigm. Nature Reviews Neurology 2014;10, 283–292

[22] Browne TR, Holmes GL. Epilepsy. N Engl J Med 2001; 344:1145-1151.

[23] Sisodiya SM. Genetics of drug resistance. Epilepsia 2005;46(Suppl 10):33–8.

[24] Kwan P, Brodie MJ. Early identification of refractory epilepsy. N Engl J Med 2000;342:314–9.

[25] Robey RW, Lazarowski A, Bates SE. P-glycoprotein - a clinical target in drug-refractory epilepsy? Mol Pharmacol. 2008;73(5):1343-6.

[26] Lazarowsk A, Czornyj L, Lubieniecki F, Vazquez S, D'Giano C, Sevlever G, Taratuto AL, Brusco A, Girardi E. Multidrug-resistance (MDR) proteins develop refractory epilepsy phenotype: clinical and experimental evidence. Curr Drug Ther 2006;1(3):291–309.

[27] Potschka H. Transporter hypothesis of drug-resistant epilepsy: challenges for pharmacogenetic approaches. Pharmacogenomics 2010;11:1427–38.

[28] Remy S, Beck H. Molecular and cellular mechanisms of pharmacoresistance in epilepsy. Brain 2006;129: 18–35.

[29] Stêpieñ KM, Tomaszewski M, Tomaszewska J, Czuczwar SJ. The multidrug transporter P-glycoprotein in pharmacoresistance to antiepileptic drugs. Pharmacological Reports 2012;64:1011-1019.

[30] Lazarowski A, Czornyj L, Lubienieki F, Girardi E, Vazquez S, D'Giano C. ABC transporters during epilepsy and mechanisms underlying multidrug resistance in refractory epilepsy. Epilepsia. 2007;48 Suppl 5:140-9.

[31] Löscher W, Sills GJ. Drug resistance in epilepsy: why is a simple explanation not enough? Epilepsia. 2007;48(12):2370-2.

[32] Löscher W. Drug transporters in the epileptic brain. Epilepsia. 2007;48 Suppl 1:8-13.

[33] Zhang L, Ong W, Lee T. Induction of P-glycoprotein expression in astrocytes following intracerebro-ventricular kainate injection. Exp Brain Res 1999;126:509–16.

[34] Seegers U, Potschka H, Loscher W. Expression of the multidrug transporter P-glycoprotein in brain capillary endothelial cells and brain parenchyma of amygdala-kindled rats. Epilepsia 2002;43:675–84.

[35] Lazarowski A, Ramos AJ, García-Rivello H, Brusco A, Girardi E. Neuronal and glial expression of the multidrug resistance gene product in an experimental epilepsy model. Cell Mol Neurobiol 2004;24(1):77–85.

[36] Rabinowicz AL, Salvat JM, Leiguarda RC, Demonty F, Salvat F, Cervio A, Manes F, Lazarowski A. Use of antiepileptic drugs in nontraumatic neurosurgical procedures. Is there any best route and time of administration? Clin Neuropharmacol. 1997;20(5): 438-41.

[37] Lazarowski A, Sevlever G, Taratuto A, Massaro M, Rabinowicz A. Tuberous sclerosis associated with MDR1 gene expression and drug-resistant epilepsy. Pediatr Neurol 1999;21:731–4.

[38] Lazarowski A, Massaro M, Schteinschnaider A, Intruvini S, Sevlever G, Rabinowicz A. Neuronal MDR-1 gene expression and persistent low levels of anticonvulsants in a child with refractory epilepsy. Ther Drug Monit. 2004;26(1):44-6.

[39] Tishler DM, Weinberg KI, Hinton DR, Barbaro N, Annett GM, Raffel C. MDR1 gene expression in the brain of patients with medically intractable epilepsy. Epilepsia 1995;36:1–6.

[40] Sisodiya SM, Heffernan J, Squier MV. Over-expression of P-glycoprotein in malformations of cortical development. Neuroreport. 1999 Nov 8;10(16):3437-41

[41] Luna-Tortós C1, Fedrowitz M, Löscher W. Several major antiepileptic drugs are substrates for human P-glycoprotein. Neuropharmacology. 2008;55(8):1364-75.

[42] Höcht C, Lazarowski A, Gonzalez NN, Auzmendi J, Opezzo JA, Bramuglia GF, Taira CA, Girardi E. Nimodipine restores the altered hippocampal phenytoin pharmacokinetics in a refractory epileptic model. Neurosci Lett. 2007 Feb 14;413(2):168-72.

[43] Höcht C, Lazarowski A, Gonzalez NN, Mayer MA, Opezzo JA, Taira CA, Girardi E. Differential hippocampal pharmacokinetics of phenobarbital and carbamazepine in repetitive seizures induced by 3-mercaptopropionic acid. Neurosci Lett. 2009 Mar 27;453(1):54-7.

[44] Chang BS, Lowenstein DH. Epilepsy. N Engl J Med 2003;349:1257-1266.

[45] Pereda AE. Electrical synapses and their functional interactions with chemical synapses. Nature Reviews Neuroscience 2014;15:250–263.

[46] Çavuş I, Romanyshyn JC, Kennard JT, Farooque P, Williamson A, Eid T, Spencer SS, Duckrow R, Dziura J, Spencer DD. Elevated basal glutamate and unchanged glutamine and gaba in refractory epilepsy. Ann Neurol. 2016 Apr 30. doi: 10.1002/ana.24673.

[47] Auzmendi JA, Orozco-Suárez S, Bañuelos-Cabrera I, González-Trujano ME, Calixto González E, Rocha L, Lazarowski A P-glycoprotein contributes to cell membrane depolarization of the hippocampus and neocortex in a model of repetitive seizures induced by pentylenetetrazole in rats. Curr Pharm Des. 2013;19(38):6732-8.

[48] Nashef L Sudden unexpected death in epilepsy: terminology and definitions. Epilepsia. 1997;38(11 Suppl):S6-8..

[49] Lazarowski AJ, García Rivello HJ, Vera Janavel GL, Cuniberti LA, Cabeza Meckert PM, Yannarelli GG, Mele A, Crottogini AJ, Laguens RP. Cardiomyocytes of chronically ischemic pig hearts express the MDR-1 gene-encoded P-glycoprotein. J Histochem Cytochem. 2005;53(7):845-50.

[50] Laguens RP, Lazarowski AJ, Cuniberti LA, Vera Janavel GL, Cabeza Meckert PM, Yannarelli GG, del Valle HF, Lascano EC, Negroni JA, Crottogini AJ. Expression of the MDR-1 gene-encoded P-glycoprotein in cardiomyocytes of conscious sheep undergo-

ing acute myocardial ischemia followed by reperfusion. J Histochem Cytochem. 2007 Feb;55(2):191-7.

[51] Auzmendi J, Merelli A, Girardi E, Orozco-Suarez S, Rocha L, Lazarowski A. Progressive heart P-glycoprotein (P-gp) overexpression after experimental repetitive seizures (ERS) associated with fatal status epilepticus (FSE). Is it related with SUDEP? Molecular & Cellular Epilepsy 2014;1:e66:1-10.

[52] Schuele SU, Widdess-Walsh P, Bermeo A, Lüders H. Sudden unexplained death in epilepsy: the role of the heart. Cleve Clin J Med. 2007;74, Suppl 1:S121-127.

[53] Devinsky O. Effects of Seizures on Autonomic and Cardiovascular Function Epilepsy Curr 2004;4:43-6.

[54] Lear-Kaul KC, Coughlin L, Dobersen MJ. Sudden unexpected death in epilepsy. A retrospective study. Am J Forensic Med Pathol 2005;26:11–17.

[55] Hocker S, Wijdicks EFM, Rabinstein AA. Refractory status epilepticus: new insights in presentation, treatment, and outcome. Neurological Research 2013;35,2:163-168.

[56] Yu L, Liao WP, Yi YH, Qiu G ABCB1 G2677T/A polymorphism is associated with the risk of drug-resistant epilepsy in Asians. Epilepsy Res. 2015 Sep;115:100-8

[57] Zhou L, Cao Y, Long H, Long L, Xu L, Liu Z, Zhang Y, Xiao B. ABCB1, ABCC2, SCN1A, SCN2A, GABRA1 gene polymorphisms and drug resistant epilepsy in the Chinese Han population. Pharmazie. 2015;70(6):416-20.

[58] Wang Y, Tang L, Pan J, Li J, Zhang Q, Chen B. The recessive model of MRP2 G1249A polymorphism decreasing the risk of drug-resistance in Asian Epilepsy: a systematic review and meta-analysis. Epilepsy Res. 2015;112:56-63.

[59] Escalante-Santiago D, Feria-Romero IA, Ribas-Aparicio RM, Rayo-Mares D, Fagiolino P, Vázquez M, Escamilla-Núñez C, Grijalva-Otero I, López-García MA, Orozco-Suárez S. MDR-1 and MRP2 Gene Polymorphisms in Mexican Epileptic Pediatric Patients with Complex Partial Seizures. Front Neurol. 2014;5:184.

[60] Manna I, Gambardella A, Labate A, Mumoli L, Ferlazzo E, Pucci F, Aguglia U, Quattrone A Polymorphism of the multidrug resistance 1 gene MDR1/ABCB1 C3435T and response to antiepileptic drug treatment in temporal lobe epilepsy. Seizure. 2015 Jan;24:124-6.

[61] Emich-Widera E, Likus W, Kazek B, Sieroń AL, Urbanek K. Polymorphism of ABCB1/MDR1 C3435T in children and adolescents with partial epilepsy is due to different criteria for drug resistance - preliminary results. Med Sci Monit. 2014 Sep 16;20:1654-61

[62] Lack of association between ABCC2 gene variants and treatment response in epilepsy. Hilger E, Reinthaler EM, Stogmann E, Hotzy C, Pataraia E, Baumgartner C, Zimprich A, Zimprich F. Pharmacogenomics. 2012 Jan;13(2):185-90. doi: 10.2217/pgs.11.143.

[63] Balan S, Bharathan SP, Vellichiramal NN, Sathyan S, Joseph V, et al. (2014) Genetic Association Analysis of ATP Binding Cassette Protein Family Reveals a Novel Associ-

ation of ABCB1 Genetic Variants with Epilepsy Risk, but Not with Drug-Resistance. PLoS ONE 9(2): e89253.

[64] Blanc F, Martinian L, Liagkouras I, Catarino C, Sisodiya SM, Thom M. Investigation of widespread neocortical pathology associated with hippocampal sclerosis in epilepsy: a postmortem study. Epilepsia 2011 52(1):10-21.

[65] Aronica E, Gorter JA, Jansen GH, van Veelen CW, van Rijen PC, Leenstra S, Ramkema M, Scheffer GL, Scheper RJ, Troost D. Expression and cellular distribution of multidrug transporter proteins in two major causes of medically intractable epilepsy: focal cortical dysplasia and glioneuronal tumors. Neuroscience 2003;118:417–29.

[66] van Breemen M, Wilms EB, Vecht CJ. Epilepsy in patients with brain tumours: epidemiology, mechanisms, and management. Lancet Neurol 20076:421–30.

[67] Lhatoo SD, Solomon JK, McEvoy AW, Kitchen ND, Shorvon SD, Sander JW. A prospective study of the requirement for and the provision of epilepsy surgery in the United Kingdom. Epilepsia 2003;44:673–676.

[68] McIntosh, A.M., R.M. Kalnins, L.A. Mitchell, G.C. Fabinyi, R.S. Briellmann and S.F. Berkovic. Temporal lobectomy: long-term seizure outcome, late recurrence and risks for seizure recurrence. Brain 2004;127:2018–30.

[69] de Tisi J, Bell GS, Peacock JL, McEvoy AW, Harkness WFJ, Sander JW, Duncan JS. The long-term outcome of adult epilepsy surgery, patterns of seizure remission, and relapse: a cohort study. Lancet 2011;378:1388–95.

[70] Lazarowski, A, F. Lubieniecki, S. Camarero, V.Cuccia and A.L.Taratuto. Stem-cell marker CD34, multidrug resistance proteins P-gp and BCRP in SEGA. Receptors & Clinical Investigation 2014;1:e53.

[71] Czornyj L, Lazarowski A. ABC-transporters as stem-cell markers in brain dysplasia/ tumor epilepsies. Frontiers in Bioscience 2014;19:1425-1435.

[72] Bauer M, Karch R, Zeitlinger M, Liu J, Koepp MJ, Asselin MC, Sisodiya SM, Hainfellner JA, Wadsak W, Mitterhauser M, Müller M, Pataraia E, Langer O. In vivo P-glycoprotein function before and after epilepsy surgery. Neurology. 2014;83(15):1326-31.

[73] Rocha L. Interaction between electrical modulation of the brain and pharmacotherapy to control pharmacoresistant epilepsy. Pharmacol Ther. 2013;138(2):211-28.